Delmar's
GERIATRIC

NURSING
CARE PLANS

3rd Edition

Delmar's
GERIATRIC
NURSING CARE PLANS

3rd Edition

SHEREE COMER, RN, MS

THOMSON
DELMAR LEARNING

Australia Canada Mexico Singapore Spain United Kingdom United States

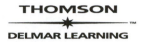

THOMSON
™
DELMAR LEARNING

Delmar's Geriatric Nursing Care Plans, 3rd Edition
by Sheree Comer

Vice President,
Health Care Business Unit:
William Brottmiller

Editorial Director:
Cathy L. Esperti

Acquisitions Editors:
Matthew Filimonov, Melissa Martin

Senior Developmental Editor:
Elisabeth F. Williams

Marketing Director:
Jennifer McAvey

Marketing Coordinator:
Kip Summerlin

Editorial Assistant:
Patricia Osborn

Technology Director:
Laurie K. Davis

Art and Design Coordinators:
Connie Lundberg-Watkins, Alex Vasilakos

Production Coordinator:
Bridget Lulay

Project Editor:
Jennifer Luck

Library of Congress Cataloging-in-Publication Data

Comer, Sheree.
   Delmar's geriatric nursing care plans.—3rd ed. / Sheree Comer
   p. ; cm.
   Rev. ed. of: Geriatric nursing care plans / Marie Jaffe. 2nd ed. 1996.
   Includes bibliographical references and index.
   ISBN 0-7668-5992-4 (alk. paper)
   1. Geriatric nursing. 2. Nursing care plans.
   [DNLM: 1. Geriatric nursing—Handbooks.
   2. Patient Care Planning—Handbooks.
WY 49 C732d 2005] I. Title: Geriatric nursing care plans. II. Jaffe, Marie S. Geriatric nursing care plans. III. Title.
   RC954.C645 2005
   610.73'65—dc21

                    2003048914

Notice to the Reader

Publisher does not warrant or guarantee any of the products described herein or perform any independent analysis in connection with any of the product information contained herein. Publisher does not assume, and expressly disclaims, any obligation to obtain and include information other than that provided to it by the manufacturer.

   The reader is expressly warned to consider and adopt all safety precautions that might be indicated by the activities described herein and to avoid all potential hazards. By following the instructions contained herein, the reader willingly assumes all risks in connection with such instructions.

   The publisher makes no representations or warranties of any kind, including but not limited to, the warranties of fitness for particular purpose or merchantability, nor are any such representations implied with respect to the material set forth herein, and the publisher takes no responsibility with respect to such material. The publisher shall not be liable for any special, consequential, or exemplary damages resulting, in whole or part, from the readers' use of, or reliance upon, this material.

CONTENTS

PREFACE

The aging of people in America is compelling all nurses to become equipped to deal with gerontological nursing and all issues that surround the care of these individuals. The need for education and skills in the care of chronic illnesses and long-term care management is essential in providing and maintaining the health and functional capabilities of aged patients. The accessibility to quality health care, cost containment for catastrophic illness and disease, patient's rights, ethical and legal decisions concerning treatment, quality of life issues, and end-of-life care are all integral parts of the trends in nursing today and for the years to come. In fact, it has been projected that by the year 2025, approximately 25% of the population will be 60 years of age or older, due, in part, to the substantial decline in the number of deaths from heart disease and stroke. Those persons aged 85 and older are expected to account for at least 18% of the population by the year 2040. Because this age bracket accounts for the highest costs, the growth in the ratio of older to younger persons will affect the already-rising health care costs, and make it even more difficult for patients to receive optimum, cost-effective health care because of fixed incomes, financial difficulties, retirement, and potential loss of a spouse, home, and independence.

Aging involves the processes of gradual and spontaneous changes from birth throughout the continuum of life, and the inevitable decline through the later ages. Aging should not necessarily be considered as a negative process because healthy aging involves minimal disease impairment and many persons are able to avoid catastrophic disease and maintain healthy, active lifestyles until their eventual death. Normal physiological function may decline but this does not mean it is always synonymous with disease. As a person ages, the potential for disability and disease increases and affects the ability to function and remain independent in activities of daily living, such as eating, dressing, personal hygiene, and ambulation.

Care of the elderly may take place in the home, hospital, long-term care facility, alternative care facility, retirement community, or outpatient clinic. Regardless of the environment or type of practitioner who delivers the required care, a compassion and sensitivity toward aging and its inherent values, capabilities, and dignity is important if one is to perform safe, meaningful care for this population.

Health care for the elderly creates the largest expenditure of a patient's economic resources if a chronic illness or disability is present, and often leads to poverty and/or deprivation of other human needs. A person may be forced to choose between having enough money to pay for food or medication. This, in turn, affects the prevention of complications or the development of additional health problems, which further compromises the physical, psychosocial, and economic needs of these individuals. Functional capabilities of the adult population over 65 are variable. New treatment options have helped to prevent, alleviate, or control disease states that previously were seen as being untreatable. Great strides have been made in pain management and the utilization of alternative medical locales, such as hospice and long-term care facilities. A broad dissemination of healthy lifestyle education has improved the quality of many elderly people's lives, which in turn improves their functional capabilities.

As the elderly population increases, so will health care costs. Currently approximately 40–50% of the hospital's revenue is from Medicare reimbursement. The amount of Medicare expenses account for more than one-fourth of all services during the elderly's last year of life, and most of that expense is incurred within the last two months of life. The decrease in Medicare reimbursement to care providers to approximately one-third of the actual cost has forced hospitals and providers to cut back on services offered, decrease pay for nurses and other care providers, and increase the workload of those who provide care for patients. The nursing shortage, as well as large volumes of nurses who leave the hospital setting due to burnout and other reasons, contributes to further cause for concern regarding the future of the elderly patient being able to obtain satisfactory health care.

CONCEPTUAL APPROACH

The nursing process serves as a learning tool for readers and as a practice and documentation format for clinicians. Based on a thorough assessment, the nurse formulates a specific plan of care for each individual patient. The care plans in this book are provided to facilitate that process for readers and practitioners. To that end, these care plans have been developed to reflect physical and functional symptomatology listed according to body systems and disease processes. Included are some of the most common problems associated with the geriatric patient. Each disorder includes, as appropriate, an overview of the disease process, medical care associated with the particular problem that may be prescribed for the condition, drug actions, diagnostic procedures, laboratory tests with expected values, essential nursing diagnosis care plans that are identified with the particular disease process, as well as discharge and outcome criteria.

Each disorder has its own pathophysiology chart that shows how the body system is affected by causative factors, pathology, complications, and resultant signs and symptoms. The essential nursing diagnoses and care plans may be cross-referenced with plans for conditions within the specific diagnosis or body system, or within a system or care plan for conditions involving other body systems if they apply. A notation for cross-referencing a care plan may be found under the listing for the nursing care plan that directs the reader to a diagnosis, where the main care plan can be found. Signs and outcomes specific to the particular condition will be notated under the diagnosis, utilizing the main care plan, with noted expansion of interventions and rationales.

It is not uncommon for the geriatric patient to have more than one condition requiring treatment and care, nor uncommon for a condition to contribute to the complication of another diagnosis. It may be necessary to combine care plans or portions of care plans that are applicable to the patient's individual case.

ORGANIZATION

Delmar's Geriatric Nursing Care Plans, 3rd edition, includes care plans by body system for disorders often seen in the elderly population. Nursing care begins with a comprehensive review and assessment of each individual patient. The data is then analyzed and a specific plan of care developed. The format of each nursing care plan in this book is summarized below.

- Nursing diagnoses as approved by the North American Nursing Diagnosis Association (NANDA) taxonomy (2003–2004); the complete NANDA listing is found in Appendix A (new to this edition).
- Related factors (etiology) for each diagnosis are suggested and the user is prompted to choose the most appropriate for the specific patient.
- Defining characteristics for each actual diagnosis are listed with prompts to the user to include specific patient data from the nursing assessment.
- Goals are related to the nursing diagnosis and include a time frame for evaluation to be specified by the user.
- Appropriate outcome criteria specific for the patient are suggested. In keeping with current practice, this edition includes a Nursing Outcome Classification (NOC) label for each nursing diagnosis. Appendix B offers a complete listing of NOC labels.
- Nursing interventions and rationales are comprehensive. They include pertinent continuous assessments and observations. Common therapeutic actions originating from nursing and those resulting from collaboration with the primary caregiver are suggested with prompts for creativity and individualization. Patient and family teaching and psychosocial support are provided with respect for cultural variation and individual needs. Consultation and referral to other caregivers is suggested when indicated.
- Nursing Intervention Classification (NIC) labels are provided in this new edition for each nursing diagnosis. These are inserted after the interventions and rationales to assist the user in becoming familiar with this classification process for nursing interventions. Appendix C provides the complete listing of the NIC labels.

- Evaluation of the patient's goal and presentation of data related to the outcome criteria is followed by consideration of the next step for the patient.

A new, descriptive introductory chapter outlines how to customize care plans for an individual patient based on the standardized care plans found in this book.

A CD is included in the back of this book which contains electronic files for all the care plans in this book.

ACKNOWLEDGMENTS

I would like to thank the many people, without whom this book would not have been possible. I am thankful for the ability and the circumstances that led to the revising of this book, for the chance to give back some of the knowledge I've been taught over the many years of nursing. I thank my husband and daughter, Allen and Ashley, for giving up their time with me, for helping run errands, and taking it all in stride when I would closet myself in the den to write. Thanks for being there for me and for all the support and love throughout all the trials and tribulations we've endured. Thanks to my dad, Miss Garver, and Uncle Joe, who always thought I was someone special, and who believed in me before I even had the ability to believe in myself. I thank Anne Lincoln for being the tireless friend she has been through really thick and thin times, and to my other friends, Beverly, Diane, and Estelle, who have taught me there are actually true friends rather than friendly acquaintances. Thanks to Dr. Paul Little for showing true caring and compassion for patients and for being one of the few doctors to still think in a holistic way about real people. Thanks to all the patients I've cared for over the years who have taught me so much about what the art of nursing can be. I especially thank people like Ken Herring, Wilbert Bruton, and Ann Carpenter, who showed strength of character and a will to survive when faced with terminal illness. Last, but certainly not least, I would like to thank all the people I've worked with at Delmar. Thanks to you all for making this book a reality.

Sheree Raye Comer, R.N., M.S.

REVIEWERS

Janet M. Dicke
Instructor RCTC
Rochester Community & Technical College
Rochester, New York

Pamela S. Covault, RN, MS
Nursing Instructor
Neosho County Community College—Ottawa
Ottawa, Canada

Carol Searls, MS, APRN, BC
Associate Professor of Nursing and Clinical Specialist
Morningside College
Sioux City, Iowa

AN INTRODUCTION TO THE USE OF THE NURSING CARE PLANS

INTRODUCTION

The benchmarks towards excellence in nursing practice are encompassed in the nursing diagnostic processes of assessment, diagnosis, planning, outcome identification, intervention, and finally, evaluation. The nursing process provides a strong framework that gives direction to the practice of nursing. Nursing care planning is the product of the application of the nursing diagnostic process. Without the planning process, quality and consistency in patient care would be lost. Nursing care plans provide a means of communication among nurses, their patients, and other health care providers to achieve health care outcomes. Nursing diagnoses provide the basis for selection of interventions to achieve outcomes for which the nurse is accountable (NANDA, 2003). "Now, as never before, today's nurse must make more complex professional decisions, determine what things to do and what things not to do for which clients. Priorities are critical: often the nurse must make hard choices between what is essential and what is merely beneficial" (Barnum, 1999). The primary purpose of the nursing diagnostic processes applied by nurses is to design a plan of care for and in conjunction with the patient that results in the prevention, reduction or resolution of the client's health problem (Harkreader, 2004).

In the current health care environment, specifically the thrust into an interdisciplinary delivery of care model, nurses are positioned for a level of accountability not seen in prior health care practice climates. In addition to requiring more independent decision making by the nurse, the current health care environment engages various disciplines in working together and jointly sharing responsibility for patient outcome achievement. The changes that are occurring offer nursing the opportunity to define its boundaries and to use the nursing process to deliver care. Nurses need the tools to assist them in accurately predicting achievable patient outcomes for a given primary condition, and they also need the skill to tailor interventions to the individual patient and his or her unique circumstances. This text is designed to provide that guidance.

NURSING CARE PLANS AND INDIVIDUAL PATIENT CARE NEEDS

This book is intended to facilitate the care planning process for nurses working with geriatric patients. The nursing diagnoses that are used throughout this book are taken from the NANDA's Taxonomy II (NANDA, 2003). The outcome statements may be made in two ways: using the Nursing Outcome Classification (NOC) or writing an outcome statement. This text also contains suggested Nursing Intervention Classifications (NIC) for each nursing diagnosis to assist the reader in applying the two classifications to the clinical setting. For each primary condition all the care plans include introductory information about the primary condition and the current medical management followed by:

1. nursing diagnoses with their related to (etiological) factors and defining characteristics
2. expected behaviorally measurable outcome criteria or patient goals
3. nursing interventions. Rationales are included for the nursing interventions to assist the nurse in building a knowledge base to apply the information, make clinical decisions, and to think how best to respond to the patient's needs.
4. evaluation, as the final piece of the nursing process. The ability of the patient to meet the evaluative criteria indicates the patient is moving toward resolution of the identified nursing diagnosis.

The nursing care plans provided in this text are intended to serve as a catalyst for reflection and a guideline to the standards of care. In order to apply them to your patient's situation you must critically think about what you know about your patient and his or her history. You must actively pursue all parts of the patient information base, examining the evidence the client has brought forth to define specific problems and then arrive at specific goals to manage those problems. You will make decisions about how to actualize those goals by choosing or selecting interventions which will assist in meeting the goals and resolving the problem. Standardized care plans provide the practitioner with minimum expectations and predictable patterns of responses. The nurse can then compare these with the patient's presentation and then move forward to design a plan of care that is responsive to that individual and also reflects current management modalities.

The process for planning individualized care involves the same steps as the nursing process.

1. Collect and review the patient assessment data. Typically, the information will be found on the standardized facility assessment sheet, the patient medication administration record, laboratory reports, and in the progress notes. Interview the patient and complete your own assessment record either from school or the focused assessment provided by the facility. After studying the health record, you need to organize the information into a summary of patient issues.

2. Identify viable nursing diagnoses and potential "risk for" situations. Review the nursing diagnoses provided by the standardized care plan. Choose those which fit the patient data base you've collected. The diagnostic process is individualized by identifying "related to" factors and "defining characteristics" which the patient has identified in the assessment process. For example: "Acute pain related to bowel cramping supported by the patient verbalizing pain at a 9 on the scale of 0–10." The patient's own words and pain rating allow the nurse to match the defining characteristics and interventions in the standardized plan to the patient's own perceptions.

3. Plan to meet specific outcomes/client goals. The goals should pertain to the specific patient interventions and move the patient toward resolution of the problem. The outcomes provided in the text will support this and allow for specific qualifiers such as time frames, target times, and patient variables to

be added to allow for individualization of the plan. "Client verbalizes pain at a level 3 or less" would be a standardized outcome. "*Within the next 24 hours*" sets an achievable target time and individualizes the plan.

4. Design interventions to meet the goal and resolve the nursing diagnosis. Choose interventions which are pertinent to the patient and are consistent with the medical orders. Ongoing evaluation of the pain level and the administration of pain medications would be examples of both independent and collaborative nursing interventions which would achieve the outcome and resolve the "Acute Pain" diagnosis.

5. Evaluate the effectiveness of the plan. By setting patient-specific, observable outcomes, the plan communicates the need for ongoing evaluation and updating. This allows for resolution of the problem or revision using the standardized care plan for potential interventions to address the problem.

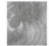

CRITICAL THINKING, THE NURSING PROCESS, AND CARE PLAN DEVELOPMENT

Critical thinking and decision making skills are used in identifying nursing diagnoses. Critical thinking entails purposeful, goal-directed thinking. It aims to make clinical judgments based on evidence (Alvaro, 2004). The nurse uses critical thinking to synthesize the information from the assessment data collection and then makes judgments about how to put the information together into a meaningful whole. In this way, the nurse applies the patient assessment information to a new clinical situation. The standardized nursing care plans in this book will allow you to review the patient assessment and history, and then assist you in formulating a new individualized nursing care plan.

The following case study illustrates how to apply individual patient data to a care plan in this book.

 GERIATRIC CASE STUDY

Peter Page is a 75-year-old retired accountant admitted to the hospital from the gastroenterologist office because of severe abdominal cramping and multiple blood-streaked diarrheal stools. The initial assessment findings include a moderately obese male who demonstrates moderate guarding of his abdomen and abdominal tenderness especially in the left lower quadrant. He rates his abdominal pain at an 8 on the scale of 0–10. His bowel sounds are hyperactive and his abdomen is slightly distended. He is experiencing episodes of nausea. His blood pressure is 170/90, pulse 115, respiratory rate 26, and temperature 102°F. The laboratory results show a WBC count of 18,000. He says he feels warm and is slightly diaphoretic. He states he has periodic constipation and takes magnesium tablets to relieve this. He has had similar episodes of pain in the past but never as severe as this. He has been in moderately good health except for emphysema and chronic bronchitis from a lifetime of smoking 1 pack of cigarettes per day and an episode of skin melanoma on the left wrist which was successfully treated. He sees his dermatologist every 6 months. He denies any drug or food allergies. He does not exercise because he has gotten "out of the habit"; in the past, he walked daily to the newsstand for the paper. He and his wife life with their daughter, which is stressful. She is a single parent with young children, and Mr. Page feels he has raised his family but "he needs to help his daughter out even though child care is very tiring." Mr. Page states he watches football and baseball and goes to the off-track betting for relaxation and distraction. He likes to eat mostly meat and potatoes and drinks a lot of milk, although he hasn't felt like eating in the past two days. He says his wife has been making him drink tea so he won't get dehydrated. When questioned about alcohol intake he stated "alcohol causes stomach cramping and bloating." His father died of stomach cancer at age 72 and his mother died of breast cancer at 74 years old.

NURSING DIAGNOSIS #1
Acute Pain

Related to: Diverticulitis, *inflammation*, infection, obstruction, spasm, sepsis, peritonitis, surgery.

Defining Characteristics: Communication of pain, fever, body aches, malaise, *abdominal pain, abdominal distention*, elevated white blood cell count, pelvic pain, dysuria, *left lower quadrant abdominal pain*, surgical wound drains, abdominal guarding, tachycardia, hypotension, bradypnea.

Outcome Criteria:

✔ The patient will verbalize: *Pain is controlled or eliminated.*

NOC: *Pain Control*

INTERVENTIONS

Assess characteristics of pain, precipitating factors, verbal and nonverbal responses, pain onset, location, severity, duration, radiation.

Assess for intermittent, cramping pain in LLQ or a steady dull pain in back or pain following meals.

Monitor vital signs during pain episode.

Monitor vital signs including pain level before and after treatment with medication.

Administer analgesic and use alternative pain reduction methods.

Administer analgesic for pain greater than 3 on scale of 0–10, Demerol 75 mg. IV ordered q4hrs; use with Phenergan 12.5mg. IV if necessary for nausea.

Encourage patient to physically rest when cramping and diarrhea are present. Provide for non-pharmacologic pain relief measures such as encouraging the client to relax by watching sports on TV.

NIC: *Pain Management*

NURSING DIAGNOSIS #2
Deficient Knowledge Therapeutic Regimen

Related to: lack of exposure to information, potential for infection, or diverticulitis.

Defining Characteristics: Request for information, cognitive limitation, noncompliance of previous instructions, *presence of preventable complications.*

Outcome Criteria:

✔ Patient will be compliant with dietary, fluid, and exercise programs.

✔ Patient will be able to avoid an exacerbation of diverticulitis.

✔ Patient will exhibit no signs and symptoms of diverticular disease.

✔ The patient/family will be able to accurately verbalize understanding of information given to them and will be able to prevent or reduce recurrences *by verbalizing how new dietary habits may aid his treatment and how exercise may reduce his stress response.*

NOC: *Knowledge: Treatment Regimen*

INTERVENTIONS

Discuss patient's willingness and readiness to learn and level of understanding.

Assess patient for knowledge of signs and symptoms of disease, and the treatment of the disease.

Assess patient for knowledge of signs and symptoms of disease, and the treatment of the disease especially the importance of a high-fiber diet and stress management techniques.

Instruct patient/family regarding risk factors associated with diverticulosis/diverticulitis.

Instruct patient regarding dietary modifications, such as eating high-fiber foods and to avoid nuts, seeds, raw fruits and vegetables.

Instruct the patient regarding dietary modifications, such as eating high-fiber foods and to avoid nuts, seeds, raw fruits and vegetables and to incorporate more cooked fruits such as prunes and to use bran for fiber in diet.

Instruct patient about connection between types of food intake and triggers for nausea and cramping such as milk and lactose intolerance.

Instruct patient in maintaining a daily exercise program.

Instruct patient in maintaining a daily exercise program by discussing exercise as a way to reduce stress and encourage client restart his daily walking regimen.

Instruct patient to avoid stressful situations.

Instruct patient to avoid stressful situations by thinking of ways to set limits on the time he provides his daughter with child care or by getting help with child care activities.

Instruct patient to maintain an adequate fluid intake of at least 2 liters/day unless contraindicated.

Instruct patient to maintain an adequate fluid intake of at least 2 liters/day, unless contraindicated, preferably water to reduce gastrointestinal symptoms.

Instruct patient to report any bleeding from the rectum, abdominal pain, especially left lower quadrant pain, alternating constipation and diarrhea or an elevation of temperature.

NIC: *Prescribed Diet, Prescribed Medication, Disease Process*

 CLINICAL PATHWAYS: A METHOD OF ACHIEVING OUTCOMES ACROSS THE CONTINUUM OF CARE

Health care participants are demanding satisfaction with the expensive services they are consuming. Health care organizations publish their outcomes and report them to state, federal, and independent agencies as a method of maintaining practice standards and attracting consumers and health care providers. The demand for the most effective and cost-efficient manner of restoring patients to health has led to the clinical pathway collaborative client care model. Clinical pathways, also known as "care maps," are care management tools that outline the expected clinical course and outcomes for a specific client type (Kelly-Heidenthal, 2003). The manner in which a pathway is constructed is usually agency specific but typically follows the patient's length of stay on a day-by-day basis for the specific disease process or surgical intervention. They are a clinical tool that organizes, directs, and times the major care activities and interventions of the entire multidisciplinary team for a particular diagnosis or procedure. Their design is intended to minimize delays, maximize appropriate resource utilization and promote quality care. "The clinical pathway describes a blended plan of care constructed by all providers, considering the subject together" (Barnum, 1999).

Clinical pathways act as the "gold standard" against which interdisciplinary outcomes and the efficiency of the care may be measured. Institutions may choose to replace the nursing care plan with a clinical pathway. The pathway then guides the nurse along a sequence of interdisciplinary interventions that incorporate standardized aspects such as patient and family teaching, nutrition, medications, activities, and diagnostic studies and treatments. The tool is developed collaboratively by all health team members and includes predictable and established time frames, usually be delineating each hospital day as an event requiring new intervention along a continuum. The issue here is to deliver consistent competent care, and a care map provides this consistency not just on a shift-by-shift basis but also throughout the entire agency. Clinical pathways also, because of their standardization of practice, allow for measuring performance improvement within an agency and between similar agencies over time.

The task here is to appreciate that clinical pathways guide rather than dictate the course of care for an individual. They do not take into account patient problems which are coexisting and are also impacting the patient's recovery process. Therefore, the process of incorporating clinical pathways and the use of this text is the same as in individualizing standard care plans. The nurse must incorporate the individualized needs that exist in conjunction with the clinical pathway. When the patient's needs vary from the outcome achievement time frame, the nurse must assess, report, and manage the variance to meet the patient's needs. The manner of reporting these variances is also frequently agency-specific. At times, the variances are documented on the clinical pathway, at other times the nursing care plan format is incorporated into the document or an individualized care plan is initiated and documentation about the variance is continued until it is resolved. Not all patients' care is incorporated into a clinical pathway model. For more complex patient care situations an individualized care plan format applying the various standardized nursing diagnoses in this text is more appropriate.

Well-designed nursing care plans and/or care maps move the patient from one level of care on the health care continuum to another. They monitor and guide the progress of the patient from the acutely ill phase of illness to the community or outpatient phase of illness. Care planning organizes and coordinates the patient care in a manner which promotes consistency, a current standard of care, and communication, and incorporates the problem solving process which integrates responsiveness to patient needs and cost efficiency.

UNIT 1

CARDIOVASCULAR SYSTEM

CHAPTER 1.1

CORONARY ARTERY DISEASE

Coronary artery disease (CAD) is a disorder in which one or more of the coronary arteries become narrowed by atherosclerosis or vasospasm, and obstruct necessary blood flow to a specific part of the heart. It had been previously shown that in autopsies of patients who are 70 years of age or older, at least 50% had an atherosclerotic obstruction in at least one artery (Beers & Berkow, 2000). CAD had been the most common cause of death in persons over the age of 65. In the past few decades, this mortality rate has decreased, and postmyocardial infarction survival rates have increased, most likely because of decreases in cholesterol levels, decreases in smoking, and better control of hypertensive risk factors.

Risk factors for CAD in the elderly population include smoking, hypertension, increases in pulse pressure, concurrent diagnosis of diabetes mellitus, obesity, inactivity, advancing age, hyperhomocysteinemia, hypertriglyceridemia, increases in total and low-density lipoprotein (LDL) cholesterol, and decreases in high-density lipoprotein (HDL) cholesterol.

Although the effectiveness of the heart's pumping action and vascular function are predisposed to changes that occur during the aging process, these changes allow the elderly to adapt and permit average activities. Chronic illnesses and changes in mobility can result in cardiac atrophy, and hemodynamic changes may cause a thickening and sclerosing of the endocardium and rigidity of the valves. To avert adverse consequences that may occur with CAD, collateral circulation development is required to compensate for the reduction in blood flow to the myocardium.

If the atherosclerosis and narrowing of the arteries is greater than the ability of collateral circulation to bypass points of obstruction, signs and symptoms of CAD appear. These depend on the extent of CAD and cerebral damage. The major abnormality resulting from CAD is angina pectoris, which may lead to myocardial infarction.

Signs and symptoms of CAD are normally supported by angiographic confirmation of coronary artery blockages or from a previously documented myocardial infarction. Electrocardiographic data may reveal patients who are in danger of new coronary events, such as, the presence of left ventricular hypertrophy, ischemic ST segment depression, left bundle branch block, conduction defects, or dysrhythmias. The prevalence of new cardiac events in the elderly is higher if the patient has CAD and complex ventricular dysrhythmias, left ventricular hypertrophy, and abnormal left ventricular ejection fractions.

MEDICAL CARE

Analgesics: morphine utilized to decrease neurotransmitter release and for myocardial infarction pain

Antianginal nitrates/nitrites: isosorbide dinitrate (Isonate, Isorbid, Isordil, Sorbitrate, Imdur), nitroglycerin (Nitroglycerin, Nitrostat, Nitrol, Tridil, Deponit, Minitran, Nitro-Bid, Nitro-Dur) used to relieve anginal pain by dilating the coronary arteries and peripheral blood vessels; also increase blood flow through the collateral coronary vasculature

Antianginal, beta-adrenergic blocker: atenolol (Tenormin), dipyridamole (Persantine), metoprolol (Lopressor), nadolol (Corgard), and propranolol hydrochloride (Inderal) used to decrease myocardial contractility, heart rate, peripheral vascular resistance, and to decrease the oxygen demands of the heart; may increase blood flow through the collateral coronary blood vasculature

Antianginal, calcium channel blocker: Amlodipine besylate (Norvasc), bepridil hydrochloride (Vascor), diltiazem hydrochloride (Cardizem), nicardipine (Cardene), nifedipine (Adalat, Procardia), and verapamil (Calan, Isoptin) used to inhibit calcium ion influx across the cardiac and smooth muscle cells, decrease myocardial contractility, decrease myocardial oxygen demand; also helps dilate coronary arteries

Stool softeners: docusate calcium or sodium (Surfak, Colace, Modane) used to decrease surface tension of the liquid contents in the bowel; water promotes softening of stool in colon for elimination without straining

Antianxieties: alprazolam (Xanax), buspirone hydrochloride (BuSpar), chlordiazepoxide (Libritabs, Librium), clorazepate dipotassium (Tranxene, Gen-XENE), diazepam (Valium, Diazepam), hydroxyzine embonate, hydrochloride, or pamoate (Atarax, Anx, Vistaril), lorazepam (Ativan, Lorazepam), meprobamate (Equanil, Miltown, Neuramate, Probate, Trancot), midazolam hydrochloride (Versed), and oxazepam (Serax) may be used for anxiety reduction by action at the limbic and subcortical levels of the CNS; some drugs may potentiate the gamma-aminobutyric acid effects; Xanax is commonly the drug used

Anticoagulants: ardeparin sodium (Normiflow), dalteparin sodium (Gragmin), danaparoid sodium (Orgaran), enoxaparin sodium (Lovenox), heparin calcium and sodium (Calciparin, Heparin), and warfarin sodium (Coumadin) used for myocardial infarction to prevent extension of thrombi and development of additional clots or deep vein thrombosis; the LMWHs binds to antithrombin III and inactivates factor Xa and thrombin and prevents the formation of clots; heparin accelerates antithrombin III–thrombin complex formation to deactivate the thrombin and prevent the conversion of fibrinogen to fibrin

Antiplatelet agent: acetylsalicylic acid (ASA, aspirin) prevents platelet aggregation; cilostazol (Pletal) decreases platelet aggregation by inhibiting phosphodiesterase III; clopidogrel bisulfate (Plavix) inhibits platelet aggregation by binding to and changing the platelet ADP receptor to inhibit ADP-mediated platelet activation and platelet aggregation; dipyridamole (Persantine) increases adenosine and inhibits platelet aggregation; eptifibatide (Integrilin) and tirofiban hydrochloride (Aggrastat) bind to the glycoprotein IIb/IIIa receptor to inhibit aggregation of platelets

Antilipidemics: atorvastatin calcium (Lipitor), cerivastatin sodium (Baycol), cholestyramine (LoCholest, Prevalite, Questran), colestipol hydrochloride (Colestid), fenofibrate (Tricor), fluvastatin sodium (Lescol), gemfibrozil (Lopid), lovastatin (Mevacor), pravastatin sodium (Pravachol), and simvastatin (Zocor) used to decrease LDL and total cholesterol in patients with elevated cholesterol levels by inhibiting 3-hydroxy-3-methylglutaryl-coenzyme A reductase which blocks cholesterol biosynthesis; some drugs inhibit lipolysis and decrease triglyceride synthesis in the level and increase HDL cholesterol levels

Thrombolytics: alteplase (tissue plasminogen activator, t-PA), anistreplase (anisolyated plasminogen–streptokinase activator complex, APSAC, Eminase), reteplase (Retavase), streptokinase (Streptase), tenecteplase (TNKase), and urokinase (Abbokinase) used to lyse the thrombi that obstruct coronary blood flow in an acute myocardial infarction; bind to fibrin and convert plasminogen to plasmin to begin local fibrinolysis

Chest X-ray: used to identify cardiac enlargement, calcifications, or pulmonary congestion

Exercise stress test (with or without radionuclides): used to show coronary artery obstruction if age allows for exercise

Electrocardiography: used to show changes indicating past myocardial infarction or changes when compared to past ECG

Positron emission tomography: used to identify ischemia and infarction

Nuclear imaging: radionuclide imaging used to show myocardial perfusion

Cardiac catheterization: used to identify presence of cardiac artery lesions, valvular defects, presence of hypertrophy, dysrhythmias, and to evaluate pressures, oxygen level, and cardiac output

Laboratory: lipid profiles used to identify elevations of cholesterol, triglycerides, and lipoproteins; cardiac enzymes used to identify damage that may occur with myocardial infarction or ischemia; CK-MB values greater than 5% of the total CK indicate myocardial necrosis, but can lack sensitivity and specificity; CK-MB isoforms are another new cardiac marker—an absolute level of CK-MB2 >1 U/L or ratio of CK-MB2 to CK-MB1 of 1.5 have increased sensitivity and specificity for the diagnosis of an MI within the first 6 hours after the onset of symptoms; the troponin complex has 3 subunits, known as troponin T, troponin I, and troponin C; troponin T and I rise less than 6 hours after the onset of ischemic changes and are the most sensitive and earliest enzyme markers; cardiac specific troponin T (cTnT) and cardiac specific troponin I (cTnI) may be present up to 7–14 days after the onset of MI; myoglobin is not a cardiac specific test, but may be detected as early as 2 hours after an MI and used in conjunction with clinical presentation and other tests; CBC may show an elevation in WBC if myocardial infarction or concurrent infection is present; electrolytes used to identify imbalances, especially in sodium, potassium, and chloride

NURSING DIAGNOSES

DECREASED CARDIAC OUTPUT

Related to: alteration in preload and afterload, inotropic changes in heart from increased systemic vascular resistance and decreased myocardial contractility, decreased coronary blood flow (ischemia) to myocardial tissue

Defining Characteristics: BP and pulse changes (initially elevated and then BP drops as cardiac output decreases and pulse increases), change in color and cold, clammy skin, oliguria, jugular vein distention, dyspnea, crackles, edema (peripheral or dependent), dysrhythmias, ECG changes in T and Q waves, and ST segment, distant heart sounds, S_3 and S_4 gallops

Outcome Criteria

✔ Patient will achieve and maintain stable vital signs and hemodynamic parameters.

✔ Patient will develop no irreversible complications associated with decreased cardiac output.

NOC: *Cardiac Pump Effectiveness*

INTERVENTIONS	RATIONALES
Assess level of cardiac functioning and existing cardiac and other conditions.	Changes associated with aging may be the cause of cardiac conditions. The existence of other factors place an additional burden on the heart.
Assess BP, pulse rate and rhythm, apical pulse, respiratory rate, depth and ease, presence of cough, hemoptysis, mentation changes, and skin color and temperature.	Indicates reduced cardiac output, vasodilation, and lower blood volume if BP is increased and pulse rate increased. Pulse decreases may be associated with digitalis toxicity. Respiratory changes or difficulties that decrease oxygen intake can

INTERVENTIONS	RATIONALES
	cause hypoxia. Preload depends on venous return of blood to the heart, afterload on the resistance against which the heart must pump blood, and contractility on the ability of the myocardium to adjust the force of contractions.
Auscultate heart sounds for S_3 or S_4 gallop or murmur; breath sounds for crackles or wheezes.	Reveals mechanical or electrical alterations in cardiac function, presence of fluid congestion in heart and/or lungs, and cardiac dysfunction. Crackles or wheezing may indicate the presence of, or impending, congestive failure and fluid overload.
Monitor for existence of dysrhythmias, changes in cardiac conduction and rhythm.	The heart conduction system controls the rhythmic contractions and relaxations of the heart and maintains its pumping efficiency, rate and rhythm which ultimately affects cardiac output. Dysrhythmias and conduction aberrations decrease cardiac output by increasing the workload of the heart and decreasing myocardial perfusion.
Assess lower extremities and sacral area for edema, distended neck veins, cold hands and feet, or oliguria.	Indicates reduced venous return to the heart and low cardiac output. Oliguria is the result of decreased venous return caused by fluid retention resulting in reduced urinary output. Distended neck veins may indicate presence of fluid overload, resulting in decreased perfusion to all body systems.
Administer cardiac glycosides, nitrates, vasodilators, antihypertensives, diuretics and electrolyte replacement as ordered.	Treats vasoconstriction, reduces heart rate and contractility, reduces blood pressure, and relaxes venous and arterial vessels, which acts to increase cardiac output and decrease work of heart.
Position in semi-Fowler's or orthopneic position.	Prevents pooling of blood in pulmonary vessels and facilitates breathing.
Weigh daily on same scale, at the same time.	Weight gain >1 lb/day may indicate fluid retention. Utilization of the same scale facilitates consistent data to ensure correct correlation with fluid status.

INTERVENTIONS	RATIONALES
Pace activities, avoiding going past point of tolerance and progress in exercise regimen as able.	Prevents undue demands on heart and protects cardiac function by preventing sudden reduction in cardiac output.
Avoid Valsalva maneuvers with straining, coughing, or moving.	Results in sudden reduction in cardiac output by increasing intra-abdominal and intrathoracic pressures, preventing blood from entering thoracic cavity with less pumped into the heart. Heart rate slows and cardiac output decreases. A sudden overload of blood to heart follows relaxation and decreased thoracic pressure results in decreased cardiac output.
Instruct patient/family in administration of prescribed medications, actions and side effects; avoid over-the-counter drugs without physician advice.	Promotes desired action and results. Prevents adverse interactions with other drugs.
Instruct patient/family in program of activities; active and passive ROM.	Promotes circulation by preserving muscle tone and strength. Heat generated by exercises promotes cellular metabolism.
Instruct patient/family in establishing pattern of bowel elimination of soft stool, proper administration of stool softener or laxative.	Promotes easy elimination without straining.
Instruct patient/family in elevation of legs when sitting, to avoid standing in one place or for long periods of time.	Promotes venous blood return.
Instruct patient/family in reporting edema, chest pain, changes in VS, output, I&O imbalance.	May indicate complications of reduced cardiac output.
Instruct patient/family in technique for taking pulse and blood pressure.	Allows for self-monitoring.

NIC: *Cardiac Care: Acute*

Discharge or Maintenance Evaluation

- BP, pulse and respirations will be within baseline levels, with clear breath sounds with optimal airflow, and absence of dyspnea
- Reduction of fatigue with increased activity tolerance will be noted.

- Patient will have warm and dry skin with palpable peripheral pulses.
- Patient will have no complaints of chest pain or complications from cardiac dysrhythmias.
- Patient will have equivalent intake and output, with no edema or weight gain over 1 lb/day.
- Patient/family will be able to accurately verbalize instructions given.
- Patient will be able to avoid preventable complications from usage of medications not prescribed by physician, such as over-the-counter medications.

 INEFFECTIVE TISSUE PERFUSION: CARDIOPULMONARY, CEREBRAL, RENAL, GASTROINTESTINAL, PERIPHERAL

Related to: reduced oxygen supply, atherosclerotic lesions, hypoperfusion, hypovolemia, myocardial infarction, angina, dysrhythmias, valvular heart disease, coexisting disease processes, age-related vascular structure changes, inactivity

Defining Characteristics: chest pain, conduction disturbances, dysrhythmias, vital sign changes, ECG changes, delayed capillary refill time, chest retractions, dyspnea, nasal flaring, use of accessory muscles, increased work of breathing, tachypnea, bradypnea, changes in mental status, weakness, paralysis, behavioral changes, abdominal distention, ileus, hypoactive or absent bowel sounds, nausea, vomiting, edema, weak or absent peripheral pulses, skin temperature changes, skin color changes, decreased peripheral tactile sensation, hematuria, oliguria, anuria, increased BUN and creatinine

Outcome Criteria

✔ Patient will have normal oxygen delivery and consumption.
✔ Patient will have systolic blood pressure at least 90 mm Hg, with normal hemodynamic parameters.
✔ Patient will have perfusion to all body systems.

NOC: *Tissue Perfusion*

INTERVENTIONS	RATIONALES
Monitor vital signs q 1 hour and prn.	Tachypnea, tachycardia, and hypotension will occur with hypoperfusion and decreased cardiac output.

(continues)

(continued)

INTERVENTIONS	RATIONALES
Administer oxygen as ordered.	Supplemental oxygen will be required as hypoxia and hypoxemia increase.
Administer IV fluids as ordered.	Fluid resuscitation may be required if blood pressure drops in order to maintain at least the minimum adequate blood flow.
Administer blood products as ordered.	May be required to increase circulating blood volume, increase oxygen-carrying capability, and to treat complications, such as anemia.
Administer vasoactive medications as needed once fluid resuscitation is tried.	Dopamine is used frequently in low doses for its ability to improve renal and splanchnic blood flow, but may be used in higher doses to support blood pressure. Dobutamine may be used for myocardial depression but should be used with caution in hypotensive patients because it also reduces SVR.
Monitor ECG for cardiac rhythm, conduction defects, and dysrhythmias, and treat per protocol.	Fluid shifting can create electrolyte imbalances and cardiac hypoperfusion that may result in cardiac rhythm irregularities. Treatment of these may be life-saving.
Auscultate lung fields and heart tones q 2–4 hours and prn. Notify physician of significant changes.	Fluid resuscitation may result in pulmonary edema, with wheezing and crackles audible. New gallops or murmurs may indicate impending cardiac failure, cardiac hypoperfusion, or impending tamponade.
Assess patient's level of consciousness and orientation.	As hypoperfusion progresses, the patient may have decreased sensorium reflecting decreasing cerebral perfusion.
Auscultate abdomen for presence and character of bowel sounds. Observe for abdominal distention.	Decreasing or absent bowel sounds may indicate presence of ileus, obstruction, or hypoperfused state.
Palpate peripheral pulses, and observe extremities for color, capillary refill, and sensation.	Hypoperfusion causes the body to shunt blood from the periphery to vital organs, leading to decreased or absent peripheral pulses, and cold extremities that are mottled or cyanotic.
Control hyperthermia with cooling blankets, antipyretics,	Hyperthermia adds to oxygen consumption and demand,

INTERVENTIONS	RATIONALES
or tepid baths.	worsening perfusion to all organs.
Avoid Trendelenburg's position for decreased blood pressure.	Position impairs gas exchange, increases pulmonary blood flow, and may decrease cerebral perfusion.
Assist with ambulation and either passive or active ROM exercises.	Assists to improve peripheral and arterial circulation, and prevents venous stasis.
Apply TED hose and remove for at least 1 hour each shift.	Helps to promote venous return. Removal allows legs to relax.
Monitor patient for orientation status. Reorient as needed.	Hypoperfusion may result in decreased sensorium, which could ultimately affect patient adversely. Reorientation helps to maintain sense of well-being and orientation to surroundings to decrease risk of injury.
Instruct patient and/or family regarding disease process.	Patient may be too ill because of hypoperfusion to be instructed. Family needs information and updates as condition changes.
Instruct family regarding all procedures, equipment, and medications.	Facilitates knowledge and helps to decrease fear.
Instruct patient/family to avoid exposure to temperature extremes.	If sensation is impaired from decreased circulation, patient may develop burns with hot baths, or cold exposure could result in vasoconstriction and decreased circulation.
Instruct patient/family regarding dietary restrictions and methods to reduce fat, cholesterol, and sodium intake.	May assist with reduction in cholesterol levels to control atherosclerosis and its effect on blood flow. Sodium restriction may also improve hypertension and edema.

NIC: *Circulatory Care*

Discharge or Maintenance Evaluation

- Patient will have vital signs within normal range.
- Patient will have peripheral pulses present with no signs of color or temperature changes to skin, no paresthesias or decreases in sensation to limbs, and capillary refill will be <3 seconds.
- Patient will be able to breathe spontaneously, with normal rate and depth, and have clear lung fields

to auscultation with oxygen saturation maintained above 90%.

IMPAIRED GAS EXCHANGE

Related to: ventilation/perfusion imbalance from ineffective breathing pattern, fluid in lungs, ineffective ventricular function, inadequate transport of oxygen and carbon dioxide, cellular respiration dysfunction, excessive mucus production

Defining Characteristics: exertional dyspnea, tachypnea, hypoxia, crackles, hypercapnia, activity intolerance, abnormal arterial blood gases, nasal flaring, use of accessory muscles, increased work of breathing, diaphoresis, mental status changes, visual changes, tachycardia, restlessness, confusion, irritability, dusky skin, changes in vital signs, dysrhythmias, inability to move secretions

Outcome Criteria

✔ Patient will achieve and maintain adequate ventilation, without adventitious breath sounds on auscultation.

✔ Patient will be able to perform activity without experiencing dyspnea or having significant abnormal changes in vital signs.

NOC: *Respiratory Status: Ventilation*

INTERVENTIONS	RATIONALES
Assess patient and establish baseline values for vital signs. Assess for coexisting disease processes.	Baseline data is crucial to help recognize age-related changes that may imitate other disease states from actual gas exchange impairment. Elderly patients usually have a shorter respiration, which decreases their maximum breathing capacity, vital capacity, functional capacity, and residual volumes. Coexisting disease processes may also impair gas exchange and cause tachypnea, tachycardias, dysrhythmias, and so forth.
Auscultate lung fields every 4 hours and prn.	Kyphosis, tracheal deviation, and dowager's hump are some of the anatomic changes which occur in elderly patients that may result in changes in breath sounds. Any abnormal breath

INTERVENTIONS	RATIONALES
	sounds that are different from baseline should be discussed with physician.
Administer oxygen as ordered. Monitor oxygen saturation as warranted, and notify physician for decreases below 90% or specified parameters.	Supplemental oxygen may be required to maintain oxygenation and prevent hypoxemia. Oxygen saturation monitoring helps to identify changes in respiratory status and potential decompensation and to allow for timely intervention. Elderly patients have an increased incidence of chronic pulmonary and cardiac diseases that can impair oxygenation.
Place patient in semi-Fowler's or high Fowler's position as tolerated.	Facilitates maximum ventilation and perfusion. In elderly patients, the muscles of the larynx and pharynx may deteriorate and these positions may be required to achieve adequate thoracic expansion.
Encourage fluids, if patient's condition allows.	Older adults may have a reduced thirst reflex that result in dehydration occurring. Dry mucous membranes may result in the inability of the patient to be able to clear secretions and can trigger the onset of a respiratory infection. Adequate hydration facilitates the liquefication of secretions in order to help the elderly individual to cough up secretions.
Instruct patient in relaxation techniques, biofeedback, and guided imagery. Discuss patient's methods of relaxation and adapt them as appropriate.	The ability of the patient to relax may enhance and facilitate reduction of oxygen demand to the tissues. Using patient's previous experiences with relaxation may enhance ability to decrease oxygen consumption and improve oxygenation.
Instruct patient in positions to use to assist when dyspnea occurs, such as high-Fowler's or orthopneic position, sitting on side of bed with arms and upper torso supported by pillows on over-the-bed table.	Because of anatomic changes in the elderly, compensation with different positions may be required to achieve maximum chest excursion and facilitate oxygenation.
Instruct patient/family to schedule rest periods between activities.	Older patients may have decreased exertional capacity and need rest periods to

(continues)

(continued)

INTERVENTIONS	RATIONALES
	conserve respiratory effort. Their alveoli are usually more fibrous and less elastic, and contain fewer functional capillaries in which to achieve oxygenation.
Instruct patient in coughing and deep breathing exercises. Blow bottles or spirometry tools may be provided.	Assist to promote and maintain mobilization of secretions and patent airway. Tools may assist with patient's ability to increase lung volume and expansion to preserve oxygenation capability.
Instruct patient/family regarding any lifestyle changes that may be required.	Patient may need to have bedroom/living area moved to first floor, be moved close to bathroom, have smaller meals more frequently, have frequent rest periods during activities, and so forth, in order to reduce exertion and oxygen demand and consumption.

NIC: *Acid-Base Management*

Discharge or Maintenance Evaluation

- Patient will be able to achieve adequate oxygenation as identified with normal ABGs within patient's own specific parameters, and with oxygen saturations above 90%, with clear breath sounds to auscultation.

- Patient will be able to perform exercises and ADLs utilizing rest periods and experience minimal fatigue.

- Patient will be able to ingest at least 2 L/day of fluid (unless contraindicated) to maintain hydration status, with no overt changes in skin turgor or weight loss >2 lbs/week.

- Patient/family will be able to accurately verbalize understanding of all instructions given.

ACUTE PAIN

Related to: myocardial ischemia, myocardial infarction, physical disability, tissue damage

Defining Characteristics: verbal communication of pain, chest pain, radiating pain to arm, jaw, or neck, clutching at chest, pain occurring after activity, facial grimacing, restlessness, irritability, self-focusing, changes in vital signs, muscle atrophy, rigidity, moan-

ing, crying, guarding, withdrawal from social contact, insomnia, dyspnea, dizziness

Outcome Criteria

✔ Patient will be free of pain or pain will be controlled to patient's satisfaction.

✔ Patient will be able to identify pain, communicate needs to caregivers, and be able to utilize methods to reduce pain adequately.

NOC: *Pain Control*

INTERVENTIONS	RATIONALES
Assess characteristics of pain, precipitating factors, verbal and nonverbal responses, pain onset, location, severity, duration, and radiation.	Pain from angina occurs when myocardial need for oxygen exceeds the ability of coronary vessels to supply needed blood flow as the lumen is narrowed by atherosclerosis and, in MI, blood flow is obstructed by thrombosis in the coronary artery causing death of myocardial tissue.
Monitor VS during pain episode.	Increases in pulse and BP are caused by anxiety and stress may precipitate angina episode. In elderly patients, dyspnea with exertion may be seen more commonly than chest pain because of increasing left ventricular end–diastolic pressures as a result of ischemia and reduced ventricular compliance. Hypotension may be a result of using nitrates in the presence of a hypovolemic state, and baroreceptor reflexes that are impaired in the elderly, make hypotension more likely to occur.
Administer nitroglycerin as ordered. (Usually can be given every 5 minutes × 3.)	Nitroglycerin dilates vasculature to improve blood flow and to reduce ischemia and pain. Nitroglycerin may be given sublingually as a tablet or spray, and is the usual drug of choice to relieve acute angina; however, if three doses do not relieve the pain, IV nitroglycerin may be used and titrated to control the pain.
Administer morphine, or analgesic as ordered prn.	Morphine frequently is the drug of choice because of its ability to decrease afterload and preload, and improve contractility.

INTERVENTIONS	RATIONALES
Administer O$_2$ at 2–4 L/min via nasal cannula as ordered.	Relieves heart muscle hypoxia.
Maintain rest during angina attack; stay with patient.	Reduces oxygen need and promotes caring attitude and trust.
Limit activity and maintain bed rest in presence of MI.	Decreases myocardial oxygen consumption and strain on heart.
Maintain quiet, calm environment, provide relaxing backrub, guided imagery, and so forth.	Reduces stimuli that increases oxygen demand.
Instruct patient to report pain lasting longer than 5 min.; review effect of medication administration.	Indicates that medication adjustment needs to be made or cardiac complication is present.
Instruct patient to maintain log of time, duration and location of angina episodes, amount of medication taken, and so forth.	Offers comparisons for physician to review.
Instruct patient to avoid activities that precipitate angina episodes such as, sudden exposure to cold, drinking cold liquids, stressful situations, large meals, straining at stools, cigarette smoking, and caffeine containing beverages.	Reduces frequency of attacks.

NIC: *Pain Management*

Discharge or Maintenance Evaluation

- Patient will exhibit no signs of discomfort and verbalize absence of pain.
- Patient will have stable vital signs within specific parameters set for patient.
- Patient will be able to identify stressors that bring on anginal attack and avoid them.
- Patient will be able to utilize medication effectively, without complication, and will be able to utilize other methods to improve pain, such as relaxation therapy and guided imagery.

ANXIETY

Related to: threat of death, life-threatening crisis of heart attack or impending heart attack, angina, limitations in activity

Defining Characteristics: communication of apprehension, sense of impending doom, fear of unspe-

cific consequences, restlessness, anxious, worried, communication of uncertainty, concerns regarding changes in life events, feelings of inadequacy, helplessness.

Outcome Criteria

✔ Anxiety level will be reduced and maintained at acceptable level.

NOC: *Anxiety Control*

INTERVENTIONS	RATIONALES
Assess changes in anxiety level during periods of pain or changes in respirations, verbalizations of fear, or sense of doom.	Anxiety results in increased oxygen demand on an already impaired heart.
Provide calm, supportive environment for expression of fears, concerns, and change in health status.	Reduces anxiety and promotes rapport, caring, and trust.
Encourage visits from family and friends.	Provides emotional support.
Speak in low voice, slowly and quietly.	Prevents additional stimuli.
Administer sedatives or anti-anxiety agents with caution.	Promotes relaxation and reduces anxiety. Elderly patients are very sensitive to effects of sedation as their metabolism is slower and the medication effects more profound.
Inform patient that angina is not a heart attack.	Allays anxiety and fear.
Instruct patient that new methods in treating MI are successful in preventing complications and dissolving clot to restore blood flow.	Reduces fear of death.

NIC: *Anxiety Reduction*

Discharge or Maintenance Evaluation

- Patient will achieve and maintain a lower level of stress and anxiety.
- Patient will be able to perform relaxation exercises when confronted with stressful situations.
- Patient will be able to avoid stress-provoking individuals, calls, or events.

ACTIVITY INTOLERANCE

Related to: imbalance between oxygen supply and demand, inadequate energy to complete activities caused by the aging process decreasing reflexes and physiologic functions, inability to perform once-normal ADLs

Defining Characteristics: chest pain, dyspnea, increased pulse and BP during activity, fatigue, weakness, decreased muscle tone, sensory deficits, behavioral changes, cognitive impairment

Outcome Criteria

✔ Patient will achieve optimal activity level with increased energy and endurance within imposed restrictions.

NOC: *Activity Tolerance*

INTERVENTIONS	RATIONALES
Assess baseline tolerance for activity, ability to adapt to limitations and/or restrictions on lifestyle.	Promotes and protects circulatory function and reduces cardiac workload.
Assess pulse, respiration, and BP 5 min before, during and after activity.	Pulse increase more than 20/min and increases in BP and respirations indicate need for reduction in activity.
If activity causes pain, administer vasodilator as ordered.	Controls pain during activity.
Provide progressive activity following bed rest to allow to use commode, sit at side of bed, sit in chair, ambulate as client is able.	Allows for activity program that increases slowly as endurance increases.
Schedule activities around rest periods.	Maintains activity below angina threshold.
Instruct patient to avoid extending activities beyond tolerance.	Conserves energy and prevents angina.
Instruct patient to avoid activity after eating, bathing, or during stress periods.	Requires additional oxygen for activities.
Instruct patient to keep medication nearby when performing activity.	Availability to administer when needed.
Inform to cease activity when pain occurs and when taking medication, to sit on chair and wait for pain to pass.	Prevents falls if feeling dizzy or faint and decreases O_2 requirement.

INTERVENTIONS	RATIONALES
Suggest cardiac rehabilitation program to establish a daily acceptable exercise plan within determined limits.	Provides necessary activity without causing increased workload to the heart and improves circulation.
Instruct patient to rest by sitting in chair rather than lying in bed, and to conserve energy during activities.	Sitting is the preferred position for resting because it prevents pooling of blood in the pulmonary vessels. Sitting upright also helps to prevent complications associated with immobility, and facilitates better chest excursion.
Instruct patient/family in use of nitrates, and when to seek medical attention.	If pain is not relieved with the administration of 3 nitroglycerin doses, or if pain persists longer than 30 minutes, patient should be taken to the nearest emergency room because pain may not be angina, and may require additional intervention to relieve ischemia to heart.

NIC: *Activity Therapy*

Discharge or Maintenance Evaluation

■ Patient will be free of pain or pain will be controlled to patient's satisfaction during activities.

■ Patient will be able to participate in ADLs, sexual activity, and exercise programs within established boundaries.

■ Patient will be able to tolerate activity utilizing rest periods.

■ Patient will be able to administer medications appropriately and identify when to seek medical assistance.

INEFFECTIVE SEXUALITY PATTERNS

Related to: knowledge deficit about alternative responses to health-related transitions, altered body function, fear of recurring MI during activity, medication regimen, perception of sexual identity, perception of changes in sexual activity that may result from chronic or acute illness or disease

Defining Characteristics: verbalization of difficulties, limitations, or changes in sexual behaviors or activities

Outcome Criteria

✔ Satisfying adjustments will be made in sexual activity that result in positive sexual experience.

NOC: *Anxiety Control*

INTERVENTIONS	RATIONALES
Assess desire and comfort in discussing concerns about sexual activity.	Patient may be embarrassed or not know how to approach the subject.
Discuss feelings of inadequacy or fear of sexual function and correct misinformation.	Patient may fear precipitating angina episode or heart attack.
Use exercise tolerance and changes in VS caused by activity as guideline to develop a plan of progressive sexual activity based on physical limits.	Provides activity without symptoms that create fear or interfere with sexual activity.
Include partner in discussion and plan.	Patient may desire to discuss alone or with partner present.
Inform patient/family about the effects of medications that affect libido and sexual function.	Medications often affect sexual function and cause unsatisfactory experience.
Instruct patient to take medications before sexual activity.	Prevents anginal episode.
Instruct patient/family that increased pulse and respiration for 15 min or longer after intercourse should be reported.	Provides for adjustments in medication, positioning, or other factors to prevent complications.
Refer to sex therapist for assistance as appropriate.	Provides alternatives for satisfying experience.
Provide patient/partner with information regarding illness and treatment.	This helps to focus on specific problems, concerns, or fears, and encourages questions from patient and significant other. People who have had an MI, angina, or with heart failure may avoid sexual activity because of misperceptions of risk for their lives. Cardiac death during sexual activity is rare. Patients are usually advised to avoid sexual activity for 8–14 weeks after an MI, whenever the patient with angina can perform the equivalent of walking up one flight of stairs without pain, and for the patient with heart failure, a 2–3 week period of abstinence is advised. Physical exercise and

INTERVENTIONS	RATIONALES
	emotional release related to sexual endeavors may actually play a part in their overall improvement. Some medications, such as those taken for hypertension, may impair sexual arousal in patients.

NIC: *Sexual Counseling*

Discharge or Maintenance Evaluation

- Patient will have vital signs within established parameters after sexual intercourse.
- Patient will experience no pain during or after sexual activity.
- Patient will be able to administer medication to avoid exertion-related pain.
- Patient/family will be able to access therapists as needed for further assistance with sexual activity if required.

▨ DEFICIENT KNOWLEDGE

Related to: CAD, lack of information and cognitive skills

Defining Characteristics: verbalization of the problem, inaccurate follow-through of instructions, request for information, apathetic behavior

Outcome Criteria

✔ Patient will be able to verbalize knowledge of medical regimen, risk factors for angina, MI, CAD, and maintain compliance with preventive regimen.

NOC: *Knowledge: Treatment Regimen*

INTERVENTIONS	RATIONALES
Assess knowledge of causes/risk factors associated with disease, methods to control angina and medical regimen for MI.	Prevents repetition of information. Promotes compliance with medical regimen to prevent extension of CAD and consequences of heart disease. Risk factors in the elderly include hypertension, increased cholesterol and triglyceride levels, cigarette smoking, diabetes mellitus, a history of physical

(continues)

(continued)

INTERVENTIONS	RATIONALES
	inactivity, obesity, and increasing homocysteine levels. Patients should be advised to alter lifestyles when possible to avoid preventable risk factors, such as by consistently taking medication for high blood pressure, stopping smoking, keeping blood glucose levels within specified parameters, and graduated exercise regimens. Modification of risk factors in the elderly can result in a greater decrease in the number of cardiac events they experience.
Write information in large letters, using black ink or simple contrasting colors.	Older patients are able to see black best and may have problems in distinguishing light colors or singular color diagrams.
Provide explanations and information in clear, simple language that is understandable. Provide limited amounts of information over periods of time rather than large amounts at one sitting.	Enhances compliance related to cognitive abilities and sensory deficits.
Use pamphlets, videotapes, and teaching aids with consideration for neurosensory deficits.	Reinforces learning and increases understanding and compliance.
Instruct patient/family regarding signs to report to physician immediately, such as chest pain that is not relieved by rest or 3 doses of nitroglycerin, dyspnea on exertion, or any increase in number of occurrences, intensity of discomfort, or length of discomfort.	In the elderly patient, dyspnea with exertion may be the most common demonstration of a myocardial event, more often than chest pain. This shortness of breath derives from a transient increase in the left ventricular end–diastolic pressure that is caused from ischemia and reduced ventricular compliance. Chest pain, if it occurs, may be described by the elderly as a tightness, heaviness, or burning discomfort substernally or in the adjacent chest area, or may be described as if the patient is choking. Angina in the elderly is frequently noted as discomfort in the back and shoulders or as a burning postprandial epigastric pain. If stable angina begins to increase in severity of symptoms, length of duration, or increase in frequency, it may indicate ischemia is proceeding into an MI.

INTERVENTIONS	RATIONALES
Instruct patient/family regarding avoidance of driving for approximately 1 month after a myocardial infarction, and for patients who have unstable angina, driving should not be allowed until all symptoms have been successfully treated with patient being stable for at least 1 month.	Sudden cardiac death is the cause for less than one out of every 1,000 collisions, but some drugs that the elderly patient may be taking, such as nitrates, can result in hypotensive episodes and syncope. Other drugs may have adverse effects on the cardiovascular system, which can also affect the patient's driving ability.
Instruct patient/family regarding dietary restrictions, such as decreasing amounts of sodium and fat, and in those patients who are obese, decreasing caloric intake while modifying food habits.	May be necessary to reduce risk of CAD and factors contributing to heart problem.
Instruct patient/family regarding the use of nutritional supplements of vitamins, especially vitamin B_6, vitamin B_{12}, and folic acid.	Homocysteine levels that are elevated may increase atherosclerosis by affecting coagulation and by changing the atherogenic properties of the LDL particles and their adherence to the vascular smooth muscle cells. Decreased B_{12} absorption can increase homocysteine levels, and conversely, high homocysteine levels deplete vitamins B_6, B_{12}, and folic acid.
Instruct patient/family regarding a specific exercise program, such as aerobic exercise, cardiac rehabilitation, or other physician-ordered exercise.	Promotes knowledge, enhances cooperation, and involves family in care. Exercise assists with promoting circulation, and when done progressively, can be performed with little risk of danger of cardiac damage or dysfunction. Exercise also help utilize and burn calories to assist in weight reduction.
Instruct patient/family regarding all medications to be taken at home, side effects to be aware of, and signs to report to physician.	Provides opportunity for questions and ensures accuracy of medication administration. Timely identification of adverse reaction to medication regime allows for prompt intervention and potential changes. Aspirin will usually be prescribed as a daily dose to reduce the risk of MI and sudden death.
Instruct patient/family to avoid all over-the-counter medications unless approved by physician.	Some medications may interact with prescribed drugs.

INTERVENTIONS	RATIONALES
When instructing patient, be sure to face patient, speak clearly, and allow time for answering questions and clarifying information.	Older patients need verification that they possess correct knowledge that is current. Age-related health changes may necessitate changes in teaching style to ensure optimal knowledge exchange.
Instruct patient/family regarding the need for PTCA, CABG, or revascularization as needed.	If patient continues to have pain after therapy has begun, and despite the use of nitrates, revascularization will be considered to prevent or limit the amount of damage of an ischemic myocardium. Non-Q wave MIs are more common in elderly patients and treatment is aimed at salvage of myocardial tissue, and prevention of death, heart failure, and cardiac dysfunction.

NIC: *Teaching: Disease Process*

Discharge or Maintenance Evaluation

■ Patient will be able to modify diet by decreasing saturated fats, decreasing sodium and using various spices to augment taste of food, and limit caloric intake within constraints of ordered dietary limitations.

■ Patient will be able to recall risk factors, methods of lowering risk, and causes of CAD accurately, and will adjust lifestyle to incorporate these modifying factors.

■ Patient/family will be able to accurately recall information regarding medication administration including dosages and times of administration.

■ Patient will be compliant with exercise program, and will be able to participate in rehabilitation without evidence of ischemia or cardiac dysfunction.

■ Patient/family will be able to seek emergent medical assistance if patient develops pain that is not relieved by rest and the use of nitrates.

Coronary Artery Disease

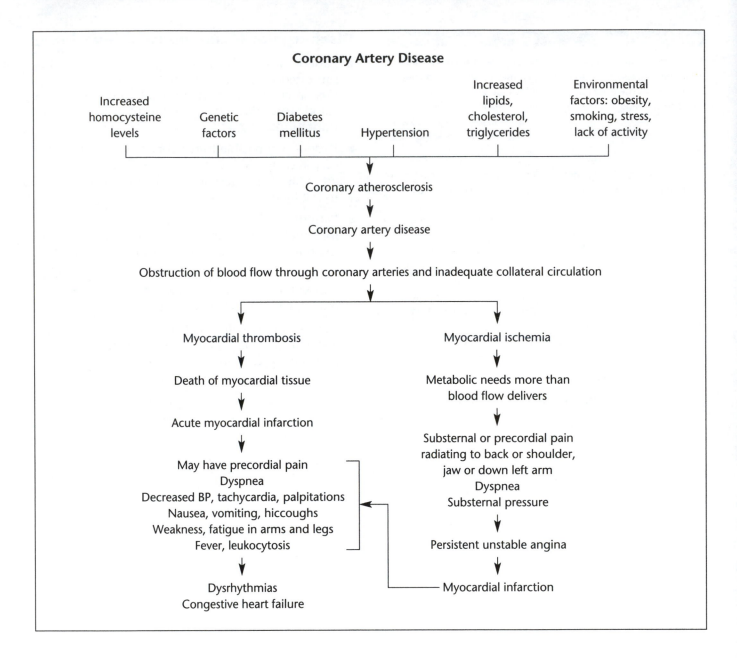

CHAPTER 1.2

HEART FAILURE

Heart failure is the inability of the heart to supply blood flow to meet physiologic demands, without utilizing compensatory changes. There may be failure involving one or both sides of the heart, which, over time, may cause the development of pulmonary and systemic congestion and complications. Congestive heart failure is a common complication following myocardial infarction and can contribute to the deaths of patients with MIs. Usually following an MI, the heart failure is left-sided as most infarctions involve damage to the left ventricle.

Heart failure usually involves some type of hindrance to the forward ejection of blood flow, such as seen with hypertension or aortic valve stenosis. It may involve the loss of cardiac muscle function that results from ischemia or infarction, or when cardiac filling is impaired, such as with ventricular hypertrophy or ventricular aneurysms. Heart failure also occurs with fluid volume overload that is seen with increased intravascular volume, valvular regurgitation, or hypermetabolic states. In the older patient, heart failure usually results either from systemic hypertension or from coronary artery disease, both of which can result in myocardial failure.

Diastolic dysfunction is responsible for approximately half the cases of heart failure among the elderly, especially in women. With diastolic dysfunction, the phase of myocardial relaxation is prolonged, and stiffness of the myocardium resulting from physiologic changes, such as increased interstitial collagen in the heart muscle, decreases the amount of blood volume as well as how quickly the heart fills with blood. This causes the left ventricular diastolic pressure to increase, which in turn, causes the amount of blood that is ejected with each heartbeat to decrease. Heart failure then occurs, even in the presence of normal systolic function, which is represented by the ejection fraction.

The elderly experience age-related cardiac changes that lower the threshold for the occurrence of heart failure, and reduce diastolic left ventricular function. Some decrease in systolic function also occurs with age. Decreases in responsiveness to beta-adrenergic stimulation damages the ability of the elderly body to respond to increased work demands and increased myocardial consumption. Their exercise capacity is decreased, and mature patients are more prone to develop heart failure as a response to stressors of systemic illness, such as infection, hypothyroidism, hyperthyroidism, anemia, renal failure, or cardiovascular events.

Heart failure can be classified as acute or chronic. In chronic heart failure, the body experiences a gradual development as the heart becomes unable to pump a sufficient amount of blood to meet the body's demands. Chronic heart failure can become acute without any overt cause.

Often, the patient will have no early symptoms of left-sided heart failure. Symptoms of decreased cardiac output will develop once the heart fails to pump enough blood into the systemic circulation. The pressure in the left ventricle increases, which in turn causes retrograde increases of pressure in the left atrium because of the increased difficulty for blood to enter the atrium from the pulmonary veins. Blood backs up in the lung vasculature, and when the oncotic pressure of the proteins in the plasma fluid exceeds the pulmonary capillary pressure, the fluid leaks into the interstitial spaces. When this fluid moves into the alveoli, shortness of breath, coughing, and crackles (rales) occur, and the patient can progress into overt pulmonary edema.

Right-sided heart failure is usually caused by left-sided heart failure, but can also be caused by pulmonary emboli, pulmonary hypertension, COPD, and the presence of right ventricular infarctions.

Common symptoms of heart failure include dyspnea, fatigue, especially with any exertion or activity, orthopnea, and dependent edema in the extremities and sacral area. Jugular vein distention and hepatojugular reflux are also frequently noted. Elderly patients may have nonspecific symptoms, such as confusion, disorientation, weakness, fatigue, and somnolence, as well as an S_3 gallop with coarse crackles in the lower lung fields. An S_4 gallop does not necessarily denote clinically substantial cardiac disease.

Treatment of heart failure usually involves attempts to improve contractility of the ventricle by use of inotropic drugs, decrease of afterload by the use of nitrates and vasodilators, and decrease of preload by the use of diuretics, nitroglycerin IV, and fluid and sodium restriction.

MEDICAL CARE

Laboratory: CBC used to identify hematologic abnormalities; platelet count used to monitor for thrombocytopenia caused by use of amrinone and other drugs; electrolyte levels to monitor for imbalances; renal profiles to monitor for kidney function problems; digoxin levels to monitor for toxicity; coagulation profiles to monitor efficacy of anticoagulation therapy; cardiac enzymes used to identify cardiac damage; albumin, prealbumin, and protein used to identify nutritional imbalance

Radiography: chest X-rays used to identify enlargement of the heart and pulmonary vein, presence of pulmonary edema, or pleural effusion

Electrocardiography: used to monitor for dysrhythmias that may occur as a result of heart failure or as a result of digitalis toxicity; may identify changes occurring from ventricular enlargement

Echocardiography: used to identify structural abnormalities, chamber size, and blood flow through the heart

Surgery: may be performed if heart failure is caused by primary valvular disease and valve replacement is warranted; coronary revascularization may be considered if coronary artery disease results in myocardial ischemia; cardiac transplantation is rarely performed in the elderly because of the limited availability of donor organs, and as such, ventricular assist devices (VADs) are used only as a bridge to transplantation

Cardiac glycosides: digitalis (Digoxin, Lanoxin) used to increase the strength and force of ventricular contractions and to decrease the conduction and rate of contractions in order to increase cardiac output; also helps to relieve heart failure symptoms and decrease the incidence of exacerbations of heart failure

Inotropic agents: inamrinone lactate (Inocor) and milrinone lactate (Primacor) used in the short-term treatment for heart failure by increasing the levels of cAMP, directly relaxes vascular smooth muscle, and produces vasodilation in patients that do not respond to other measures; IV dobutamine (Dobutrex) and dopamine (Intropin) are sometimes used in severe heart failure patients by increasing the myocardial contractility and stroke volume; also can decrease afterload, preload, and assist with AV node conduction which ultimately results in increased cardiac output

Vasodilators: cyclandelate (Cyclan, Cyclandelate, Cyclospasmol), dipyridamole (Persantine), hydralazine (Apresoline), isosorbide dinitrate (Isordil), minoxidil (Loniten, Minodyl), and tolazoline (Priscoline) used to increase stroke volume by facilitating blood ejection, decreasing preload and afterload, decreasing oxygen demand, decreasing systemic vascular resistance, and increasing venous capacitance by relaxing arterial and venous smooth muscle; combination of Isordil and Apresoline noted to reduce morbidity in patients who have systolic heart failure

ACE inhibitors: benazepril hydrochloride (Lotensin), candesartan cilexetil (Atacand), captopril (Capoten), enalapril (Vasotec), eprosartan mesylate (Teveten), fosinopril sodium (Monopril), irbesartan (Avapro), losartan potassium (Cozaar), moexipril hydrochloride (Univasc), perindopril erbumine (Aceon), quinapril hydrochloride (Accupril), ramipril (Altace), telmisartan (Micardis), trandolapril (Mavik), and valsartan (Diovan) used to prevent the conversion of angiotensin I to angiotensin II by inhibiting the angiotensin converting enzyme (ACE) to enable the decrease in vasoconstriction, preload, and afterload; angiotensin II receptor blockers inhibit angiotensin II at the end-organ receptor level and tend to have less incidence of coughing

Calcium channel blockers: depending on the drug used, may worsen heart failure and increase mortality; those with negative inotropic effects can exacerbate symptoms, with the exception of amlodipine (Norvasc), and use of this drug with severe left ventricular failure patients decreases mortality in patients without known CAD; verapamil (Calan, Isoptin) and diltiazem (Cardizem) can exacerbate symptoms or precipitate heart failure, but in some patients who have diastolic heart failure, these drugs may decrease symptoms in patients, especially those with hypertrophic cardiomyopathy

Beta-blockers: bisoprolol (Zebeta), carvedilol (Coreg), and metoprolol (Lopressor, Toprol XL) used in patients with severe systolic left ventricular failure to reduce symptoms and mortality after MI; should not be utilized with patients who are critically symptomatic, who have class IIIS or IV heart failures, or who have COPD or significant conduction dysfunction

Antidysrhythmics: drugs such as adenosine (Adenocard), amiodarone (Cordarone, Pacerone), bretyllium tosylate (Bretylol), esmolol hydrochloride (Brevibloc), or ibutilide fumarate (Corvert), may be required to restore sinus rhythm in patients who develop atrial fibrillation or other dysrhythmias; type I antiarrhythmic drugs should be avoided in patients with heart failure unless they have an implanted defibrillator because mortality rates are high if their ejection fraction is <40%; elderly patients depend on atrial contractions for adequate ventricular filling pressures and volume, so drugs may be required to maintain an intrinsic sinus rhythm

Anticoagulants: enoxaparin sodium (Lovenox), heparin calcium and sodium (Calciparin, Heparin), and warfarin (Coumadin) may be used for patients who have atrial fibrillation or previous history of emboli; elderly patients have an increased risk for adverse consequences from these drugs

COMMON NURSING DIAGNOSES

 ## DECREASED CARDIAC OUTPUT (see CAD)

Related to: alteration in preload and afterload, inotropic changes in heart, accumulation of blood in lungs or systemic venous system

Defining Characteristics: BP and pulse changes, fatigue, cold, clammy skin, cyanosis, dependent edema, dyspnea, orthopnea, cough, crackles, ascites, hepatomegaly, splenomegaly, frothy, bloody sputum, confusion, nocturia, restlessness

 ## IMPAIRED GAS EXCHANGE (see CAD)

Related to: ventilation/perfusion imbalance from fluid in alveoli, reduced area for exchange in left sided failure

Defining Characteristics: hypoxia, restlessness, somnolence, confusion, altered mentation, hypercapnia, cyanosis, dyspnea, crackles, activity intolerance, abnormal arterial blood gases

ADDITIONAL NURSING DIAGNOSES

 ## EXCESS FLUID VOLUME

Related to: compromised regulatory mechanisms of heart's failure to act as a pump and maintain cardiac output

Defining Characteristics: edema, weight gain, effusion, dyspnea, orthopnea, crackles, oliguria, change in respiratory pattern, ascites, peripheral edema, hepatomegaly, splenomegaly, cyanosis, frothy, blood-tinged sputum, confusion, restlessness

Outcome Criteria

✔ Blood pressure will be maintained within normal limits and edema will be absent or minimal in all body parts.
✔ Fluid volume will be stabilized with balanced intake and output.

NOC: *Fluid Balance*

INTERVENTIONS	RATIONALES
Monitor vital signs. Notify physician of significant abnormalities.	Fluid volume excess will cause increases in blood pressure, and those changes will be reflected from the development of pulmonary congestion and heart failure.
Auscultate lung fields for the presence of crackles (rales), or other adventitious breath sounds. Observe for presence of cough, increased dyspnea, tachypnea, orthopnea, or paroxysmal nocturnal dyspnea.	May indicate pulmonary edema from cardiac decompensation and pulmonary congestion. Pulmonary edema symptoms reflect left-sided heart failure. Right-sided heart failure may have a slower onset, but symptoms of dyspnea, orthopnea, and cough are more difficult to reverse.
Observe for jugular vein distention and dependent edema. Note presence of generalized body edema (anasarca).	May indicate impending congestive failure and fluid excess. Peripheral edema begins in feet and ankles, or other dependent areas, and ascends as failure progresses. Pitting will usually

(continues)

(continued)

INTERVENTIONS	RATIONALES
	occur only after ten or more pounds of excess fluid are retained. Anasarca will be seen only with right-sided heart failure or bi-ventricular failure. Edema is the excess accumulation of interstitial fluid in the tissues or organs caused by increased capillary pressure or permeability associated with decreased resistance to flow through the arterioles, increased resistance to flow through the venules, or loss of capillary wall integrity, or by decreased osmotic pressure to move fluid from the tissues back into the capillaries.
Investigate abrupt complaints of dyspnea, air hunger, feelings of impending doom, or suffocation.	Excessive fluid buildup can promote other complications, such as pulmonary edema or pulmonary embolus, and intervention must be immediate.
Determine fluid balance by measuring intake and output, and observing for decreases in output and concentrated urine.	Decreased cardiac output leads to decreased renal perfusion and impairment with excessive fluid volume, which causes sodium and water retention and oliguria.
Weigh daily and notify physician of >2 lb/day increase.	Abrupt changes in weight usually indicate excess fluid. Weight gains of 5 pounds usually reflect approximately 2 liters of fluid accumulation.
Provide patient with adequate fluid intake of up to 2 L/day, unless fluids are ordered to be restricted.	Fluids maintain hydration of cellular tissues, but may need to be restricted because of cardiac decompensation if excessive intravascular or intracellular fluid accumulations are present.
Administer diuretics as ordered.	Drugs may be required to correct fluid overload, depending on emergent nature of problem. Diuretics increase urine flow rate and may inhibit reabsorption of sodium and chloride in the renal tubules.
Monitor lab work for electrolyte imbalances. Note increasing lethargy, hypotension, or muscle cramping.	Hypokalemia can occur with the administration of diuretics. Signs of potassium and sodium deficits may occur from fluid shifts with diuretic therapy.

INTERVENTIONS	RATIONALES
Place patient in semi-Fowler's or high Fowler's position.	Diuresis may be enhanced by recumbent position caused by increased glomerular filtration and decreased production of ADH. Position may facilitate ease of breathing.
Auscultate bowel sounds and observe for abdominal distention, anorexia, nausea, or constipation. Provide small, easily-digestible meals.	CHF progression can impair gastric motility and intestinal function. Small, frequent meals may enhance digestion and prevent abdominal discomfort while allowing patient time to rest to facilitate improvement of breathing.
Measure abdominal girth every shift, if warranted.	Progressive right-sided heart failure can cause fluid to shift into the peritoneal space and cause ascites.
Palpate abdomen for liver enlargement and note any right upper quadrant tenderness or pain.	Progressive heart failure can lead to venous congestion, abdominal distention, liver engorgement, and pain. Liver function may be impaired which can impede drug metabolism.
Reposition patient every 2 hours or more often. Elevate legs, and pad bony prominences.	Edematous tissue interferes with movement and is more susceptible to injury from pressure. Edematous tissues are not well oxygenated and lack circulation of necessary nutrients and increased waste products. Bed rest reduces oxygen and cardiac demands and can help to enhance renal perfusion and excretion of excess fluids. Repositioning facilitates improved breathing, mobility of secretions, and decreases risk of pressures sores.
Instruct patient/family regarding dietary limitations such as lowering sodium and potassium intake, foods to avoid, and seasonings that can be substituted to improve palatability.	Decreases in sodium can reduce fluid and electrolyte retention. Information regarding dietary choices can facilitate compliance postdischarge.
Instruct patient in medications, effects, side effects, and symptoms of which to notify physician.	Provides knowledge, facilitates compliance with medication regimen, and helps to identify adverse effects that may require prompt intervention.
Instruct patient to weigh daily on same scale, at same time, with	Utilization of same scale provides consistent data that will accurately

INTERVENTIONS	RATIONALES
same clothing if possible, and to notify physician of significant gains or losses (>2 lb/wk change).	reflect fluid balance/imbalance. Identification of changes may require intervention by physician or change in medical regimen.
Instruct patient to avoid restrictive clothing and shoes.	Edema may result in tightness and cause pressure and injury to tissues.
Instruct patient to avoid prolonged standing, excessively hot environment, and to change positions slowly when rising from a sitting or lying position.	Orthostatic hypotension may occur as a result of medications or prolonged position. Heat increases dilatation of superficial vasculature and may contribute to hypotension.

NIC: *Hypervolemia Management*

Discharge or Maintenance Evaluation

■ Patient will have no dependent or generalized edema, nor have fluid excess as exhibited by weight gain over 1 lb/day.

■ Patient will maintain fluid balance, with equivalent intake and output, and vital signs will be within normal parameters.

■ Patient will have clear lung fields to auscultation, with no adventitious breath sounds.

■ Patient/family will be able to accurately verbalize understanding of all instructions, medications, and dietary restrictions.

■ Patient/family will be able to modify dietary lifestyle to reduce the presence and recurrence of preventable heart failure.

CONSTIPATION

Related to: less than adequate fluids, dietary intake and bulk, anorexia, gastrointestinal distress

Defining Characteristics: decreased appetite, abdominal pain, hepatomegaly, nausea, hard-formed stool, reduced frequency, absence of stools

Outcome Criteria

✔ Patient will have normal elimination pattern reestablished and maintained.

NOC: *Bowel Elimination*

INTERVENTIONS	RATIONALES
Determine patient's bowel habits, lifestyle, ability to sense urge to defecate, painful hemorrhoids, and history of constipation.	Assists with identification of an effective bowel regimen and/or impairment, and need for assistance. GI function may be decreased as a result of decreased digestion. Functional impairment related to muscular weakness and immobility may result in decreased abdominal perstalsis and difficulty with identification of the urge to defecate. Identifying other conditions the patient may also have can assist in discovering potential contributory factors to constipation.
Assess patient's stool frequency, characteristics, presence of flatulence, abdominal discomfort or distention, and straining at stool.	Age-related changes in the elderly patient, such as decreased rectal compliance, impairment of rectal sensation, and delayed colonic transit predispose the older patient to constipation. The elderly patient also has decreased anal and sphincter pressures that may affect continence.
Auscultate bowel sounds for presence and quality.	Abnormal sounds, such as high-pitched tinkles, suggest complications like ileus.
Monitor diet and fluid intake.	Adequate amounts of fiber and roughage provide bulk and adequate fluid intake (at least 2 L/day) is important in keeping stools soft.
Monitor for complaints of abdominal pain and abdominal distention.	Gas, abdominal distention, or ileus could be a factor. Lack of peristalsis from impaired digestion can create bowel distention and worsen to the point of ileus.
Monitor patient for mental status changes, syncope, chest pain, or transient ischemic attacks. Notify physician if these symptoms occur.	Undue straining may have harmful effects on arterial circulation that can result in cardiac, cerebral, or peripheral ischemia.
Assess for rectal bleeding.	Excessive straining may produce hemorrhoids, rectal prolapse, or anal fissures, with resultant pain and bleeding.
Provide bulk, stool softeners, laxatives, suppositories, or enemas as warranted.	May be required to stimulate evacuation of stool. Up to 60% of elderly patients use laxatives routinely and constipation is more common in this population. Osmotic laxatives

(continues)

(continued)

INTERVENTIONS	RATIONALES
	that contain magnesium should be used on a short-term basis only and in patients who do not have renal insufficiency.
Remove fecal impaction prn as ordered.	Impaction may result in complications, such as intestinal obstruction, colonic ulceration, or paradoxical diarrhea. Impaction is more probable in patients who have limited mobility or decreased mental capacity.
Assess for urinary retention and urinary tract infection.	These conditions frequently occur together with fecal impaction.
Provide high-fiber diet, whole grain cereals, breads, and fresh fruits.	Improves peristalsis and promotes elimination.
Monitor medications that may predispose patient to constipation.	Analgesics, anesthetics, anticholinergics, antidepressants, antihypertensives, diuretics, iron, anti-Parkinson drugs, and anticonvulsant drugs are some medications that are known to cause constipation, which are frequently taken by the elderly.
Determine pre-existing habits of laxative/enema usage.	Laxative dependence can predispose patient to constipation.
Instruct patient to avoid frequent use of enemas.	Promotes enema dependence and causes fluid loss that results in more difficult elimination.
Instruct patient/family in activity or exercise programs within limits of disease process.	Activity promotes peristalsis and stimulates defecation. Exercises help to strengthen the abdominal muscles that aid in defecation.
Instruct patient and help establish bowel regime, such as trying to move bowels in early morning after breakfast.	Colonic motor activity is highest at this time and facilitates elimination.

NIC: *Constipation/Impaction Management*

Discharge or Maintenance Evaluation

- Patient will have improved dietary and fluid intake.
- Patient will achieve bowel elimination pattern establishment and be able to maintain elimination of soft, formed stool without cramping or straining.

- Patient will be able to use dietary modifications, increased fluids, and activity to improve bowel habits, and avoid laxative and enema dependence.
- Patient will be able to maintain daily exercise within parameters of disease process.
- Patient will avoid impaction, urinary retention, and urinary tract infections.

DISTURBED SLEEP PATTERN

Related to: internal factors of illness from heart failure

Defining Characteristics: interrupted sleep, restlessness, irritability, verbal complaints of not feeling rested, paroxysmal nocturnal dyspnea, inability to function, difficulty awakening, difficulty staying asleep, insomnia, nighttime awakenings, daytime napping

Outcome Criteria

- ✔ Patient will be able to sleep without interruption and will express feelings of being rested.
- ✔ Patient will be able to perform techniques to promote sleep.

NOC: *Sleep*

INTERVENTIONS	RATIONALES
Assess patient's sleep pattern and changes, naps, amount of activity, awakenings and frequency, and patient's complaints of lack of rest.	Provides information to alleviate sleep deprivation in relation to age-related changes and to identify and establish plan of care.
Monitor for complaints of pain, dyspnea, discomfort, and nocturia.	Identification of causative factors of frequent awakenings helps facilitate changes in sleep pattern.
Provide calm, quiet environment, closing curtains, adjusting lighting, and so forth.	Helps to promote conducive atmosphere for restful sleep. External stimulus may interfere with going to sleep and increase awakenings in the elderly patient because sleep is usually of less intensity.
Administer medications to promote normal sleep patterns as ordered.	Medication may be required to achieve rest during hospitalization. Hypnotics induce sleep, while tranquilizers reduce anxiety.
Provide warm drinks, extra cover, warm bath prior to bedtime, and so forth.	Ritualistic procedures may prevent breaks in established routines and promote comfort and

INTERVENTIONS	RATIONALES
	relaxation prior to sleep. Snacks that are high in protein and milk contain L-tryptophan which helps promote sleep.
Instruct patient to avoid stimulants, such as caffeinated drinks, stressful activity, and so forth prior to sleep.	Overstimulation prevents patient from falling asleep.
Instruct patient in relaxation techniques, guided imagery, muscle relaxation, meditation, and so forth.	Relaxation techniques frequently help promote sleep.
Instruct patient/family regarding adverse reactions of medications that may disturb sleep.	Antipsychotics sometimes result in behavior disturbances and frequent awakenings. Beta-blockers can result in nightmares resulting from alterations in CNS effects, and patients with asthma or COPD may have nocturnal wheezing and dyspnea. Diuretics can cause nocturia, and cause patients to be unable to resume sleep. Histamine blockers may create delirium in the elderly patient. Some bronchodilators increase stimulation of the CNS and cause insomnia.
Instruct patient to avoid using alcohol at bedtime.	Although alcohol may initially cause sleepiness, it interrupts sleep later in the night.

NIC: *Sleep Enhancement*

Discharge or Maintenance Evaluation

- Patient will identify factors that prevent restful sleep or disrupt sleep.
- Patient will be able to achieve and maintain an adequate amount of sleep to facilitate maximal functioning.
- Patient will be able to establish a sleep pattern.
- Patient/family will be able to accurately verbalize understanding of instructions given, and will comply with avoidance of substances that cause disruption of sleep.

FATIGUE

Related to: decreased capacity for physical activity, sense of exhaustion, intolerance of activity, decreased cardiac output, increased metabolic demand

Defining Characteristics: drowsiness, failure of sleep to restore energy level, lack of energy, inability to maintain routines, decreased concentration, lethargy, listlessness, decreased performance, perceived need for additional energy to accomplish tasks, increase in physical complaints, dyspnea, increased work of breathing, alteration in mental status

Outcome Criteria

✔ Patient will have increased energy and be able to participate in normal activities.

NOC: *Activity Tolerance*

INTERVENTIONS	RATIONALES
Assess/observe patient for signs of activity intolerance, such as dyspnea, extreme fatigue, lethargy, or vital sign changes.	Provides baseline information so that identification of problem and interventions may be planned. Elevations in pulse, blood pressure, and respiratory rate may indicate physiologic intolerance of activity and fatigue.
Provide periods of rest or sleep alternating with periods of activity as patient can tolerate.	Prevents excessive fatigue and increases stamina.
Avoid scheduling patient for two or more energy-draining procedures on same day, if possible.	Conserving energy helps to avoid overexertion and potential for exhaustion.
Schedule patient's daily routine based on specific needs and desires.	Encourages compliance with treatment regimen and reduces fatigue.
Encourage food high in iron and minerals, unless disease process contraindicates.	Helps to avoid anemia and demineralization that can affect fatigue. Low red blood cell counts can affect a patient's oxygenation as oxygen molecules are carried throughout the body via the hemoglobin molecules.
Provide small, easily digestible meals.	Frequent small meals conserve energy and encourage increased intake of nutritive sustenance.
Instruct patient regarding effects of fatigue on daily activity and personal lifestyle.	Helps to increase patient compliance and allows for planning schedule for activity and rest.
Instruct patient to schedule rest periods between activities.	Helps to decrease fatigue and increase stamina.
Instruct patient and help him to establish a regular sleeping pattern.	Adequate amounts of sleep each night will help decrease fatigue.

NIC: *Energy Management*

Discharge or Maintenance Evaluation

- Patient will be able to identify methods of reducing fatigue and will be able to modify lifestyle to incorporate these methods.
- Patient will be able to have reduced fatigue and will be able to prevent further episodes of fatigue.
- Patient will be able to accurately recall information regarding energy conservation techniques.

INEFFECTIVE COPING

Related to: multiple life changes, loss of independence, limitations on lifestyle, chronic disease

Defining Characteristics: inability to meet basic needs, dependency, chronic fatigue, worry, anxiety, poor self-esteem, verbalization of inability to cope

Outcome Criteria

✔ Patient will be able to achieve increased independence in activities and decision-making process.

✔ Patient will be able to adapt to lifestyle changes necessitated by current illness or disease process.

NOC: *Coping*

INTERVENTIONS	RATIONALES
Assess coping methods, use of defense mechanisms, feelings about lifestyle changes, any losses associated with illness, and ability to ask for help.	Allows for interventions that promote control over life and ability to cope with long-term illness.
Assist to identify positive defense mechanisms and promote their use.	Use of defense mechanisms that have worked in past increases ability to cope and promotes self-esteem.
Provide environment that allows for free expression of concerns and fears.	Encourages trust and relieves anxiety and worry.
Assist to set short- and long-term goals; provide positive feedback regarding progress and focus on abilities rather than disabilities.	Promotes self-worth and responsibility.
Inform patient that compliance with treatment regimen reduces risk factors.	Maintains health status by preventing recurrence of acute episode.
Refer to support group or counseling if appropriate; involve family members if client desires.	Provides information and support from others with similar experiences.

INTERVENTIONS	RATIONALES
Teach relaxation techniques.	Reduces stress and anxiety.
Teach problem solving approaches and new ways or methods to adapt to chronic illness.	Promotes coping ability with life style changes.

NIC: *Mutual Goal-Setting*

Discharge or Maintenance Evaluation

- Patient will be able to use appropriate coping mechanisms and problem-solving methods to adapt to functional losses.
- Patient will be able to ask for assistance when needed.
- Patient will be able to achieve a level of independence that is appropriate with his activity limitations and coping ability.
- Patient will be able to access community resources postdischarge.

DEFICIENT KNOWLEDGE

Related to: lack of information on dietary, activity and drug therapy

Defining Characteristics: verbalization of the problem, request for information, noncompliance with medical regimen

Outcome Criteria

✔ Patient will be compliant with low sodium diet, drug therapy, and exercise regimen.

NOC: *Knowledge: Treatment Regimen*

INTERVENTIONS	RATIONALES
Assess knowledge of proper diet for low sodium intake, administration of cardiac glycosides, diuretics, and other drugs ordered.	Provides basis for teaching and avoids repetition of information.
Utilize booklets, pictures, tapes, and charts in teaching client and family.	Aids in teaching by use of visual adjuncts.
Provide clear explanations and instruction in medication names, action, dosage, frequency, storage, how to take and expected results.	Enhances compliance as complexity and number of medications increase.

INTERVENTIONS	RATIONALES
Instruct patient/family to report side effects of anorexia, nausea, vomiting, diarrhea, headache, fatigue, blurred vision, or irregular and slow pulse.	May indicate symptoms of digitalis toxicity.
Instruct patient/family to take pulse before taking cardiac glycoside, omit dose and report if pulse below 60/min (50/min if taking beta-blocking drug).	Bradycardia leads to dysrhythmias or other cardiac complications.
Instruct patient/family to avoid use of table salt, commercially prepared or convenience foods, cheese, snack foods, soy sauce, pickled foods, sodas, or antacids that contain salt.	Reduces salt intake and fluid retention as increased sodium levels decrease movement of fluid from cell to capillary circulation.
Instruct patient/family to include citrus juices, bananas, broths, and whole grains in diet.	Foods that contain potassium may be helpful for replacement if diuretic therapy given.
Instruct patient/family to season foods with lemon and spices.	Replaces salt as seasoning.
Instruct patient to report weakness, palpitations, fatigue, leg cramps, excessive thirst, or 2 lb/day weight loss.	May indicate symptoms of hypokalemia if on diuretic therapy.

INTERVENTIONS	RATIONALES
Refer to dietician if weight loss plan needed.	Overweight increases workload of heart.
Instruct patient to modify activities to meet rest needs.	Prevents fatigue and increased oxygen need.

NIC: *Teaching: Individual*

Discharge or Maintenance Evaluation

- Patient will be able to administer medications accurately and appropriately.

- Patient will be able to identify signs and symptoms indicating changes in cardiac status and report them to physician.

- Patient will be compliant with dietary restrictions.

- Patient will be compliant with weight loss program, if needed.

- Patient will be able to accurately verbalize information received and will be able to avoid preventable complications.

Heart Failure

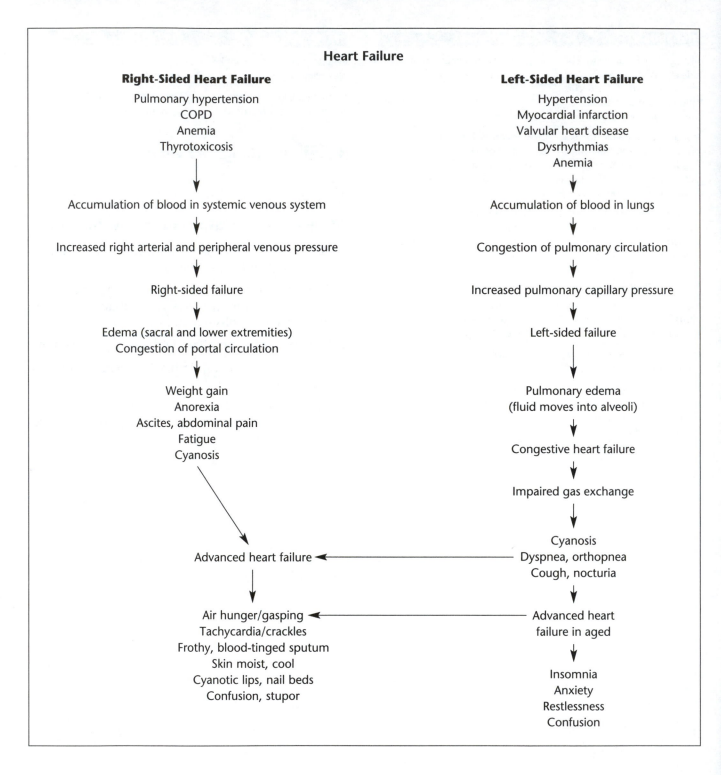

Right-Sided Heart Failure

Pulmonary hypertension
COPD
Anemia
Thyrotoxicosis

↓

Accumulation of blood in systemic venous system

↓

Increased right arterial and peripheral venous pressure

↓

Right-sided failure

↓

Edema (sacral and lower extremities)
Congestion of portal circulation

↓

Weight gain
Anorexia
Ascites, abdominal pain
Fatigue
Cyanosis

Advanced heart failure ←

↓

Air hunger/gasping ←
Tachycardia/crackles
Frothy, blood-tinged sputum
Skin moist, cool
Cyanotic lips, nail beds
Confusion, stupor

Left-Sided Heart Failure

Hypertension
Myocardial infarction
Valvular heart disease
Dysrhythmias
Anemia

↓

Accumulation of blood in lungs

↓

Congestion of pulmonary circulation

↓

Increased pulmonary capillary pressure

↓

Left-sided failure

↓

Pulmonary edema
(fluid moves into alveoli)

↓

Congestive heart failure

↓

Impaired gas exchange

↓

Cyanosis
Dyspnea, orthopnea
Cough, nocturia

↓

Advanced heart
failure in aged

↓

Insomnia
Anxiety
Restlessness
Confusion

CHAPTER 1.3

HYPERTENSION

Essential, or primary hypertension, is an elevated blood pressure of unknown origin, but may be the result of changes in the elderly in their pressor and depressor functions that regulate arterial pressure. Secondary hypertension, which is an elevated blood pressure resulting from a known cause, will cause inflammation and necrosis in the arterioles, which then results in decreased blood flow to vital body organs, and places stress on the heart and vessels.

Conditions that may trigger hypertension include renal syndromes, such as renal artery stenosis, chronic glomerulonephritis, polycystic renal disease, or renal neoplasms, endocrine dysfunction, such as thyroid disorders, pheochromocytoma, primary aldosteronism, or Cushing's disease, or the use of medications, such as tricyclic antidepressants, monoamine oxidase inhibitors, phenylpropanolamine, and other vasoconstrictors. Secondary hypertension can additionally be induced by cocaine use, excessive alcohol intake, licorice, or coarctation of the aorta.

Uncontrolled hypertension is associated with permanent damage to body systems. Atherosclerosis may predispose elderly patients to isolated systolic hypertension when artery compliance is decreased.

Blood pressure elevation is considered to be hypertension if the systolic pressure is greater than 140 mm Hg or the diastolic pressure is greater than 90 mm Hg, and is classified based on the severity from a high normal to malignant hypertension. Hypertensive crisis is defined as a sustained increase in diastolic blood pressure above 120 mm Hg, which is high enough to cause irreversible damage to organs and tissue death.

More than half the elderly American population over the age of 65 have some degree of elevated systolic and/or diastolic pressure (Beers & Berkow, 2000). Elevations of systolic pressure can be noted as a cause of cardiovascular problems, and actually increase morbidity. Untreated, hypertension in the elderly population may result in death resulting from cerebrovascular accident, congestive heart failure, intracerebral hemorrhage, coronary artery disease, peripheral vascular disease, dissecting aneurysms, or kidney failure.

Hypertension may result from several origins—adrenal origin (as in pheochromocytoma, Cushing's disease, brain tumors, etc.), renal origin (as in pyelonephritis), cardiovascular origin (as in atherosclerosis or coarctation of the aorta, etc.), or unknown origin, which accounts for the majority of all known hypertension cases.

Systolic blood pressure is the pressure that the heart pumps against to force blood from the left side of the heart to the aorta and to major arteries. Diastolic blood pressure is the pressure required to permit filling of the ventricles before the next systole cycle. The pulse pressure, which is the value of the difference between the systolic and diastolic pressures, may be used to indicate perfusion problems. The mean arterial pressure, or MAP (or MABP) is the average pressure attempting to push the blood through the circulatory system and should be greater than 60 mm Hg in order to adequately perfuse organs.

Elevated blood pressure may occur as a result of emotional stress with as much as a 40 mm Hg increase, and may also result from ventilatory insufficiency, post-seizures, electroconvulsive therapy, intracerebral injury, CNS disorders caused by the massive stimulation of catecholamines, coronary artery bypass surgery, myocardial infarction, heart failure, renal insufficiency, endocrine disorders, and some drugs.

A pseudohypertension that occurs in elderly patients is a result of stiffening of the arteries, so it is essential that blood pressure measurements be taken with appropriate techniques, with correct sizes of cuffs, and in both arms. Occlusive atherosclerotic disease in the subclavian or brachial arteries can reduce the systolic blood pressure unilaterally.

Risk factors include: ages between 30 and 70 years of age, race (black), use of birth control pills, obesity, familial history, smoking, stress, diabetes mellitus, and sedentary lifestyle. Treatment is aimed at lowering blood pressure by use of antihypertensive medications, diuretics to increase urinary output, and by eliminating factors that promote the elevation of blood pressure.

In the elderly, a conscious decision should be exercised about utilizing medication therapy and the potential for side effects from the drugs. A "stepped care" regimen is used most often, with step one involving the use of thiazide diuretics and calcium ion antagonists; step two involves the supplemental use of beta-adrenergic blockers, used with caution in the elderly except in cases of postmyocardial infarction; step three includes vasodilators; and step four involves guanethidine.

MEDICAL CARE

Laboratory: CBC used to identify anemias and fluid losses; renal profiles to identify renal dysfunction; lipid panels used to identify elevations in cholesterol, triglycerides, or lipoproteins that may increase the risk of atherosclerosis; electrolyte profiles used to identify imbalances, especially hypokalemia and/or hypernatremia, caused by diuretic use; plasma renin and angiotensin levels are usually decreased in elderly patients with essential hypertension; urinalysis and creatinine clearance tests are used to identify infection and renal dysfunction; urine VMA used to identify elevation of catecholamine metabolites which may be indicative of pheochromocytoma; glucose levels used to identify potential causes of hypertension; thyroid profiles used to identify hyperthyroidism which may lead to vasoconstriction and hypertension; aldosterone level used to identify primary aldosteronism

Radiography: chest X-rays used to identify cardiac enlargement, pulmonary congestion, or infiltrates; IVP may be used to identify the presence of kidney disease; renal arteriogram may be used to show renal artery stenosis or other causes of hypertension

Electrocardiography: used to monitor for changes in rate and rhythm, conduction abnormalities, left ventricular hypertrophy, ischemia, electrolyte abnormalities, drug toxicity, and the presence of dysrhythmias

Diuretics: chlorthalidone (Hygroton, Thalitone), hydrochlorothiazide (Esidrix, Ezide, HydroDiuril, Microzide, Oretic), Indapamide (Lozol), and metolazone (Mykrox, Zaroxolyn) are thiazide-acting diuretics that increase sodium and water excretion by

inhibiting reabsorption of sodium in the cortical diluting site of the ascending loop of Henle, or inhibit sodium and chloride reabsorption in the distal segment of the nephron; amiloride hydrochloride (Amiloride, Midamor), spironolactone (Aldactone), and triamterene (Dyrenium) are potassium-sparing diuretics that inhibit sodium reabsorption and potassium and hydrogen excretion caused by the action on the distal tubules; both promote diuresis and elimination of acebutolol hydrochloride sodium

Vasodilators: hydralazine (Apresoline), minoxidil (Loniten), and nitroprusside sodium (Nitropress) are used to relax smooth muscle in the arterioles that help to reduce peripheral resistance

Beta-adrenergic blockers: (Sectral), atenolol (Tenormin), betaxolol (Kerlone), bisoprolol fumarate (Zebeta), carteolol hydrochloride (Cartrol), carvedilol (Coreg), metoprolol (Lopressor), nadolol (Corgard), penbutolol (Levatol), pindolol (Visken), propranolol (Inderal), and timolol maleate (Blocadren) used to decrease blood pressure by inhibiting the impulse through the sympathetic pathways and to decrease cardiac output, sympathetic stimulation, and renin secretion by the kidneys

Alpha-adrenergic blockers: doxazosin mesylate (Cardura), fenoldopam mesylate (Corlopam), labetalol hydrochloride (Normodyne, Trandate), phentolamine mesylate (Regitine), prazosin hydrochloride (Minipress), and terazosin hydrochloride (Hytrin) used to reduce blood pressure by acting on the peripheral vasculature to generate vasodilatory action and to decrease peripheral vascular resistance

Calcium channel blockers: diltiazem (Cardizem), felodipine (Plendil), isradipine (DynaCirc), nicardipine (Cardene), nifedipine (Procardia), nisoldipine (Sular), and verapamil (Calan, Isoptin) used to reduce blood pressure by the inhibition of calcium ion influx across the smooth muscle and cardiac cells which reduces arteriolar resistance

Angiotensin-converting enzyme (ACE) inhibitors: benazepril hydrochloride (Lotensin), candesartan cilexetil (Atacand), captopril (Capoten), enalapril maleate (Vasotec), eprosartan mesylate (Teveten), fosinopril sodium (Monopril), moexipril hydrochloride (Univasc), perindopril erbumine (Aceon), quinapril hydrochloride (Accupril), ramipril (Altace), telmisartan (Micardis), and trandolapril (Mavik) used to lower blood pressure by inhibiting ACE which prevents the conversion of angiotensin I to angiotensin

II, which is a strong vasoconstrictor; the reduction in angiotensin II helps to reduce the peripheral arterial resistance and decreases aldosterone secretion, which effectively reduces the water and sodium retention to lower blood pressure

Angiotensin II receptor blockers: irbesartan (Avapro), losartan potassium (Cozaar), and valsartan (Diovan) used to reduce blood pressure by blocking the binding of angiotensin II to the receptor sites in the vascular smooth muscle to help inhibit the pressor effect of the renin-angiotensin-aldosterone system

Central-acting adrenergics: clonidine hydrochloride (Catapres), guanabenz acetate (Wytensin), guanfacine hydrochloride (Tenex), hydralazine hydrochloride (Apresoline), lisinopril (Prinivil, Zestril), and methyldopa hydrochloride (Aldomet) used to help decrease sympathetic outflow to the heart, kidneys, and peripheral vessels to decrease peripheral vascular resistance, heart rate, and blood pressure

COMMON NURSING DIAGNOSES

EXCESS FLUID VOLUME (see HEART FAILURE)

Related to: increased sodium and water retention, decreased organ perfusion, compromised regulatory mechanisms, decreased cardiac output, increased ADH production

Defining Characteristics: edema, weight gain, intake greater than output, increased blood pressure, increased heart rate, shortness of breath, dyspnea, orthopnea, crackles (rales), S_3 gallop, oliguria, jugular vein distention, pleural effusion, specific gravity changes, altered electrolyte levels

ADDITIONAL NURSING DIAGNOSES

DECREASED CARDIAC OUTPUT (see CAD)

Related to: vasoconstriction, increased preload, increased afterload, ischemia

Defining Characteristics: elevated systolic and/or diastolic blood pressure, cardiac output <4 L/min, cardiac index <2.5 L/min/m^2, decreased stroke volume, increased peripheral vascular resistance >250 dynes/second/cm^{-5}, increased systemic vascular resistance >1400 dynes/second/cm^{-5}

RISK FOR DEFICIENT FLUID VOLUME

Related to: fluid loss, use of diuretics

Defining Characteristics: increased urinary output greater than intake, weight loss (sudden), hypokalemia, dry skin and mucous membranes, decreased skin turgor, thirst, hypotension, oliguria, anuria

Outcome Criteria

✔ Patient will achieve and maintain a normal and balanced fluid volume status and be hemodynamically stable, as evident by weight maintenance, equivalent intake and output, and vital signs within the patient's normal parameters.

NOC: *Fluid Balance*

INTERVENTIONS	RATIONALES
Monitor vital signs every 2–4 hours, and prn.	Tachycardia, hypotension, and decreases in pulse quality may indicate fluid shifting has resulted in volume depletion. Temperature elevations with diaphoresis may result in increased insensible fluid loss.
Monitor I&O every hour, and notify physician of significant fluid imbalances in which output is greater than intake.	Continuing negative balances may result in volume depletion.
If patient has wounds with significant amounts of drainage, use drainage bags to measure output, or weigh dressings.	Excess wound drainage can result in major fluid imbalances. Dressings that weigh 1 kg represent approximately 1 L of fluid.
Weigh daily, on same scale, at same time, when possible.	Changes in weight from day to day may correlate to fluid shifts that may occur. Utilizing the same scale provides for consistent and accurate data.
Observe skin turgor and hydration status.	Decreases in skin turgor, tenting of skin, and dry mucous membranes may indicate fluid volume deficits.
Administer IV fluids as ordered.	Replaces fluids and maintains circulating volume.
Monitor lab work, especially electrolytes, hematocrit and hemoglobin, and specific gravity of urine.	Diuretic therapy may result in hypokalemia and hyponatremia from rapid fluid loss. Increased specific gravity may indicate dehydration, as do increases in hemoglobin and hematocrit.

(continues)

(continued)

INTERVENTIONS	RATIONALES
Instruct patient regarding the importance of continuing fluid intake, measuring intake and output, and daily weights.	Provides knowledge and encourages the patient to participate in own care, thus, giving feeling of self-control.
Obtain consultation with dietician for assistance with patient's dietary needs, such as restriction of fluids, sodium, potassium, or protein.	Preferred foods and beverages may allow patient to prevent volume depletion while maintaining dietary restrictions. Excessive sodium and potassium will increase fluid retention, and protein may cause renal insufficiency if renal perfusion is already impaired.

NIC: *Fluid/Electrolyte Management*

Discharge or Maintenance Evaluation

■ Patient will have stable vital signs within parameters specific to patient.

■ Patient will achieve normal fluid balance, with equivalent intake and output.

■ Patient will be able to accurately verbalize importance of fluid intake and understanding of dietary restrictions and monitoring for imbalances.

■ Patient will have urine output within normal limits for amount and specific gravity.

■ Patient will have lab work within normal parameters, with no signs or symptoms of electrolyte imbalances.

RISK FOR INJURY

Related to: decreased compliance of arteries caused by aging, decreased plasma renin activity, decreased angiotensin II levels, nephrosclerosis from decreased renal blood flow and increased intrarenal vascular resistance with aging, vascular changes within the brain and extremities

Defining Characteristics: orthostatic hypotension, syncope, visual blurring, sustained hypertension, fatigue, dysrhythmias, palpitations, chest pain, dyspnea with exertion, orthopnea, peripheral edema, paresthesias, headache, speech impediments, retinal hemorrhages, papilledema, arterial bruits

Outcome Criteria

✔ Patient will have no trauma or injury.
✔ BP will be returned to and maintained at baseline parameters for age.

NOC: *Risk Control*

INTERVENTIONS	RATIONALES
Assess gradual changes in vision that includes blurring and vision loss.	Decreased blood flow to the retina in long term hypertension results in impaired visual acuity.
Assess for dizziness, faintness when changing position (lying to upright), and changes in BP in lying, sitting, or standing positions at 2–3 min intervals for 15 min periods.	Abrupt drops in BP occur with quick changes to standing position as blood pools in the lower part of body. Cardiac output decreases and blood flow to the brain is reduced. As blood volume falls, BP also falls. Condition is common with age and decreased baroreceptor sensing activity.
Assess mental function and memory impairment.	As blood flow to the brain decreases, mentation is affected and compliance in medication is affected, resulting in over or under medication and BP instability.
Administer antihypertensives and adjunct medications accurately as prescribed.	Lowers and regulates BP gradually and safely.
Maintain clear pathways, proper lighting, and have articles within reach or orient to placement. Walking aids, such as a cane or walker may be required.	Prevents trauma from bumping into furniture, falls from reaching or from the lack of hand rails or walking aids.
Assist with ADLs as needed, if vision is impaired.	Provides care that client is unable to perform until modifications are made for self-care.
Assist to change positions slowly to standing; check BP and allow to stand for 3–4 min.	Prevents orthostatic hypotension, causing weakness and dizziness in the elderly, as cerebral blood flow is affected by falls in systolic pressure.
Instruct patient in the use of a cane or walker to assist with ambulation.	Ambulation aids help to promote stability when patient is walking and helps prevent falls.
Instruct patient in taking blood pressure and pulse on the same arm in a lying and standing	Assists to monitor blood pressure response to therapy and correlates data for physician to monitor

INTERVENTIONS	RATIONALES
position. Patient is to report increases over 170 mm Hg systolic or 100 mm Hg diastolic to physician.	efficacy of current antihypertensive treatment. Obtaining blood pressures in standing and lying positions allow for identification of potential orthostatic hypotension.
Instruct patient/family that when patient arises, to first roll to side of the bed, and then slowly assume a sitting position by pushing with arm on the bed, sitting on edge of the bed for several minutes, and then rising.	Assists to cope with orthostatic hypotension by allowing circulatory system to adjust.
Instruct patient to avoid hot environment, drinking alcohol, excessive exercising, hot baths, or use of jacuzzi.	Causes excessive vasodilatation and fainting.
Instruct patient to wear girdle or support hose.	Prevents blood pooling in abdomen or lower extremities. Reduces potential for deep vein thrombosis, which could result in further complications, such as pulmonary emboli, CVA, or MI.
Instruct patient in daily exercise regimen.	Inactivity decreases venous tone and blood return to the heart, resulting in orthostatic hypotension.

NIC: *Risk Identification*

NIC: *Surveillance: Safety*

Discharge or Maintenance Evaluation

- Patient will have no falls or injuries related to visual acuity dysfunction or orthostatic hypotension.

- Patient will be able to administer correct medication and dosage to maintain blood pressure at set parameters, and will be able to report significant alterations to physician.

- Patient will be able to participate in exercise regimen with no adverse effects.

- Patient will have few to no symptoms of orthostatic hypotension during standing process.

- Patient will be able to avoid preventable complications, such as DVTs.

NONCOMPLIANCE WITH MEDICAL REGIMEN

Related to: health beliefs, refusal to modify health practices, refusal to accept medical regimen, inability to practice specified health behaviors

Defining Characteristics: inability to achieve blood pressure stabilization, failure to keep appointments, failure to progress in achievement of medical treatment plan, presence of exacerbations of disease process

Outcome Criteria

✔ Patient will be able to comply with dietary, medication, and activity regimen with achievement of desired results.

✔ Patient will be able to use support systems to help modify noncompliant behavior.

NOC: *Compliance Behavior*

INTERVENTIONS	RATIONALES
Assess patient's reasons for noncompliance, health beliefs, and cultural influences.	Listening to patient's reasons may identify concerns and help to establish a plan of care.
Recognize patient's perceptions regarding disease and treatment plan, and talk to patient in a nonjudgmental approach.	Promotes acceptance of patient and allows for clarification of information and misperceptions.
Assist patient to plan a treatment approach that is acceptable and appropriate for lifestyle and belief system.	Assists with compliance if treatment plan is realistic and includes input from patient and family.
Encourage patient to monitor own blood pressure and weight, take own medications, and plan own meals.	Involves patient in care, and promotes independence, control, and compliance.
Acknowledge that patient has a right to choose not to follow approved treatment plan.	Patient's rights must be valued unless control over action is required to prevent harm to the patient or to others.
Assist patient to develop and record in log information to report to physician or referral personnel.	Provides comparison needed to continue or adjust regimen.

(continues)

(continued)

INTERVENTIONS	RATIONALES
Suggest support groups for smoking cessation, weight control, fitness, and so forth.	Encourages and supports compliance of regimen that contributes to risk factors for heart disease.
Instruct patient in reasons for compliance with treatment (avoidance of complications, avoidance of coronary or cerebral events, and avoidance of death).	Promotes understanding of reduction of risk factors to prevent complications, and may assist with patient's compliance.
Attempt to utilize contracting with patient to observe behavior that does not contribute to significant complications.	Contracting may induce patient to utilize control and involves both the caregiver and the patient in a formal promise, which may achieve the goal of having the patient accept a portion of his treatment regimen.
Identify if lack of financial means is an element of his noncompliant behavior, and if so, consult with community resources to help patient meet costs of medical treatment or other financial concerns.	Assisting the patient to meet financial obligations may improve compliance. Frequently, with the elderly who are on a fixed income, or who may have lost financial backing because of loss of a spouse, the ability to comply with a medication regimen is not valid. Often, the patient must choose between food and medication.

NIC: *Behavior Modification*

Discharge or Maintenance Evaluation

- Patient will follow the plan to control blood pressure.
- Patient will be able to access and utilize community resources adequately.
- Patient will be able to identify reasons for noncompliance, and with assistance, be able to formulate strategies to effectively maintain prescribed treatment.
- Patient will be able to adhere to any contract made.
- Patient will be able to avoid preventable complications by complying with treatment program.

DEFICIENT KNOWLEDGE

Related to: lack of information on disease process and risk of cardiovascular disease, dietary sodium restriction, weight loss, and/or medication administration

Defining Characteristics: verbalization of the problem, inaccurate follow-through of instruction, request for information, misconceptions related to cognitive ability, lack of initiative of learning about disease and/or treatment, or incorrect information previously given, lack of improvement of previous regimen, development of preventable complications

Outcome Criteria

✔ Patient will exhibit appropriate knowledge of medical regimen prescribed to control hypertension with gradual reduction in BP to prescribed ranges.

NOC: *Knowledge: Disease Process*

INTERVENTIONS	RATIONALES
Assess patient's knowledge of causes/risk factors associated with disease and methods to control and stabilize BP.	Prevents repetition of information and promotes compliance of treatments necessary to maintain a stable BP.
Inform patient of potential for cardiovascular disease, CVA, renal failure, CAD, and effect to vital organs with sustained hypertension.	Hypertension predisposes the elderly to cardiovascular disease, caused in part by reduced beta-adrenergic responsiveness, deposits of collagen and other substances in the myocardium, and the reduction of myocardial contractility. Hypertension in the elderly also predisposes them to renal dysfunction resulting from a decrease in renal blood flow, increased intrarenal vascular resistance, and a decreased glomerular filtration rate.
Provide explanations and information in clear and simple language that is understandable; provide limited amounts of information over periods of time rather than large amounts at one sitting.	Reduces potential for noncompliance of medical regimen related to decreased cognitive ability to understand.
Instruct patient/family regarding low-sodium, low-fat, and low-cholesterol diet. Provide consultation with dietician as warranted.	Assists in reducing blood pressure by decreasing fluid retention and by reducing risk for atherosclerosis. Dietician may be able to facilitate patient's eating habits and lifestyle into prescribed diet so that patient will not feel as if all favorite foods have been forever banned. Alternate choices and methods of improvement of taste may facilitate compliance.

INTERVENTIONS	RATIONALES
Instruct patient in isotonic exercises, such as walking, swimming, or bicycling. Caution patient to avoid isometric exercises, such as weight lifting.	Isotonic exercises help to promote weight loss and muscle tone while reducing blood pressure. Isometric exercises can actually increase hypertension.
Instruct patient in medications, effects, side effects, and signs and symptoms to report to physician.	Promotes knowledge and helps to ensure that patient is compliant with dosage regimen. Identification of adverse reactions from medications will allow for prompt and timely intervention.
Instruct patient to avoid over-the-counter medications unless approved by physician.	Some medications may interact with prescribed drugs and actually worsen blood pressure.
Instruct patient to report headache, memory loss, nausea, vomiting, or tremors to physician.	May indicate uncontrolled hypertension and allows for potential medication alteration.

INTERVENTIONS	RATIONALES
Instruct patient to keep all appointments with physician.	Promotes compliance for monitoring of efficacy of diet and therapy, as well as need for adjustments to treatment plan.

NIC: *Teaching: Disease Process*

Discharge or Maintenance Evaluation

■ Patient will be able to identify and utilize appropriate dietary items to comply with dietary restrictions.

■ Patient will be able to maintain weight within set parameters, or will be able to reduce weight if necessary.

■ Patient will be able to perform exercises effectively and without change in hemodynamic status as evident by stable vital signs and absence of chest pain, dyspnea, or other complication.

■ Patient will be able to accurately verbalize understanding of medications, effects, side effects, and symptoms to report to physician.

■ Patient will be able to prevent complications.

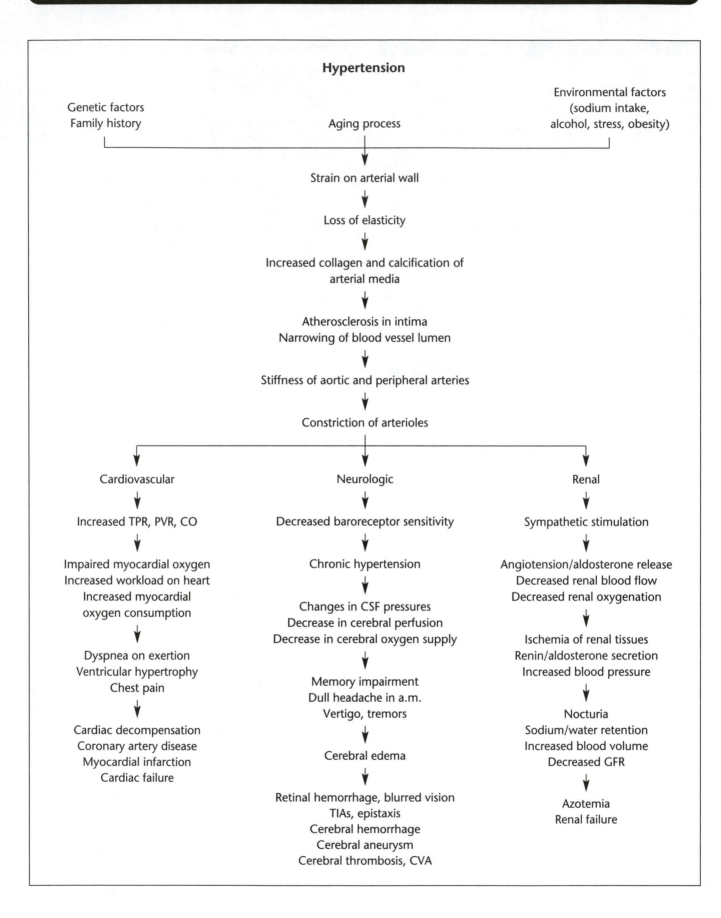

Hypertension

Genetic factors
Family history

Aging process

Environmental factors
(sodium intake,
alcohol, stress, obesity)

Strain on arterial wall

Loss of elasticity

Increased collagen and calcification of
arterial media

Atherosclerosis in intima
Narrowing of blood vessel lumen

Stiffness of aortic and peripheral arteries

Constriction of arterioles

Cardiovascular

Increased TPR, PVR, CO

Impaired myocardial oxygen
Increased workload on heart
Increased myocardial
oxygen consumption

Dyspnea on exertion
Ventricular hypertrophy
Chest pain

Cardiac decompensation
Coronary artery disease
Myocardial infarction
Cardiac failure

Neurologic

Decreased baroreceptor sensitivity

Chronic hypertension

Changes in CSF pressures
Decrease in cerebral perfusion
Decrease in cerebral oxygen supply

Memory impairment
Dull headache in a.m.
Vertigo, tremors

Cerebral edema

Retinal hemorrhage, blurred vision
TIAs, epistaxis
Cerebral hemorrhage
Cerebral aneurysm
Cerebral thrombosis, CVA

Renal

Sympathetic stimulation

Angiotension/aldosterone release
Decreased renal blood flow
Decreased renal oxygenation

Ischemia of renal tissues
Renin/aldosterone secretion
Increased blood pressure

Nocturia
Sodium/water retention
Increased blood volume
Decreased GFR

Azotemia
Renal failure

CHAPTER 1.4

PERIPHERAL VASCULAR DISEASE

Peripheral vascular disease (PVD) involves occlusion of the blood supply to arteries, veins, and lymphatics in the extremities by atherosclerotic plaques, which are also known as atheromas. Changes in the peripheral vasculature are frequently age-related, and compare to the atherosclerotic changes seen in the cerebral and coronary arteries. Also known as arteriosclerosis obliterans, this disease develops slowly and without overt symptomatology for many years, and even then, the vessel involved is normally at least 70% occluded before warning signs are recognizable.

The classic sign of peripheral atherosclerosis is intermittent claudication, involving pain, tightness, or weakness in an exercising muscle caused by the decrease in blood supply. Other clinical symptoms may occur and are dependent upon the speed with which the occlusion develops, the amount of intrusion into the vasculature, and the specific vessel involved. With intermittent claudication, pain occurs initially only upon walking and is relieved with rest. Pain is normally exacerbated by walking uphill or walking briskly. Once the disease progresses, pain occurs more frequently in less time and distance spent walking, and can evolve to ischemic type pain even at rest. Elderly patients who are inactive may initially complain with foot pain at rest. With time and progression, the patient may experience decreased perfusion of tissues and potential for necrosis and gangrene. When foot pain is present, blood flow is normally diminished below 10% of normal flow. Pulses become weaker and/or absent, and the potential for ischemia, necrosis, and gangrene is increased. If the patient is diabetic, with peripheral neuropathic changes, gangrene may occur without much pain because of poor circulation from diabetic changes within the vasculature. When a posterior tibialis pulse is absent, it usually always indicates peripheral arterial disease.

Acute ischemia occurs when an artery is abruptly and suddenly occluded by an embolism, an arteriosclerotic plaque, an aneurysm, or an acute thrombosis with pre-existing atherosclerotic disease. The extremity has a sudden onset of severe pain, coldness, pallor, and numbness. Pulses are absent. Treatment of this condition includes surgical intervention with arterial bypass surgery to help prevent amputation by restoring tissue perfusion. In some elderly patients, amputation is a better choice than arterial bypass surgery, with less risk for those with concurrent cardiac disease. Bypass graft patency usually lasts approximately 5 years following surgery.

Thrombophlebitis occurs when a clot forms in a vein secondary to inflammation or when the vein is partially occluded from some disease process. As a general rule, two out of the following three factors occur prior to the formation of a thrombus—blood stasis, injury to the vessel, and/or alterations in blood coagulability.

Deep vein thrombosis (DVT) pertains to clots that are formed in the deep veins and may result in complications such as pulmonary embolism, postphlebotic syndrome, or chronic venous insufficiency. This can be a residual effect of thrombophlebitis in which the veins are partially occluded or valves within the vessels have been damaged. Immobility and a sedentary lifestyle may preclude elderly patients to this condition as a result of venous stasis. This chronic insufficiency may cause increased venous pressure and fluid accumulation in the interstitial tissues, which results in edema, tissue fibrosis, and induration.

When blood viscosity is increased because of an increase in hematocrit, the potential for clotting and precipitation of DVTs is also increased. DVT normally occurs in the veins within the leg, with a resultant one-sided limb enlargement and dependent edema, and frequently with pain, erythema, and warmth to the area. The potential for complications occur when the embolism dislodges and moves to a crucial organ, such as the heart, lungs, or brain.

Treatment of thrombophlebitis includes controlling thrombotic development, relieving pain, improving of blood flow, and preventing of complications.

MEDICAL CARE

Laboratory: lipid profile used to identify potential for atherosclerosis; homocysteine levels used to identify elevations that may be a risk factor for early atherosclerotic disease by acceleration of atherosclerosis by influencing coagulation and increasing atherogenesis; vitamin B_{12} levels, vitamin B_6 levels, and folate levels used to identify factors that may contribute to increased homocysteine levels; CBC used to identify concurrent infective processes and anemia; coagulation profiles used to identify abnormalities and to monitor anticoagulant therapy

Beta-adrenergic blockers: acebutolol ·hydrochloride (Sectral), atenolol (Tenormin), betaxolol (Kerlone), bisoprolol fumarate (Zebeta), carteolol hydrochloride (Cartrol), carvedilol (Coreg), metoprolol (Lopressor), nadolol (Corgard), penbutolol (Levatol), pindolol (Visken), propranolol (Inderal), and timolol maleate (Blocadren) used in the treatment of patients with intermittent claudication to decrease sympathetic outflow to peripheral vasculature, and only rarely do any of these drugs exacerbate the peripheral claudication

Drug therapy: pentoxifylline (Trental) and cilostazol (Pletal) used because of their ability to inhibit platelet aggregation, vasodilatory action, and the ability to improve capillary blood flow by lowering blood viscosity; cilostazol is a phosphodiesterase inhibitor and should not be used in patients who also have heart failure or other cardiovascular conditions; dipyridamole (Persantine) or acetylsalicylic acid (Aspirin, ASA) used to increase blood flow and inhibit platelet aggregation to prevent intravascular coagulation, but usually aspirin is not used as a prophylactic measure for DVT

Anticoagulants: enoxaparin sodium (Lovenox), heparin calcium and sodium (Calciparin, Heparin), and warfarin (Coumadin) may be used for patients who have DVTs by interfering with the synthesizing coagulation factors in the liver, preventing the extension of an existing clot, and prevention of new clots from developing; elderly patients have an increased risk for adverse consequences from these drugs

Thrombolytics: alteplase (tissue plasminogen activator, t-PA), anistreplase (anisolyated plasminogen-streptokinase activator complex, APSAC, Eminase), reteplase (Retavase), streptokinase (Streptase), tenecteplase (TNKase), and urokinase (Abbokinase) used to lyse the thrombi that obstructs blood flow in patients who have severe venous thrombosis and who are at high risk for chronic venous insufficiency; these drugs bind to fibrin and convert plasminogen to plasmin to begin local fibrinolysis, but benefits versus risks should be weighed prior to usage in the elderly because of their greater risk of bleeding; these drugs usually more likely to be effective if used within the first 3 days of the clot formation

Vitamin supplementation: vitamin B_6, vitamin B_{12}, and folic acid used to supplement deficiencies in each particular vitamin; folic acid helps to lower high homocysteine levels, shown to increase the risk of peripheral vascular disease, and can also be used for anemia; homocysteine increases the rate of atherosclerosis by interfering with blood coagulation and increasing the aggregating properties of LDL to the vascular smooth muscle cells; vitamin B_6 and B_{12} deficiencies noted in patients who have hyperhomocysteinemia

Doppler ultrasonography: used to identify blood flow velocity in extremities and vascular system

Venography: used to identify venous blood flow and vein competency, filling capacity of vein, and location of clot in deep vein thrombosis

Impedence plethysmography: reveals changes in volume and rate of blood flow, degree of obstruction, venous flow in deep veins, incompetent valves, size and dilatation of veins

Oscillometry: measures the amplitude of arterial pulses

^{125}I *Fibrinogen uptake test:* radioactive scan performed after radioactive fibrinogen is injected, and concentrates in the area of clot formation; not sensitive to thrombi high on the iliofemoral region or with inactive thrombi

Surgical interventions: ligation of saphenous veins and removal of the affected smaller veins may be required if venous insufficiency not controlled; endarterectomy may be required to surgically remove placque from the affected vessels; bypass grafts used to restore blood flow by the anastomosis of synthetic or vein grafts to distal and proximal parts of the affected vessel after removal of the diseased portion accomplished; insertion of an inferior vena caval filter (Greenfield filter, umbrella filter) may be performed based on likelihood of movement of DVT into the pulmonary vasculature and is often used if clot is located in the iliofemoral veins; amputation may be necessary if condition requires removal of a toe, foot, or portion of the leg in the presence of severe disease and gangrene

Percutaneous transluminal angioplasty: balloon catheter insertion into the artery used to dilate vessel and remove obstruction; also done with laser

COMMON NURSING DIAGNOSES

ACTIVITY INTOLERANCE (see CAD)

Related to: physiologic changes associated with the aging process, generalized weakness, fatigue, chronic illness, bed rest, immobility, thrombophlebitis, intermittent claudication

Defining Characteristics: communication of fatigue or weakness, presence of circulatory impairment, claudication on ambulation, changes in heart rate and blood pressure in response to activity, dysrhythmias, dyspnea on exertion

ADDITIONAL NURSING DIAGNOSES

INEFFECTIVE TISSUE PERFUSION: PERIPHERAL

Related to: disruption of arterial flow caused by atherosclerosis, disruption of venous flow caused by immobility, coagulopathy, venous stasis, increased venous pressure, thrombus formation, or vein inflammation

Defining Characteristics: intermittent claudication, absent or weak peripheral pulses, decreased capillary refill, chronic pain or pain at rest, cold feet, dependent edema of legs, erythema of skin, pallor to legs upon elevation, thick nails on feet, ischemic lesions on extremity, gangrene, necrosis, deformed dilated varicosities, aching pain in legs, heaviness of legs with prolonged standing, edema, skin discoloration, positive Homan's sign, positive Pratt's sign, pain and deep muscle tenderness, swelling and warm at affected area, stasis ulcers, stasis dermatitis, hyperhomocysteinemia, abnormal coagulopathy

Outcome Criteria

✔ Patient will be free of pain, with adequate perfusion to extremities.

✔ Patient will have strong, palpable peripheral pulses, with no color or temperature changes to extremities.

✔ Patient will be able to maintain tissue perfusion and oxygenation to extremities with no overt complications noted.

NOC: *Tissue Perfusion: Peripheral*

INTERVENTIONS	RATIONALES
Monitor vital signs, cardiac rhythm, and peripheral pulses at least every 2 hours, and prn. Notify physician of significant changes.	Irregular tachycardias may result in decreased cardiac output and perfusion. Lack of peripheral pulses requires emergent treatment and notification of physician because a loss of pulses indicates lack of arterial blood flow and perfusion. The posterior tibialis pulse is sometimes difficult to palpate if the patient has edema or prominent and bony malleoli. With age, the pulse of patent arteries normally becomes more pronounced because of the loss of smooth muscle and elastic tissue. Changes in respiratory rate, pulse, and blood pressure may indicate the presence of pulmonary embolism.
Auscultate lung fields every 4 hours and prn. Notify physician of significant changes.	Adventitious breath sounds, or absent breath sounds may occur if patient develops pulmonary embolism.
Observe patient for new cough, shortness of breath, or hemoptysis.	May indicate presence of pulmonary embolism that results from mobilization of deep vein thrombosis.
Assess skin color, temperature, and quality every 4 hours and prn.	Mottling may occur if tissue perfusion is decreased, also causing skin to become cooler and skin texture changes. The nurse should elevate the foot above heart level for at least 20 seconds and then lower it to a dependent position. If the pallor lasts longer than 30 seconds, or a rubor becomes visible, blood flow is less than 10% of normal. Rubor is usually more pronounced in the toes and increases in surface area at

(continues)

(continued)

INTERVENTIONS	RATIONALES
	different levels. If necrosis or gangrene is present, surgical intervention will most likely be required.
Auscultate abdomen, groins, and carotid areas for bruits.	Presence of bruits heard over these areas indicates the presence of an aneurysm or narrowing of vasculature.
Measure size of calves and document every 4 hours.	Changes in size may indicate fluid shifts, edema, venous pooling, and stasis.
Apply antiembolic hose as indicated. Remove for 1 hour every shift.	Hose may help to increase venous return, but can result in edema from constant constriction. Removal for an interval every shift helps to minimize this.
Elevate extremity unless contraindicated.	Elevation of leg helps to increase venous return, but the use of the bed knee gatch or pillows under the knees may obstruct venous return.
Administer vasoactive drugs as ordered.	These medications may assist in dilating vasculature to improve circulation and perfusion, but these drugs work only if the vessels are capable of dilating.
Administer anticoagulants as ordered.	Thrombus formation can promote further reduction in circulation and decrease tissue perfusion, and medication helps to prevent clot formation.
Observe patient for bleeding from gums, nose, IV sites, and presence of petechiae.	May indicate presence of complications from anticoagulation therapy.
Instruct patient/family in disease process. Allow for ample time to provide instruction and for questions to be asked.	Promotes knowledge and facilitates compliance. Extra time may be required for the elderly to process information, as well as consideration of how narrowing of the vasculature may impede adequate perfusion and thought processes.
Instruct patient/family to use caution or avoid using heating pads, electric blankets, and so forth to involved areas.	Decreased perfusion states alter sensation and the elderly may not be able to recognize temperature extremes that may result in tissue injury.
Instruct patient to avoid crossing legs or knees.	Crossing legs at the knees or ankles may impede circulation to an already-impaired vasculature, and furthers venous stasis and pooling of blood.

INTERVENTIONS	RATIONALES
Instruct patient regarding activity, especially to avoid standing in one position for lengthy times.	Ambulation encourages venous blood flow by active muscle compression, while standing promotes venous stasis.
Instruct patient/family in use of antiembolic stockings: how to put on, to remove every 8 hours at least for 1 hour, and so forth.	Proper positioning of stockings is imperative to produce the desired results. Information provides knowledge and allows the patient and family to take an active role in the treatment plan for the patient.
Instruct patient/family regarding medications, especially anticoagulants. Be specific regarding the need to notify the physician for bleeding noted in mouth, on body, or in body fluids. Inform patient/family of need to reduce amounts of green, leafy vegetables while on oral anticoagulants.	Promotes knowledge and facilitates prompt identification of adverse reaction of medication. Leafy vegetables contain vitamin K, which interacts and reduces anticoagulation effect.
Instruct patient/family regarding need for appropriate foot care and foot wear.	Because of decreased perfusion and altered sensation, too-tight shoes may further impede circulation and cause tissue damage and necrosis. Provision of foot care allows for observation and prevention of complications.
Instruct patient/family in relaxation techniques, guided imagery, biofeedback, and so forth.	Relaxation helps to enhance vasodilation and prevent vasoconstriction that may be a result of anxiety.
Instruct patient/family to notify physician for any signs of wound formation to extremities.	In the elderly, wounds frequently heal poorly, and skin is extremely prone to breakdown, which can result in deterioration to cellulitis, infection, necrosis, or gangrene. Gangrene initially is demonstrated by the presence of ecchymosis that is rapidly followed by blackening of the involved part, and gangrene may occur without patient's complaint of pain.
Prepare patient/family for surgical procedures as indicated.	If arterial circulation is compromised, or if necrosis has resulted in gangrene, surgical intervention may be the only recourse for patient. Knowledge of what to expect decreases anxiety and facilitates compliance.

NIC: *Circulatory Care*

NIC: *Circulatory Precautions*

Discharge or Maintenance Evaluation

- Patient will be free of pain, or pain will be controlled to patient's satisfaction.
- Patient will have palpable pulses to all areas.
- Patient will exhibit no signs or symptoms of decreased perfusion to extremities or cerebrum.
- Patient will have stable vital signs, with no abnormalities on electrocardiogram.
- Patient will have coagulation profiles within specific set parameters, and will exhibit no bleeding complications or hemorrhage.
- Patient/family will be able to accurately verbalize and demonstrate appropriate foot care, use of antiembolic stockings, and signs for which physician is to be notified.
- Patient's wounds/ulcerations will heal and patient will exhibit no signs of necrosis or gangrene.
- Patient will have perfusion restored if surgical procedures become necessary, and will suffer no adverse complications from surgery.
- Patient will exhibit no signs or symptoms of pulmonary embolism.

CHRONIC PAIN

Related to: intermittent claudication, physical disability, impaired venous emptying, inflammation, thrombophlebitis

Defining Characteristics: verbal report of pain for more than 6 months, altered ability to continue previous activities, physical withdrawal, social withdrawal, guarded behavior, protective behavior of affected limb, facial grimacing, crying, moaning, atrophy of muscle, irritability, restlessness, hypersensitivity, depression, fatigue, insomnia, weight gain, weight loss

Outcome Criteria

✔ Patient will exhibit a reduction and control of pain.

NOC: *Pain Level*

INTERVENTIONS	RATIONALES
Assess patient's level of pain complaints, correlation between activity and pain, and physical signs of pain. Assess calf pain, swelling, edema, deep muscle tenderness, temperature over	Correlation of pain and activity may assist in developing plans of care to modify activities. Presence of any of these symptoms may indicate potential venous thrombus and inflammation. Venous

INTERVENTIONS	RATIONALES
affected area, and for positive Pratt's and Homan's signs.	impairment will determine the amount of edema present.
Assess patient for complaints of leg heaviness or deep aching pain after prolonged standing.	May indicate venous insufficiency from venous stasis and/or varicosities.
Assess patient's pain at rest or with ambulation, and note the amount of activity that precipitates pain.	Arterial insufficiency reduces oxygen and nutrients to the tissues and results in pain when these needs increase as a direct result of activity.
Assist with and encourage a progressive daily walking regimen.	Helps to promote collateral circulation development in the presence of arterial insufficiency and prevents venous stasis pain.
Provide bed cradle over legs.	Prevents pain from pressure of bed linens on legs, and reduces potential for tissue damage and decreases pain.
Administer pain medication as ordered.	Relieves pain that is caused by claudication or inflammation.
Apply warm compresses to area, if applicable and appropriate.	Increases the blood flow to the area, decreasing pain and inflammation.
Instruct patient/family in providing rest periods between activities.	Rest periods help prevent severe arterial insufficiency by providing oxygen and nutrients to tissues, and thereby, reduces pain.
Instruct patient/family in relaxation techniques, guided imagery, massage, and so forth.	These methods may be used as an adjunct to analgesics and may decrease the amount of medication required. These techniques also allow the patient and family to work together toward the patient's plan of care and helps to encourage independence.
Instruct patient to elevate legs for 1 hour throughout the day.	Promotes pain relief by assisting in venous return.
Instruct patients to avoid prolonged standing, sitting, or crossing of legs.	Increases venous pressure and leads to feelings of heaviness, pain, and aching to legs.
Instruct patient to avoid wearing constrictive clothing or shoes.	Decreases venous return and may cause increased venous pressure, tissue damage, and pain. Constrictive clothing and shoes decrease circulation to the extremities causing pain during ambulation.
Provide consultation with counselors, pain management clinic, or other community resources.	Provides for post discharge assistance for patient and family.

NIC: *Pain Management*

Discharge or Maintenance Evaluation

- Patient will verbalize that pain has been controlled by rest and/or analgesia to his satisfaction.
- Patient will be able to regain ability to pursue activities within limitations, by use of rest periods and other techniques.
- Patient will be able to accurately verbalize methods to decrease pain.
- Patient will be able to access community resources as needed for chronic pain once discharged.

RISK FOR INJURY

Related to: decreased tactile sensation, decreased temperature sensation, lack of awareness of environmental dangers, anticoagulant usage

Defining Characteristics: inability to sense pain, inability to sense hot and cold temperatures to extremities, easy bruising, trauma to extremities, changes in mobility, confusion, disorientation, poor nutritional status, changes in mental status, inability to perform activities of daily living, falls, accidents, altered coagulation, hemorrhage

Outcome Criteria

- ✔ Patient will experience no injury, trauma, or fall.
- ✔ Patient will avoid injury to extremities from environmental hazards.

NOC: *Safety Status: Physical Injury*

INTERVENTIONS	RATIONALES
Assess patient's mobility and stability status, muscular weakness, cognitive limitations, balance, and gait difficulties.	Provides information for baseline data to establish plan of care. Falls are common in the elderly patient and may result from muscle weakness and skeletal support dysfunction. Claudication may result at different times dependent on the weather, incline of walking, or rapidity with which the patient ambulates.
Assess patient's sensor deficits and perceptual changes.	Changes in visual and auditory acuity, changes in thought processes and orientation, and perception of tactile stimuli are frequently altered in elderly patients and may contribute to falls and other trauma. Sensitivity

INTERVENTIONS	RATIONALES
	to pain may be decreased and paresthesias may promote tissue injury and damage. As peripheral atherosclerosis increases, a sense of coolness may occur in one leg, or paresthesias may increase after resting and may indicate arterial insufficiency.
Assess patient for mentation status, orientation, vertigo, and syncope.	Assists to identify situations that may promote injury. Neurologic changes may indicate movement of the DVT into the systemic circulation and potential lodging within the brain, lungs, or heart, leading to decreased perfusion.
Identify environmental hazards, such as poor lighting, cluttered pathways, high beds, articles placed out of reach, and absence of safety aids.	Potential safety hazards should be repaired/removed to prevent possibility of injuries. Paresthesias associated with claudication may result in patient having injury without feeling pain or having knowledge of injury.
Maintain bed in lowest position, with side rails raised at all times.	Helps to prevent falls, or reduces extent of injury if patient attempts to get out of bed without assistance.
Assist patient with ambulation and use assistive devices, such as walkers or canes.	Helps to promote safety and prevent falls if patient is too weak or impaired to walk alone. Patient may experience sudden weakness with arterial insufficiency and claudication.
Stay with patient, especially if patient complains of dizziness or faintness.	Reduces potential for injury from falls if fainting does occur, and provides reassurance for the patient.
Instruct patient/family regarding environmental safety, to avoid use of throw rugs, to move furniture against walls, to have adequate lighting and night lights, and to use nonslip footwear when ambulating.	Changing patient's environment reduces risk of falls and injury. Sturdy shoes with nonslip soles prevents stumbling and slipping, especially if circulatory status is impaired and paresthesias occur.
Instruct patient/family regarding use of ambulation aids.	Assists patient to continue with mobility in a safe manner.
Instruct family to avoid allowing patient to drive if patient is not capable.	Cognition may be decreased in the elderly patient, and decreased tissue perfusion and sensory alterations may cause injury to patient and to others. Claudication causing paresthesias, as well as potential DVT mobility may make driving an unsafe activity.

INTERVENTIONS	RATIONALES
Instruct patient/family regarding need to change position slowly.	Orthostatic hypotension from rapid changes in position may cause dizziness and fainting that may result in falls and injury.
Instruct patient/family in medications, side effects, reactions to report to physician.	Provides knowledge, promotes compliance, involves family in care, and helps to identify potential problems to allow for timely intervention.
Instruct patient/family in signs of bleeding from gums, mouth, nose, GI tract, urinary tract, or other areas to report to physician.	May indicate altered coagulopathy and potential for hemorrhage if anticoagulants are used.

NIC: *Surveillance: Safety*

Discharge or Maintenance Evaluation

- Patient will experience no fall or injury from dangerous objects.
- Patient will experience no injury from medication usage.
- Patient will be able to engage in social activity and ambulation within limitations with adequate safety aids utilized, and hazardous environment adapted to a safer atmosphere.
- Patient will exhibit no signs of hemorrhage from anticoagulant use.
- Patient will be free of any injury related to claudication or vascular insufficiency.

 RISK FOR IMPAIRED SKIN INTEGRITY

Related to: vascular changes related to the aging process, pressure on skin surfaces, bed rest, immobility, intermittent claudication, alteration in arterial and venous circulation, alterations in tissue perfusion

Defining Characteristics: thin, dry skin on extremities, redness to pressure areas, edema, ulcerations or lesions to extremities, dermatitis, pigmentation to legs, mottling, cyanosis, pallor, decreased or absent pulses, warmth to area, disruption of skin surface, excoriation of skin, decreased tactile sensation

Outcome Criteria

✔ Patient will experience intact skin status, and skin will be free of irritation or trauma.

NOC: *Tissue Integrity: Skin and Mucous Membranes*

INTERVENTIONS	RATIONALES
Assess patient's skin status every 4 hours and prn. Observe for changes in color and temperature to extremities and to bony prominences.	Identifies potential disruption of skin surfaces that may result from pressure, friction, or shearing forces.
Assess for skin dryness, lack of subcutaneous tissue, edema, presence of varicose veins, and discoloration of lower extremities.	Identifies potential circulatory insufficiency that may lead to skin breakdown as perfusion of oxygen and nutrients are reduced.
Assess patient's mobility status and ability to move in bed. Turn patient at least every 2 hours and prn.	Immobility is the most common cause of skin impairment. Unrelieved pressure to skin and soft tissues reduces circulation and may predispose patient to skin breakdown.
Apply padding to bony prominences and other susceptible body parts without circulation.	Helps to promote circulation and comfort, and prevents skin breakdown.
Remove splints, antiembolic hose, and other devices at least every shift and examine skin. Apply lotion unless contraindicated.	Skin irritation may be present under appliance or hose, and elderly patients frequently lack tactile sensation to signal that a problem may exist. Examination of skin helps to prevent excoriation and lotion provides moisture to avoid cracking dry skin that may predispose patient to skin breakdown.
Perform/assist patient with foot care daily; trim nails per hospital protocol; use heel protectors as warranted.	Assists patient to maintain good foot care, and helps to prevent excessive friction on delicate tissues that are already circulatory impaired.
Elevate head of bed no more than 30 degrees when feasible.	Higher degrees may promote pressure and friction from a sliding effect.
Provide range of motion exercises every 4 hours and prn.	Helps to maintain mobility of joints and prevent contractures and atrophy. Helps to maintain skin integrity by preventing complications that might lead to further tissue damage.
Instruct patient/family to always test water temperature prior to bathing or soaking feet.	Temperatures higher than 115° F may cause burns and elderly patient who has an impaired tactile sensation may not be able to recognize temperature danger.
Instruct patient/family to avoid exposure of feet to temperature extremes and to avoid going barefoot.	Prevents trauma to feet if circulation or sensation is impaired.

(continues)

(continued)

INTERVENTIONS	RATIONALES
Instruct patient/family to avoid bumping against furniture.	May create breaks in fragile, dry, thin skin.
Instruct patient/family to avoid use of over-the-counter products for calluses and corns.	Some commercial products contain harsh chemicals that may injure already-compromised skin.
Instruct patient/family to maintain activity and avoid prolonged sitting or standing in one position.	Helps to maintain circulation and prevents pressure on tissues.
Instruct patient/family in the use of oils and lotions to skin and nails.	Helps to prevent skin dryness that may result in a predisposition to skin breakdown.
Instruct patient/family in daily inspection of skin and routine care using a nonirritating soap, patting skin dry rather than rubbing, and reporting signs of breakdown to physician.	Daily maintenance program will help to protect the older patient's skin integrity and involves family in care. The elderly, especially those who have chronic health problems and immobility, are at a higher risk of pressure ulcerations. Physiologic changes with aging also cause increased

INTERVENTIONS	RATIONALES
	exposure to problems that are connected to dry skin.
Instruct patient/family regarding need to maintain adequate nutrition. Discuss use of supplements, dietary sources of increased protein, and dietary restrictions.	Sound nutrition helps maintain appropriate tissue perfusion, oxygenation, and nourishment to prevent skin breakdown. With impaired tissue integrity, a patient may require increased calories for increased metabolic demands.

NIC: *Skin Surveillance*

Discharge or Maintenance Evaluation

■ Patient will have intact skin that is free from redness, irritation, bruises, and rashes.

■ Patient and family will be able to prevent pressure-related skin breakdown or damage.

■ Patient will maintain adequate nutrition.

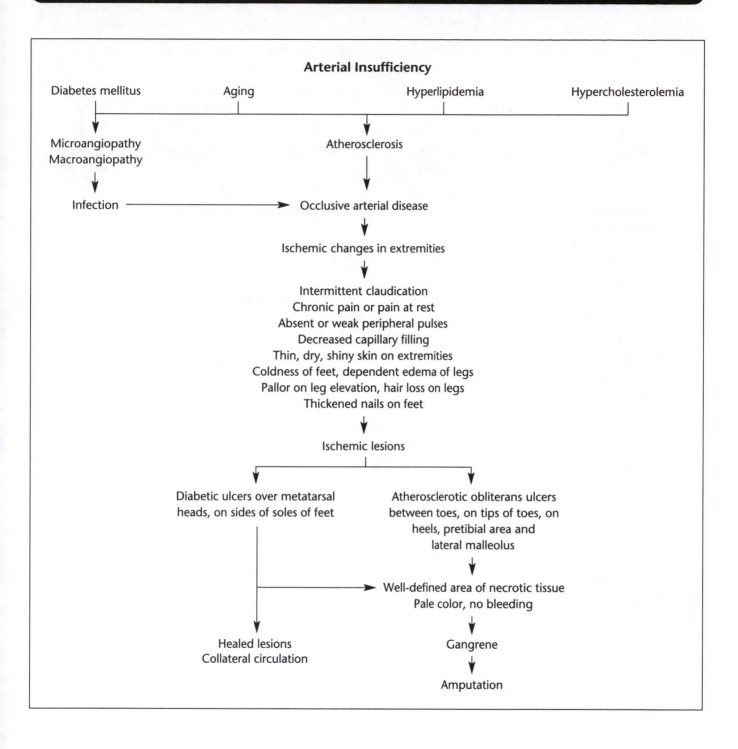

Arterial Insufficiency

Diabetes mellitus   Aging   Hyperlipidemia   Hypercholesterolemia

Microangiopathy   Atherosclerosis
Macroangiopathy

Infection ⟶ Occlusive arterial disease

Ischemic changes in extremities

Intermittent claudication
Chronic pain or pain at rest
Absent or weak peripheral pulses
Decreased capillary filling
Thin, dry, shiny skin on extremities
Coldness of feet, dependent edema of legs
Pallor on leg elevation, hair loss on legs
Thickened nails on feet

Ischemic lesions

Diabetic ulcers over metatarsal   Atherosclerotic obliterans ulcers
heads, on sides of soles of feet   between toes, on tips of toes, on
                                        heels, pretibial area and
                                        lateral malleolus

                                        Well-defined area of necrotic tissue
                                        Pale color, no bleeding

Healed lesions   Gangrene
Collateral circulation

                                        Amputation

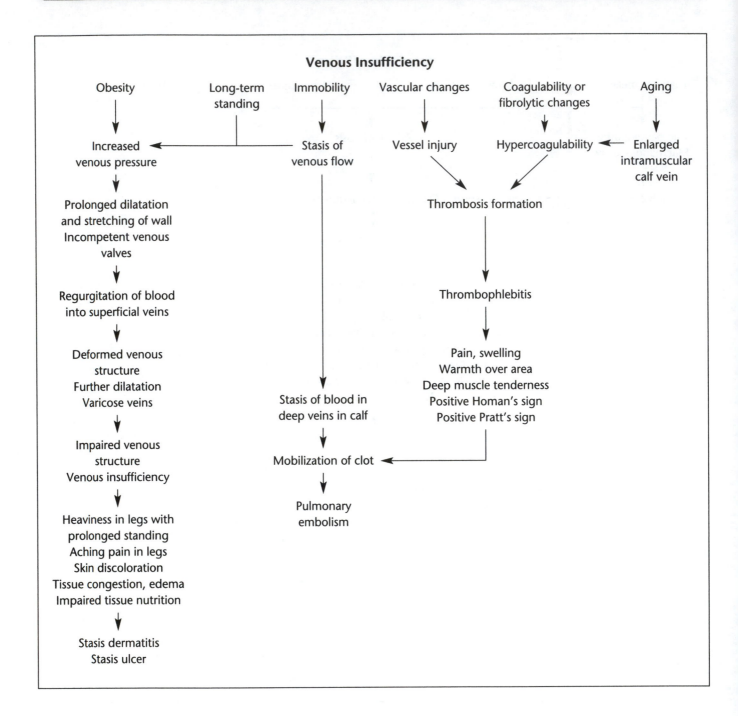

Venous Insufficiency

Obesity

Long-term standing

Immobility

Vascular changes

Coagulability or fibrolytic changes

Aging

Increased venous pressure

Stasis of venous flow

Vessel injury

Hypercoagulability

Enlarged intramuscular calf vein

Prolonged dilatation and stretching of wall
Incompetent venous valves

Thrombosis formation

Regurgitation of blood into superficial veins

Deformed venous structure
Further dilatation
Varicose veins

Thrombophlebitis

Impaired venous structure
Venous insufficiency

Stasis of blood in deep veins in calf

Pain, swelling
Warmth over area
Deep muscle tenderness
Positive Homan's sign
Positive Pratt's sign

Heaviness in legs with prolonged standing
Aching pain in legs
Skin discoloration
Tissue congestion, edema
Impaired tissue nutrition

Mobilization of clot

Pulmonary embolism

Stasis dermatitis
Stasis ulcer

CHAPTER 1.5

PACEMAKERS

Artificial cardiac pacemakers are used to provide an electrical stimulus to depolarize the heart and cause a contraction to occur at a controlled rate. The function of the pacemaker, or pacer, is to maintain the heart rate when the patient's own intrinsic system is unable to do so. Over 85% of patients who receive pacemakers are over the age of 65 (Beers & Berkow, 2000), and the use of pacers in the elderly population has significantly reduced the morbidity that was related to high-grade heart blocks. The stimulus of the pacer is produced by a pulse generator and delivered via electrodes/leads that are implanted in the epicardium or endocardium. The electrodes may be unipolar or bipolar, and the proximal end attaches to a pulse generator that is placed in the chest or abdomen.

Pacemakers are used for varying degrees of heart block, sick sinus syndrome, sinus node dysfunction, overriding of some cardiac dysrhythmias, prophylactically during diagnostic testing, myocardial infarctions, congestive heart failure caused by rhythm disturbances, after open heart surgery, or in congenital anomalies of the heart.

Sick sinus syndrome is prominently found in the elderly patient, with pathologic changes distinguished by fibrotic changes in the sinus node and conduction system. In over 50% of elderly patients over the age of 70, amyloidosis is present in the heart, and myofilament calcium activation from preceding systoles may result in a prolonged isovolumetric relaxation, both of which may provoke dysrhythmias that require pacer supplementation.

Problems associated with permanent pacemakers are uncommon, but when they do occur, are major. Battery failure, myocardial perforation, pacer lead fracture, dislodgement of the lead, or fibrosis surrounding the catheter site can result in an abrupt loss of pacing and, depending on how dependent the patient may be on the pacemaker for his heart rhythm, may result in bradydysrhythmias, or even asystole. Occasionally cardiac tamponade may occur as a result of right ventricle perforation from the catheter electrode, and there may be instances in some patients who have scant subcutaneous tissue, that the generator or pacer wires may erode through the skin.

MEDICAL CARE

Radiography: chest X-rays used to identify and evaluate placement of lead wires, potential dislodgement, pulmonary complications, cardiac size, and hypertrophy

Electrocardiography: used to monitor pacemaker function, heart rhythm problems, dysrhythmias, and potential dysfunction or complication from pacer

Surgery: required for placement of permanent pacemaker, although normally done in interventional cardiac catheter lab in most hospitals; also required for battery or lead replacement

Reprogramming: used to change settings of pacemaker in response to patient needs

Antimicrobials: used to prevent infection to surgical site

COMMON NURSING DIAGNOSES

 DECREASED CARDIAC OUTPUT (see CAD)

Related to: alteration in cardiac rate and rhythm, conduction defects, insufficient blood to the heart, complications from catheter lead fracture, failing batteries, or erosion through skin, inappropriate pacemaker function

Defining Characteristics: ECG changes, dysrhythmias, heart block, sick sinus syndrome, inappropriate pacing or sensing, chest pain, coughing, dyspnea, adventitious breath sounds, wheezing, fatigue, syncope, restlessness, cold, clammy skin, decreased peripheral pulses, jugular vein distention, skin color changes, pallor, cyanosis, changes in blood pressure, edema, cardiac gallops, changes in mental status, disorientation, hiccoughs

 ## ACUTE PAIN (see CAD)

Related to: pacemaker insertion, pacemaker malfunction, chest pain, decreased perfusion

Defining Characteristics: communication of pain, facial grimacing, restlessness, changes in pulse and blood pressure

 ## ACUTE PAIN (see CAD)

Related to: pacemaker insertion, pacemaker malfunction, cardiac ischemia, chest pain, decreased perfusion.

Defining Characteristics: communication of pain, facial grimacing, restlessness, changes in pulse and blood pressure, diaphoresis, dysrhythmias

 ## ANXIETY (see CAD)

Related to: threat to body image, threat to role functioning, pain, change in health status, fear of death

Defining Characteristics: restlessness, insomnia, anorexia, increased respirations, increased heart rate, increased blood pressure, difficulty concentrating, dry mouth, poor eye contact, decreased energy, irritability, crying, feelings of helplessness

 ## DEFICIENT KNOWLEDGE (see CAD)

Related to: lack of understanding about pacemakers, lack of understanding about disease processes, lack of recall, new health crisis

Defining Characteristics: questions regarding problems, inadequate follow-up on instructions given, misconceptions, lack of improvement of previous regimen, development of preventable complications, withdrawal from family and friends

ADDITIONAL NURSING DIAGNOSES

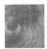 ## INEFFECTIVE TISSUE PERFUSION: CARDIOPULMONARY, CEREBRAL

Related to: cardiac dysrhythmias, heart blocks, tachydysrhythmias, decreased blood pressure, decreased cardiac output, pacemaker battery failure

Defining Characteristics: decreased blood pressure, decreased heart rate, decreased cardiac output <4 L/min, cardiac index <2.5 L/min/m^2, decreased stroke volume, increased peripheral vascular resistance >250 dynes/second/cm^{-5}, increased systemic vascular resistance >1400 dynes/second/cm^{-5}, changes in level of consciousness, mental changes, cold, clammy skin, cardiopulmonary arrest, inappropriate pacing or sensing

Outcome Criteria

✔ Patient will be free of dysrhythmias with an adequate cardiac output to perfuse all body organs.

NOC: *Tissue Perfusion: Cardiac, Pulmonary, Cerebral*

INTERVENTIONS	RATIONALES
Monitor ECG for change in rhythm, rate, and presence of dysrhythmias. Treat as indicated.	Observation for pacemaker malfunction promotes prompt treatment. Pacer electrodes may irritate ventricle and promote ventricular ectopy.
Obtain and observe rhythm strip every 4 hours and prn. Notify physician of abnormalities.	Identifies proper functioning of pacemaker, with appropriate capture and sensing.
Monitor vital signs every 15 minutes until stable, then every 2 hours, and prn.	Assures adequate perfusion and cardiac output.
Monitor for signs of failure to sense patient's own rhythm, and correct problem.	Potential causes are lead dislodgment, battery failure, low sensitivity, catheter wire fracture, or improper placement of catheter.
Monitor for signs of failure to pace, and correct problem.	Potential causes are battery failure, lead dislodgment, disconnection of temporary pulse generator, or catheter lead fracture.
Ensure that all electrical equipment is grounded. Avoid touching equipment and patient at the same time.	Prevents potential for microshock and accidental electrocution. Electric current seeks the path of least resistance, and the potential for stray current to travel through the electrode into the patient's heart may precipitate ventricular fibrillation.
Monitor for muscle twitching or hiccoughs.	May indicate pacer lead has dislodged and migrated to chest wall or diaphragm after perforation of the heart.

INTERVENTIONS	RATIONALES
Monitor for sudden complaints of chest pain, and auscultate for pericardial friction rub or muffled heart tones. Observe for JVD and pulsus paradoxus.	May indicate perforation of the pericardial sac, and impending or present cardiac tamponade.
Monitor patient for complaints of dizziness, syncope, weakness, pronounced fatigue, edema, chest pain, palpitations, pulsations in neck veins, or dyspnea.	During ventricular pacing, AV synchrony may cease and cause a sudden decrease in cardiac output. May indicate "pacemaker syndrome" or failure of the pacer to function which results in decreased perfusion.
Limit movement of the extremity involved near insertion site as ordered.	Prevents accidental disconnection and dislodgment of lead wires immediately after placement.
Monitor patient for low blood-sugar levels, use of glucocorticoids or sympathomimetics, mineralocorticoids, or anesthetics.	May impair the pacemaker stimulation thresholds.
Protect patient from microwave ovens, radar, diathermy, electrocautery, TENS units, and so forth.	Environmental electromagnetic interference may impair demand pacemaker function by disrupting the electrical stimulus.
If patient arrests, and requires defibrillation, attempt to avoid pacemaker battery location as site for defibrillation. If patient is successfully resuscitated, prepare for potential reprogramming of pacemaker.	Defibrillatory shock may result in pacemaker damage and potential diversion of electrical current. Pacemaker may be damaged or settings may be altered by application of electrical current required to resuscitate patient.
Instruct patient on need for pacemaker, procedures involved, expected outcomes, and so forth.	Provides knowledge, decreases fear and anxiety, and provides baseline for further instruction.
Instruct patient in checking pulse rate every day for 1 month, then every week, and to notify physician if rate varies more than 5 beats/minute.	Provides patient with some control over situation. Assists in promoting a sense of security. Allows for prompt recognition of deviations from preset rate and potential pacemaker failure.
Instruct on activity limitations: avoid excessive bending, stretching, lifting more than 5 pounds, strenuous exercise, or contact sports.	Full range of motion can be recovered in approximately 2 months after fibrosis stabilizes pacemaker lead. Excessive activity may cause lead dislodgment.
Instruct to avoid shoulder-strap purses, suspenders, or firing rifle resting over generator site.	May promote irritation over implanted generator site.
Instruct to wear a medic-alert bracelet with information about	Provides information about the patient, condition, and pacemaker

INTERVENTIONS	RATIONALES
type of pacemaker and rate.	should patient be incapacitated and unable to speak for self.
Instruct patient to notify physician if radiation therapy is needed, and to wear a lead shield if it is required.	Radiation therapy can cause failure of the silicone chip in the pacer with repeated radiation treatment.
Instruct patient/family regarding avoiding electromagnetic fields, magnetic resonance imaging, radio transmitters, arc welding equipment, large running motors, or large ungrounded power tools. If patient notices dizziness or palpitations, patient should try to move away from the area, and if symptoms persist, to seek medical attention. Late-model microwave ovens are no longer thought to be a threat because of tighter seals preventing leakage of energy.	May affect the function of the pacemaker and alter the programmed settings. Sometimes these magnetic fields will affect the pacemaker function only if direct contact is made and once distance is placed between the patient and the equipment, normal function of the pacemaker resumes. If programmed settings are altered, the pacer will require reprogramming. Hyperbaric oxygen chambers may also affect pacer function.

NIC: *Dysrhythmia Management*

Discharge or Maintenance Evaluation

- Patient will be free of dysrhythmias and able to maintain cardiac output within normal limits.
- Patient will be able to recall accurately all instructions given.
- Patient will be able to recall and adhere to all activity restrictions.
- Permanent pacemaker function will be without complication, with no lead dislodgment or competitive rhythms noted.

IMPAIRED SKIN INTEGRITY

Related to: insertion of permanent pacemaker, alteration in activity, changes in mobility, aging process, loss of elasticity of skin

Defining Characteristics: disruption of skin tissue, insertion sites, destruction of skin layers

Outcome Criteria

✔ Patient will have healed wound sites without signs or symptoms of infection.

NOC: *Wound Healing: Primary Intention*

INTERVENTIONS	RATIONALES
Inspect pacemaker insertion site for redness, edema, warmth, drainage, or tenderness.	Prompt detection of problems promotes prompt treatment.
Change dressing daily, or per hospital protocol, using sterile technique.	Allows for observation of the site and detection of inflammation or infection. Sterile technique is recommended because of the close proximity of the portal to the heart, increasing the potential for systemic infection.
Instruct on wound care to pacer site and to avoid taking showers for 2 weeks after insertion.	Promotes compliance with care to decrease potential for infection. Moisture can promote bacterial growth.
Instruct patient/family to observe for and report to physician the following symptoms: redness to site, drainage, temperature greater than 100° F, pain or tenderness to site, or swelling at site.	Provides for prompt recognition of complications and facilitates timely treatment.
Instruct patient to avoid wearing constrictive clothing until site has healed completely.	May cause discomfort at incision site from pressure and rubbing against skin.
Instruct patient/family regarding pacemaker use, need for removal/replacement, and signs and symptoms to report to physician.	Pulse generators may require removal for battery replacement, fracture of lead wires, pacemaker failure, and so forth. Knowledge of potential problems can help facilitate timely identification, notification of physician, and appropriate care.

NIC: Wound Care

Discharge or Maintenance Evaluation

- Patient will have well-healed incision with no signs or symptoms of infection.
- Patient will be able to accurately recall all instructions given.
- Patient will be able to demonstrate appropriate wound care prior to discharge.

RISK FOR INJURY

Related to: pacemaker failure, puncture or perforation of heart tissue, bleeding, lead migration, lung perforation, skin erosion

Defining Characteristics: decreased cardiac output <4 L/min, cardiac index <2.5 L/min/m^2, decreased stroke volume, increased peripheral vascular resistance >250 dynes/second/cm^{-5}, increased systemic vascular resistance >1400 dynes/second/cm^{-5}, hemorrhage, diaphoresis, hypotension, restlessness, dyspnea, cyanosis, chest pain, muscle twitching, hiccoughs, muffled heart tones, jugular vein distention, pulsus paradoxus, skin breakdown, drainage, redness to skin, hemothorax, pneumothorax, deviated mediastinum, decreased breath sounds

Outcome Criteria

✔ Patient will be free of life-threatening complications that may be associated with pacemaker insertion.

NOC: Risk Detection

INTERVENTIONS	RATIONALES
Monitor patient for bleeding at pacemaker site. Apply pressure dressings as warranted.	Bleeding at incisional site may occur based on the patient's coagulation status. Pressure dressings or manual pressure may be required to control bleeding. The elderly patient's skin is more fragile than younger patients and more prone to bleeding.
Monitor for presence of pulses at site distal to the pacer insertion.	Hemorrhage may promote tissue edema and compression to arterial blood flow resulting in diminished or absent pulses.
Monitor vital signs; observe for diaphoresis, dyspnea, and restlessness.	Hypotension and these other signs may indicate puncture of the subclavian vasculature and potential hemothorax.
Monitor for dyspnea, chest pain, pallor, cyanosis, absent or diminished breath sounds, tracheal deviation, and patient's feeling of impending doom.	May indicate puncture of the lung and presence of pneumothorax, requiring immediate treatment.
Monitor patient for presence of muscle twitching and hiccoughs. Notify physician.	May indicate perforation of the heart with pacing to the chest wall or diaphragm.
Observe for signs and symptoms of cardiac tamponade—pericardial friction rub, pulsus paradoxus, muffled heart tones, and JVD.	May indicate perforation of the pericardial sac and impending cardiac tamponade which requires immediate medical attention.

INTERVENTIONS	RATIONALES
Instruct patient in signs and symptoms, such as restlessness, syncope, chest pain, or dyspnea, of which to notify nurse and physician.	Provides for prompt identification of potential complication and allows for timely treatment. May indicate malposition of lead irritating heart muscle tissue, which can then be promptly treated.
Instruct patient/family to notify physician for redness, swelling, or drainage at site of pacer battery insertion.	Provides for potential identification of infection and allows for prompt treatment with antimicrobials to reduce possibility of sepsis.

NIC: *Surveillance: Safety*

Discharge or Maintenance Evaluation

- Patient will be free of hemorrhage or infection.
- Patient will have no complications associated with pacemaker insertion.
- Patient will have clear breath sounds, with adequate oxygenation, and exhibit no signs of dyspnea.

RISK FOR INFECTION

Related to: invasive procedure, pacemaker insertion

Defining Characteristics: redness and heat at site, pain at site, swelling and fluid collection at site

Outcome Criteria

✔ Patient will exhibit no signs of infection at site of catheter or permanent battery.

NOC: *Risk Detection*

INTERVENTIONS	RATIONALES
Assess presence of hematoma, redness and swelling at site, temperature elevation, and/or skin erosion.	Indicates presence of infection or potential for skin breakdown.
Administer antimicrobials as ordered.	Prevents or treats wound infection.
Empty drainage device, if present.	Promotes wound drainage and healing.
Apply sterile dressing until wound heals. Avoid dislodging of catheter during site care.	Maintains sterility of wound.

INTERVENTIONS	RATIONALES
Instruct patient of signs to observe indicating infection, and to notify physician.	Provides for measures to take and information to report for prompt treatment.
Instruct patient in method to take temperature.	Monitors for potential elevation associated with infection.
Instruct patient in technique to change dressing.	Sterility can be maintained if proper technique used.

NIC: *Infection Protection*

NIC: *Incision Site Care*

Discharge or Maintenance Evaluation

- Site will be free of infection, intact, and healed.
- Patient will be able to accurately demonstrate wound care.
- Patient will be able to accurately verbalize understanding of signs and symptoms to report to physician.

IMPAIRED PHYSICAL MOBILITY

Related to: pain, limb immobilization

Defining Characteristics: inability to move as desired, imposed restrictions on activity, decreased muscle strength, decreased muscle coordination, pain, limited range of motion

Outcome Criteria

✔ Patient will regain optimal mobility within limitations of disease process, and will have increased strength and function of limbs.

NOC: *Mobility Level*

INTERVENTIONS	RATIONALES
Evaluate patient's perception of his degree of immobility.	Psychological and physical immobility are interrelated. Psychological immobility is used as a defense mechanism when the patient has no control over his body, and this can lead to disproportionate fear and concern. If pacemaker insertion was an emergent procedure, patient may have misperceptions

(continues)

(continued)

INTERVENTIONS	RATIONALES
	regarding movement and be afraid that any movement may result in death. Changes in body image promote psychological immobility and may result in emotional handicaps, rather than actual physical ones. Identification of patient's perceptions will help establish a treatment plan.
Maintain bed rest following pacemaker insertion for 24–48 hours, or per physician protocol.	Provides time for stabilization of leads and decreases potential for dislodgment.
Immobilize extremity proximal to pacer insertion site with arm board, sling, and so forth.	Prevents potential for dislodgment of lead caused by movement.
Resume range of motion exercises 5 days after permanent pacer insertion to affected extremity. Provide ROM to unaffected extremity immediately after pacer insertion, as warranted.	Promotes gradual increase of activity. Stretching should be avoided until lead wire has been secured in heart by fibrotic changes. ROM prevents stiffness of shoulders and joint immobility.
Encourage extension/dorsiflexion exercises to feet every 1–2 hours.	Promotes venous return, prevents venous stasis, and decreases potential for thrombophlebitis.
Monitor patient for progression and improvement in stiffness/pain.	Physical therapy may be required if immobility results are severe.
Apply trapeze bar to bed.	Allows for easier movement by allowing patient to assist with movement in bed with unaffected extremity.
Reposition every 2 hours and prn.	Prevents potential for immobility hazards, such as pressure areas and atelectasis.
Instruct patient regarding deep breathing exercises to be done every 1–2 hours, and to avoid forceful coughing.	Facilitates lung expansion and decreases potential for atelectasis. Coughing may dislodge pacemaker lead.
Instruct patient/family regarding need for immobilization of arm immediately post-pacemaker insertion, and how long immobility is to be expected.	Provides knowledge, and decreases fear that patient may be immobilized for long periods of time.

NIC: *Physical Restraint*

Discharge or Maintenance Evaluation

- Patient will regain optimal mobility of all joints with no signs or symptoms of complications.

- Patient will be able to demonstrate and recall instructions regarding deep breathing and range of motion exercises.
- Patient will exhibit no signs or symptoms of lead dislodgement.

DISTURBED BODY IMAGE

Related to: presence of pulse generator and battery, loss of control of heart function, disease process

Defining Characteristics: fear of rejection, fear of reaction from others, negative feelings about body, refusal to participate in care, refusal to look at wound, withdrawal from social contacts, withdrawal from family

Outcome Criteria

✔ Patient will recognize physical change in body image and deal appropriately with situation.

NOC: *Body Image*

INTERVENTIONS	RATIONALES
Evaluate level of patient's knowledge about disease process, treatment, and anxiety level.	May identify extent of problem and interventions that will be required.
Evaluate the extent of loss to the patient/family, and what it means to them.	Depending on the time frame for patient teaching prior to the insertion of the pacemaker, the patient may not have received adequate information, and may have difficulty dealing with changes in his body appearance, as well as generalized health condition and loss of control.
Assess patient's stage of grieving.	Provides recognition of appropriate versus inappropriate behavior. Prolonged grief may require further care.
Observe for withdrawal, manipulation, noninvolvement with care, or increased dependency. Set limits on dysfunctional behaviors and help patient to seek positive behaviors that will assist with recovery.	May suggest problems with adjustment to health condition, grief response to the loss of function, or worry about others accepting patient's new body status. Patients may deal with crises in the same manner as previously and may need redirection in behaviors to facilitate recovery and acceptance.
Provide positive reinforcement during care and with instruction	Promotes trust and establishes rapport with patient, as well as

INTERVENTIONS	RATIONALES
and setting goals. Do not give false reassurance.	provides an opportunity to plan for the future based on reality of situation.
Provide opportunity for patient to take active role in wound care.	Promotes self-esteem and facilitates feelings of control of body and health.
Provide reassurance that pacemaker will not alter sexual activity.	Promotes knowledge and decreases fear.
Discuss potential for mood changes, anger, grief, and so forth, after discharge, and to seek help if persisting for lengthy time.	Facilitates identification that feelings are not unusual and must be recognized in order to deal with them effectively.
Identify support groups for patient/family to contact.	Provides ongoing support for patient and family and allows for ventilation of feelings.

INTERVENTIONS	RATIONALES
Consult counselor/therapist, as warranted.	May be required for further interventions to resolve emotional or psychological issues.

NIC: *Body Image Enhancement*

Discharge or Maintenance Evaluation

- Patient will be able to effectively deal with body image disturbances in present situation.
- Patient will be able to talk with family, therapist, or others about emotional or psychological problems.
- Patient will be able to problem-solve and identify short- and long-term goals within reasonable expectations of clinical situation.

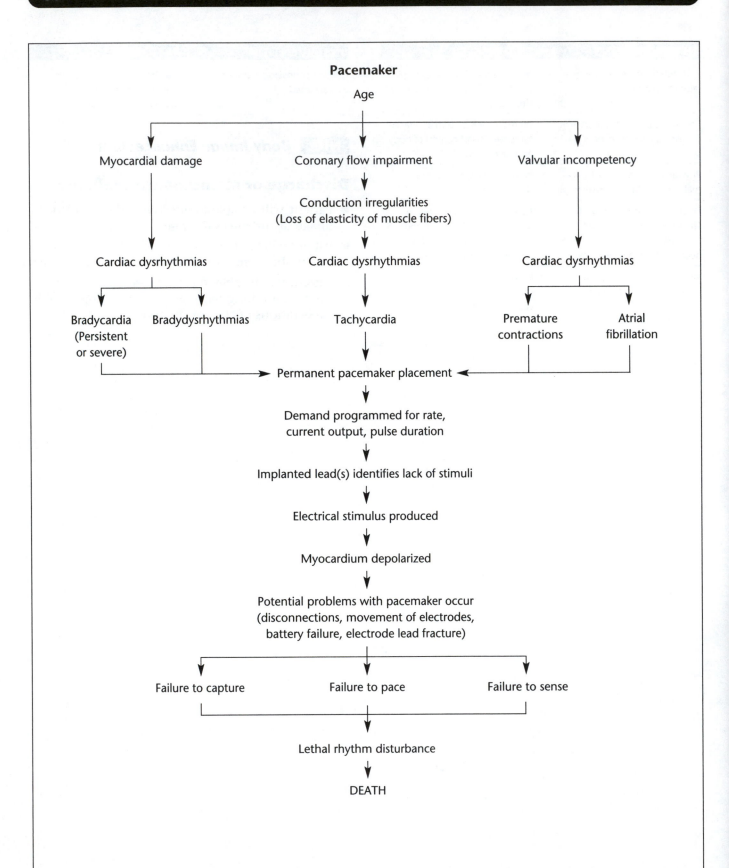

UNIT 2
RESPIRATORY SYSTEM

CHAPTER 2.1

CHRONIC OBSTRUCTIVE PULMONARY DISEASE

Chronic obstructive pulmonary disease (COPD) is an irreversible condition in which the airways become obstructed and the resistance to airflow is increased during expiration when airways collapse. COPD is also known as chronic obstructive lung disease (COLD). COPD is usually further subdivided into other diseases such as bronchitis and emphysema, and actually the term, COPD, refers to these simultaneous disease entities.

COPD is the most common cause of pulmonary disability in the elderly population and includes asthma, emphysema, and chronic bronchitis. Changes in the respiratory system associated with aging, such as loss of elasticity of connective tissue and muscle, decreased strength of muscles used in breathing, decreased rib mobility and chest expansion, and reductions in the reflex ability of coughing caused by muscle tone contribute to the progressive severity of these diseases. In the past 20 years, COPD has escalated more quickly than any of the other leading causes of death, and now ranks second only to coronary artery disease as a compensated disability, and fourth leading cause of death in the United States (Beers & Berkow, 2000).

Emphysematous changes include enlarging of the air spaces distally to the terminal bronchioles, and concurrent changes in alveolar walls. Capillary numbers decrease in the remaining walls and may sclerose. Gas exchange is decreased by the reduction in available alveolar surfaces as well as decreased perfusion to nonventilated areas. Ventilation/perfusion mismatching occurs and functional residual capacity is increased. The anteroposterior diameter of the chest is often enlarged by the loss of elasticity and increased air trapping in the airway supportive structures. These type A patients are often called "pink puffers" because of the increased response to hypoxemia. Symptoms include dyspnea and an increase in breathing effort, which result in a well-oxygenated, or pink, patient who displays overt dyspnea, or puffing.

Bronchitis is usually associated with prolonged exposure to lung irritants, which results in inflammatory changes and thickening of bronchial walls, and increases in mucus production. The patient exhibits a chronic productive cough caused, in part, by the increase in size of mucus glands and decrease in cilia. A true diagnosis of bronchitis is distinguished by a productive cough occurring most of the time for at least 3 months out of each year for 2 consecutive years. Patients who have chronic bronchitis have a greater amount of mucus glands, smooth muscle hyperplasia, and the structural support of their airways is decreased. These type B patients are often called "blue bloaters" because their response to hypoxemia is reduced, with increasing $PaCO_2$ levels and cyanosis. These patients frequently have bouts of cor pulmonale, or right-sided heart failure, resulting in peripheral edema, leading to death, so elderly "blue bloaters" are rare.

The most common precipitating factors for COPD include cigarette smoking, air or environmental pollution, allergic response, autoimmunity, and genetic predisposition. The most universal symptoms of COPD include coughing, increase in sputum production, dyspnea, and wheezing. These symptoms tend to deteriorate rapidly in elderly patients. Dyspnea usually begins after age 50, and worsens more and more with time. Exacerbations of bronchitis with COPD patients frequently occur as a direct result from viral infections, such as *Haemophilus influenza* or *Streptococcus pneumoniae*. Hypoxemia or hypercapnia associated with confusion and restlessness because of brain swelling and dysfunction, may be misdiagnosed as an age-related change.

Treatment is aimed at avoidance of respiratory allergens and irritants, controlling bronchospasms, and improving airway clearance. There is no cure for COPD, but quality of life can be improved and reduced numbers of exacerbations can occur if the patient is compliant with therapy and reconditioning rehabilitation programs.

MEDICAL CARE

Laboratory: cultures used to identify causative organisms and determine appropriate antimicrobial therapy; CBC used to identify presence of infection with elevated white blood cell count, and to monitor for increases in RBCs and hematocrit as the body tries to compensate for oxygen transport requirements; alpha$_1$-antitrypsin levels used to identify deficiency that may be present if patient has hereditary predisposition; theophylline levels used to monitor for therapeutic and toxic levels

Radiography: chest X-rays used to identify hyperinflation of lungs, flattened diaphragm, or pulmonary hypertension; used to identify barotraumas that may occur, increased anteroposterior chest diameter, large retrosternal air spaces, or secondary cardiovascular complications with right-sided heart failure; used to identify thickened bronchial walls and potential right ventricular hypertrophy with patients who have chronic bronchitis; used to identify rib fractures that may occur with severe coughing in the presence of osteoporosis

Electrocardiography: used to identify dysrhythmias associated with this disease; tall P waves in inferior leads, vertical QRS axis, atrial dysrhythmias, right ventricular hypertrophy, sinus tachycardia, and right axis deviation

Pulmonary function studies: used to evaluate pulmonary status and function, and to identify airway obstruction, increased residual volume, total lung capacity, compliance, decreased vital capacity, diffusing capacity, and expiratory volumes with emphysema patients and are usually done prior to and after administration of an aerosol bronchodilator; increased residual volume, decreased vital capacity, and FEV with normal static compliance and diffusion capacity are noted with bronchitis patients; normal aging results in a gradual reduction of the FEV$_1$ and a slight increase in functional residual capacity and residual volume; an increased dead space is frequently noted in patients with COPD

Oxygen: used to improve hypoxemia; liter flow should be low in order to maintain the patient's respiratory drive; PaO$_2$ may be acceptable at 55–60 mm Hg to avoid hypoventilation and maintain function

Arterial blood gases: used to identify acid–base disturbances, presence of hypoxemia and hypercapnia, and to evaluate responses to therapies; hypoxemia results from ventilation/perfusion mismatching caused by bronchospasm, airway collapse, destruction of alveoli, presence of bronchial mucus, or from a reduction in the alveolar oxygen pressure when accompanied by hypoventilation; if hypoventilation occurs, hypercapnia also transpires; hypoxemia diagnosed in the elderly population requires attention to detail because the normal values for the aged are less than those for younger persons

Bronchodilators: albuterol (Proventil, Ventolin, Volmax), aminophylline (Aminophylline, Phyllocontin, Truphylline), ephedrine sulfate (Pretz-D), epinephrine (Adrenalin Chloride, Epi-Pen, Sus-Phrine, Vaponefrin, Primatene, Bronkaid) ipratropium bromide (Atrovent), isoproterenol hydrochloride (Isuprel, Medihaler-Iso), levalbuterol hydrochloride (Xopenex), metaproterenol sulfate (Alupent, Metaproterenol), oxtriphylline (Choledyl SA), pirbuterol acetate (Maxair), salmeterol xinafoate (Serevent), terbutaline sulfate (Brethaire, Brethine, Bricanyl), and theophylline (Aerolate, Aquahyllin, Lanophyllin, Elixophyllin, Slo-Phyllin, Theolair, Theostat 80) are some of the drugs used to relieve bronchospasm and help to promote clearance of mucoid secretions by relaxing bronchial smooth muscle by stimulation of beta$_2$-receptors; anticholinergics are used to relax larger central airways; some drugs help to block the release of mediators that affect allergens within the mast cells inside the respiratory tract; others inhibit phosphodiesterase

Antiasthmatics: beclomethasone dipropionate (Beclovent, Vanceril), cromolyn sodium (Crolom, Gastrocrom, Intal, Nasalcrom), flunisolide (AeroBid), nedocromil sodium (Tilade), triamcinolone acetonide (Azmacort), zafirlukast (Accolate), and zileuton (Zyflo) are used to prevent allergic reactions by stabilizing the mast cells and preventing the release of the inflammatory mediators after exposure to specific antigens, which may predispose the patient to an asthmatic attack

Expectorants: guaifenesin (Anti-Tuss, Hytuss, Naldecon, Robitussin, Uni-tussin) used to stimulate bronchial secretory cells to increase the production of respiratory tract secretions and to irritate the gastric mucosa to stimulate gastric reflex and production of respiratory secretions

Mucolytics: acetylcysteine (Mucomyst, Mucosil) used to liquefy thick, tenacious mucus for easier removal and mobilization by coughing

Corticosteroids: budesonide (Pulmicort Turbuhaler), flunisolide (AeroBid), fluticasone propionate (Flovent), triamcinolone acetonide (Azmacort), and oral prednisolone (Prednisone) are used for their anti-inflammatory action and to bolster the body's defenses when exposed to potential infections or allergic reactions; used to decrease secretions in the lungs; use of steroids is controversial

Antimicrobials: used to treat respiratory infections, and should be based upon culture sensitivity for appropriate drug use

IV fluids: used to maintain hydration and for administration of medical therapeutics and emergency drugs

Chest physiotherapy: percussion and postural drainage are used to facilitate mobilization of the secretions and promote clearance of the airways

COMMON NURSING DIAGNOSES

 ### IMPAIRED GAS EXCHANGE (see CAD)

Related to: bronchospasm, mucus production, edema, inflammation to bronchial tree, hypoxemia, fatigue, ventilation/perfusion imbalance

Defining Characteristics: dyspnea, tachypnea, hypoxia, hypoxemia, hypercapnia, confusion, restlessness, cyanosis, inability to move secretions, tachycardia, dysrhythmias, abnormal arterial blood gases, decreased oxygen saturation

 ### INEFFECTIVE BREATHING PATTERN (see TB)

Related to: fear of suffocation, pain, decreased lung expansion, tracheobronchial obstruction, inflammatory process, inadequate oxygenation, respiratory muscle weakness, respiratory center depression

Defining Characteristics: dyspnea, tachypnea, bradypnea, apnea, cough, nasal flaring, cyanosis, shallow respirations, pursed-lip breathing, changes in inspiratory/expiratory ratio, use of accessory muscles, diminished chest expansion, barrel chest, abnormal arterial blood gases, fremitus, anxiety, decreased oxygen saturation, adventitious breath sounds, increased

anteroposterior chest diameter, decreased energy, fatigue, assumption of a three-point position

 ### ACTIVITY INTOLERANCE (see CAD)

Related to: fatigue, weakness, increased effort and work of breathing, inadequate rest, hypoxia, hypoxemia

Defining Characteristics: dyspnea, decreased oxygen saturation levels with movement or activity, increased heart rate and blood pressure with movement or activity, feelings of tiredness, weakness

 ### ANXIETY (see CAD)

Related to: threat of death, change in health status, life-threatening crises, chronic nature of disease and effect on lifestyle

Defining Characteristics: fear, restlessness, muscle tension, helplessness, communication of uncertainty and apprehension, feeling of suffocation, feelings of inadequacy

RISK FOR INFECTION (see TB)

Related to: inadequate primary defenses, decrease in ciliary action, stasis of body fluids, chronic disease process, inability to move secretions, immunosuppression, poor nutrition

Defining Characteristics: increased temperature, chills, elevated white blood cell count, inability to move secretions, depression of cough reflex, reduced pulmonary macrophages, loss of respiratory defense mechanisms over long term or impairment of their efficacy

INEFFECTIVE COPING (see HEART FAILURE)

Related to: multiple life changes caused by COPD disease process, limitations imposed on lifestyle, inadequate coping methods, fear of death, inadequate support system, continual dyspnea

Defining Characteristics: inability to meet role expectations, inability to meet basic needs, constant worry, apprehension, fear, inability to problem-solve, anger, hostility, aggression, inappropriate defense mechanisms, low self-esteem, insomnia, depression, destructive behaviors, vacillation when choices are required, delayed decision-making, muscle tension, fatigue, withdrawal from society

ADDITIONAL NURSING DIAGNOSES

 ### INEFFECTIVE AIRWAY CLEARANCE

Related to: bronchospasm, fatigue, thick secretions, infection, obstruction, decreased energy

Defining Characteristics: dyspnea, tachypnea, bradypnea, bronchospasms, increased work of breathing, use of accessory muscles, increased mucus production, cough with or without productivity, adventitious breath sounds, abnormal arterial blood gases, fatigue, obstruction, infection, elevated WBC count, shift to the left on differential

Outcome Criteria

✔ Patient will achieve the return of and ability to maintain patent airways and respiratory status baselines.

NOC: *Respiratory Status: Airway Patency*

INTERVENTIONS	RATIONALES
Observe patient and assess energy level and endurance, and how these affect respiratory status.	Energy ability decreases with age and more than one chronic disease state further compromises the ability to maintain ventilation.
Assess respiratory status for rate, depth, ease, use of accessory muscles, and work of breathing.	Changes may vary from minimal to extreme caused by bronchial swelling, increased mucus secretions caused by oversecretion of goblet cells and tracheobronchial infection, bronchospasms narrowing air passageways, and presence of other disease states.
Auscultate lung fields for the presence of wheezes, crackles (rales), rhonchi, or decreased breath sounds.	Wheezing results from squeezing of air past the narrowed airways during expiration which is caused by bronchospasms, edema, and obstructive secretions. Crackles (rales) result from consolidation of leukocytes and fibrin in the lung causing an infection or by fluid accumulation in the lungs. Decreased breath sounds may indicate alveolar collapse with little to no air exchange in the lung area being auscultated, and usually results in poor ventilation.

INTERVENTIONS	RATIONALES
Administer oxygen as ordered. Monitor oxygen saturation by pulse oximetry, and notify physician of readings <90% or as prescribed by physician.	Provides supplemental oxygen to benefit patient. Low flow oxygen delivery systems use some room air and should be used in patients with COPD so as to not depress their respiratory drive. High levels of oxygen may cause severe damage to tissues, oxygen toxicity, increases in A-a gradients, microatelectasis, and ARDS. Oxygen by itself may not always correct hypoxia of tissues and restore perfusion. Oximetry readings of 90 correlate with PaO_2 of 60 mm Hg, and levels below 60 mm Hg do not allow for adequate perfusion to tissues and vital organs. Oximetry uses light waves to identify difference between saturation and reduced hemoglobin of the tissues and may be inaccurate in low blood flow states or in the elderly.
Assess patient for pallor or cyanosis, especially to nail beds and around mouth.	May indicate hypoxemia, but is not a reliable indicator of the loss of airway patency because cyanosis will not occur until a level of 5 grams of reduced hemoglobin/100 ml of blood in the superficial capillaries is reached, and this does not occur until late in chronic respiratory disease.
Monitor patient for cough and production of sputum, noting amount, color, character, patient's ability to expectorate secretions, and patient's ability to cough.	Mucus color from yellow to green may indicate the presence of infection. Tenacious, thick secretions require more effort and energy to cough up and remove, and may actually create an obstruction and stasis that leads to infection and respiratory changes.
Position patient in high Fowler's or semi-Fowler's position, if possible.	Promotes maximal lung expansion.
Turn patient every 2 hours and prn.	Repositioning promotes drainage of pulmonary secretions and enhances ventilation to decrease potential for atelectasis.
Administer bronchodilators as ordered.	Promotes relaxation of bronchial smooth muscle to decrease spasm, dilates airways to improve ventilation, and maximizes air exchange.

(continues)

(continued)

INTERVENTIONS	RATIONALES
Encourage fluids, up to 3–4 L/day, unless contraindicated.	Provides hydration and helps to thin secretions for easier mobilization and removal.
Perform postural drainage and percussion as ordered.	Postural drainage utilizes gravity to help raise secretions and clear sputum. Percussion and/or vibration may assist with movement of secretions away from bronchial walls and enable patient to cough them up and increase the force of expiration. Some positions utilized during chest physiotherapy may be contraindicated in the elderly patient, and the aged may not be able to tolerate intense percussion because of fragility of bones and skin.
Encourage deep breathing and coughing exercises every 2 hours.	Assists in lung expansion, as well as dislodgment of secretions for easier expectoration.
Suction patient if warranted.	Patient may be too weak or fatigued to remove own secretions.
Instruct patient/family regarding splinting abdomen with pillow during cough efforts.	Promotes increased expiratory pressure and helps to decrease discomfort. Forceful coughing in the elderly may predispose patients who have osteoporosis to rib fractures.
Instruct patient/family on alternative types of coughing exercises, such as quad thrusts, if patient has difficulty during coughing.	Minimizes fatigue by assisting patient to increase expiratory pressure and facilitates cough.
Instruct patient on deep-breathing exercises and use of incentive spirometry.	Promotes full lung expansion and decreases anxiety.
Instruct patient/family to avoid using milk, milk products, caffeine drinks, and alcohol.	Milk and milk products thicken mucus, caffeine reduces the effect of some bronchodilators, and alcohol increases cell dehydration and bronchial constriction.
Instruct patient to avoid excessively hot or cold fluids or environmental temperature extremes.	May predispose patient to coughing spells, creating dyspnea and bronchospasms.
Instruct patient to seek help and stop smoking if patient is a smoker.	Smoking causes increased mucus, vasoconstriction, increased blood pressure, inflammation of the lung lining, and decreased numbers of macrophages in the airways and mucociliary blanket.

INTERVENTIONS	RATIONALES
Instruct patient/family to avoid crowds and persons with upper respiratory infections when possible.	Prevents possible transmission of an infection to the patient who already is immunocompromised.
Instruct patient/family in the use of inhalers, nebulizers, and medications.	Provides knowledge, and promotes the correct administration of medication for optimal effect.

NIC: *Airway Management*

Discharge or Maintenance Evaluation

- Patient will achieve and maintain a patent airway.
- Patient will have clear breath sounds to auscultation, and will have respiratory status parameters with optimal air exchange.
- Patient will be compliant and be able to accurately administer medications on a daily basis, preventing exacerbations of disease process.
- Patient will be able to cough up secretions and perform coughing and deep-breathing exercises.

 IMBALANCED NUTRITION: LESS THAN BODY REQUIREMENTS

Related to: inability to take in enough food, increased metabolism caused by hypermetabolic disease state, decreased level of consciousness, inability to absorb nutrients because of biologic or psychological factors

Defining Characteristics: actual inadequate food intake, altered taste, altered smell sensation, weight loss, body weight 20% or more under ideal for height and frame, anorexia, absent bowel sounds, decreased peristalsis, muscle mass loss, decreased muscle tone, changes in bowel habits, nausea, vomiting, abdominal distention, lack of interest in food, satiety immediately after ingesting food, abdominal pain or discomfort, sore, inflamed buccal cavity, depression, anxiety, social isolation, difficulty in feeding self, changes in mental status, fatigue from work of breathing, shortness of breath, changes in oxygen saturation with activity, altered arterial blood gases

Outcome Criteria

✔ Patient will have adequate nutritional intake with no weight or muscle mass loss.

NOC: *Nutritional Status: Nutrient Intake*

INTERVENTIONS	RATIONALES
Evaluate patient's ability to eat.	Provides information regarding factors associated with reduced intake of nutrients. Lack of activity in the elderly patient contributes to anorexia, and increased work of breathing results in fatigue, which prevents adequate ingestion of food.
Weigh patient every day, on same scale, at same time if possible.	Provides information regarding weight loss or gain. Continued weight loss will result in catabolic metabolism and impaired respiratory function. Consistent use of same scale provides accurate data from which to base changes in care.
Observe for muscle wasting.	May indicate muscle store depletion, which can impair respiratory muscle function.
Observe for nausea, vomiting, abdominal distention and palpability, and stool characteristics.	Patients with severe respiratory disease may develop GI dysfunction from analgesics/sedatives, bed rest, trapped air, and stress, which may result in ileus formation.
Obtain calorie count and assessment of metabolic demands based on disease process.	Establishes imbalances between actual nutritional intake and metabolic needs, and enables a plan of care to be established with regard to provision of adequate nutritive consumption.
Assess patient's mouth and condition of teeth, fit of dentures, and presence of food left in mouth.	Provides information regarding patient's ability to chew foods without difficulty. The elderly may not be able to tolerate food selections that would benefit their condition because of lack of ability to ingest foods properly. Alterations in consistency of foods may be an option.
Monitor medication side effects and food interactions with medications being taken.	Some medications impair nutritional intake by causing nausea or vomiting, or inhibiting absorption of nutrients.
Monitor patient for effort expended to perform physical functions of eating.	Fatigue impairs the ability to chew and swallow foods, and further impairs respiratory function.
Provide diet of smaller, more frequent meals per day with high-protein and high-carbohydrate	Smaller meals may be able to be consumed with less fatigue, and actual intake may increase. May

INTERVENTIONS	RATIONALES
foods that are easily chewed and swallowed, unless contraindicated.	assist in maintaining nutritional status while preventing further muscle wasting.
Provide and encourage high-caloric liquid supplements.	Provides additional protein and caloric intake. Some liquid supplements contain additional amounts of fat, which help to reduce the carbon dioxide levels that are seen with COPD patients and facilitate improved respiratory status.
Administer vitamin/mineral supplementation as ordered.	Provides adequate vitamin inclusion in diet for proper body function.
Position patient in upright position for meals, and maintain this position for at least 30 minutes after eating.	Prevents aspiration and promotes movement of food by gravity and peristalsis.
Provide rest periods for patient during meal. Ensure proper oral hygiene prior to and after meals.	Enhances appetite and reduces difficulty if dyspnea or reflux is present.
Assist patient with meal when needed. Do not rush patient.	Promotes independence and adequate intake without choking.
Provide thickened fluids if patient has difficulty handling liquids.	Thicker substances are easier to swallow.
If patient is unable to ingest adequate nutrition, administer tube feedings or parenteral nutrition, as ordered.	May be required for alternate methods of providing required nutrition.
Determine patency of enteral feeding tube at least every 8 hours. Flush with 20–30 cc of water every 8 hours, before and after medication administration via the tube, and prn.	Oral or nasal tubes may migrate with coughing, resulting in improper placement and potential for aspiration. Flushing of the tube maintains patency.
Aspirate gastric residuals every 4–8 hours, and decrease or hold feedings per hospital policy.	Increasing residuals may indicate decreased or absent peristalsis and lack of absorption of required nutrients which may require another form of nutritional support.
Use food coloring to tint feedings. Do not use red food coloring.	Helps to identify aspiration of feedings when suctioned. Be aware that the food coloring may cause false readings on occult blood tests on stools. Red coloring should be avoided because of similarity of blood color and this may impair ability to differentiate bleeding problems. Some facilities avoid using

(continues)

(continued)

INTERVENTIONS	RATIONALES
	food coloring because of potential bacterial contamination.
If feeding tube becomes occluded, instill warm cranberry juice, carbonated cola, or mixture of monosodium glutamate and water into tube per hospital policy. Notify physician if tube is occluded.	Helps to dissolve clogged particulate matter to maintain patency of tube. If occlusion is not able to be removed, tube must be replaced in order to facilitate administration of nutritive substances.
Administer antidiarrheal medications as warranted/ordered.	Osmolality imbalances may result in diarrhea, requiring antidiarrheals for control. Changing strengths or types of feeding solutions may be helpful.
Administer metoclopramide as ordered.	Medication helps to stimulate gastric motility and may be helpful to increase absorption.
Administer parenteral alimentation fluids as warranted via infusion pump.	Provides complete nutritional support without dependence on GI function for absorption. Additives are based upon lab work and patient requirements. Increases in protein and nitrogen may be prescribed for increased metabolic demands of the patient.
Administer intralipids as ordered, if not admixed with TPN solution.	Provides additional caloric benefits as well as a source of essential fatty acids. Lipids may be utilized for respiratory failure to help decrease CO_2 retention.
Change solution at least every 24 hours, as well as tubing.	Some additives may be unstable after 24 hours, and prolonged infusion with the same solution may promote bacterial growth.
Do not stop TPN abruptly; taper over several days/hours per protocol.	Rebound hypoglycemia may result if dextrose concentrations are abruptly changed.
Monitor lab work per hospital protocol: general chemistry, renal profiles, CBC, urine or blood glucose levels.	Requirements for electrolyte replacement or alteration in formula may be changed based on this information. High dextrose content in TPN solutions may require additions of insulin to meet metabolic demands if pancreatic disease, hepatic disease, or diabetes are present.

INTERVENTIONS	RATIONALES
Instruct patient in need for supplemental nutritional support, procedures to be performed, and tests that will be required.	Promotes knowledge, decreases fear of the unknown, and facilitates cooperation with procedures. Provides opportunity for patient to make an informed choice.
Instruct patient regarding insertion of nasogastric tube. Use small weighted tube and obtain chest X-ray or KUB X-ray post-insertion.	Smaller lumen tubes are less irritating to nasal mucosa, and decrease the incidence of gastroesophageal reflux. Radiographic confirmation of placement is necessary because of the potential for aspiration when the patient may have an impaired gag reflex.
Instruct patient and assist with placement of central venous catheter for TPN administration. Obtain chest X-ray post-insertion.	Centrally-placed intravenous lines may enable higher concentrations of amino acids to be utilized. Radiographic confirmation of placement as well as ruling out hemo- or pneumothorax postprocedure, is mandatory.

NIC: *Gastrointestinal Intubation*

NIC: *Nutrition Therapy*

NIC: *Total Parenteral Nutrition (TPN) Administration*

Discharge or Maintenance Evaluation

- Patient will maintain baseline weight with no loss of muscle mass.
- Patient will maintain adequate nutritional status with use of nutritional support, and will experience no complications from support.
- Patient will show no signs of malnutrition status.
- Patient will be able to accurately recall and verbalize understanding of instructions and be compliant with procedures and testing.
- Patient will maintain a normal nitrogen balance and immunity will not be compromised.

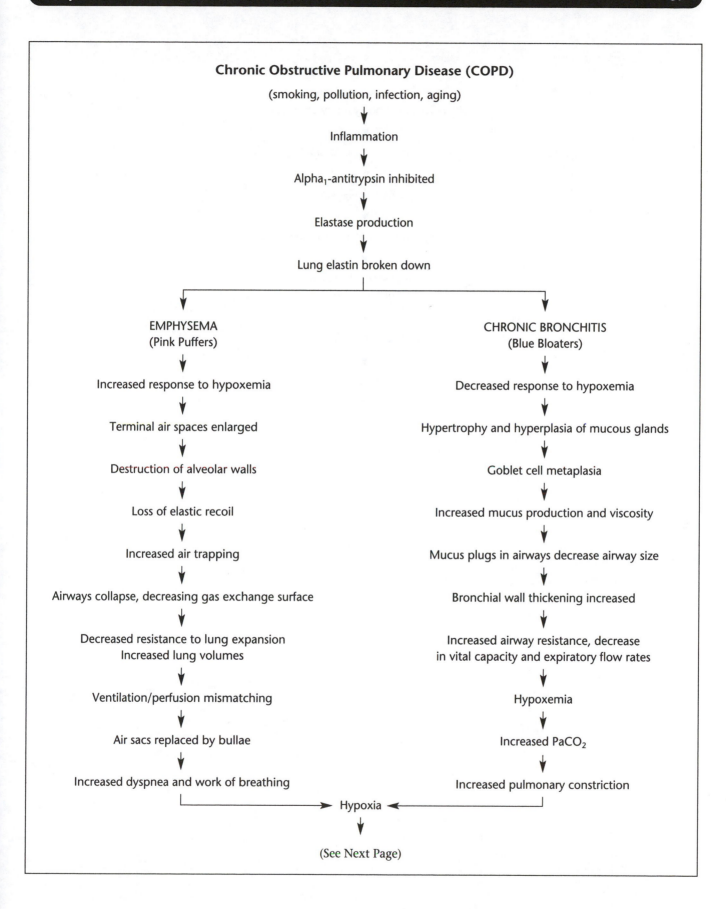

Chronic Obstructive Pulmonary Disease (COPD)

(smoking, pollution, infection, aging)

↓

Inflammation

↓

Alpha$_1$-antitrypsin inhibited

↓

Elastase production

↓

Lung elastin broken down

EMPHYSEMA (Pink Puffers)	CHRONIC BRONCHITIS (Blue Bloaters)
Increased response to hypoxemia	Decreased response to hypoxemia
Terminal air spaces enlarged	Hypertrophy and hyperplasia of mucous glands
Destruction of alveolar walls	Goblet cell metaplasia
Loss of elastic recoil	Increased mucus production and viscosity
Increased air trapping	Mucus plugs in airways decrease airway size
Airways collapse, decreasing gas exchange surface	Bronchial wall thickening increased
Decreased resistance to lung expansion Increased lung volumes	Increased airway resistance, decrease in vital capacity and expiratory flow rates
Ventilation/perfusion mismatching	Hypoxemia
Air sacs replaced by bullae	Increased PaCO$_2$
Increased dyspnea and work of breathing	Increased pulmonary constriction

→ Hypoxia ←

↓

(See Next Page)

COPD (continued)

Further pulmonary constriction
Increased pulmonary artery pressures

↓

Pulmonary hypertension

↓

Right ventricular strain

↓

Right ventricular hypertrophy

↓

Right ventricular failure
Cor Pulmonale

↓

Left ventricular failure

↓

Circulatory collapse

↓

DEATH

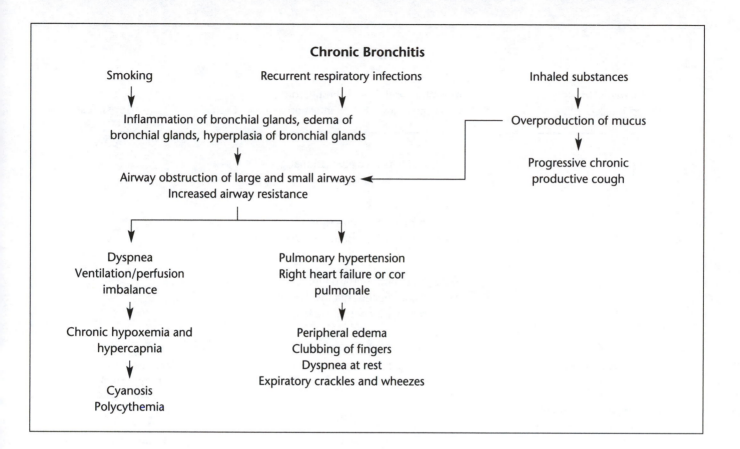

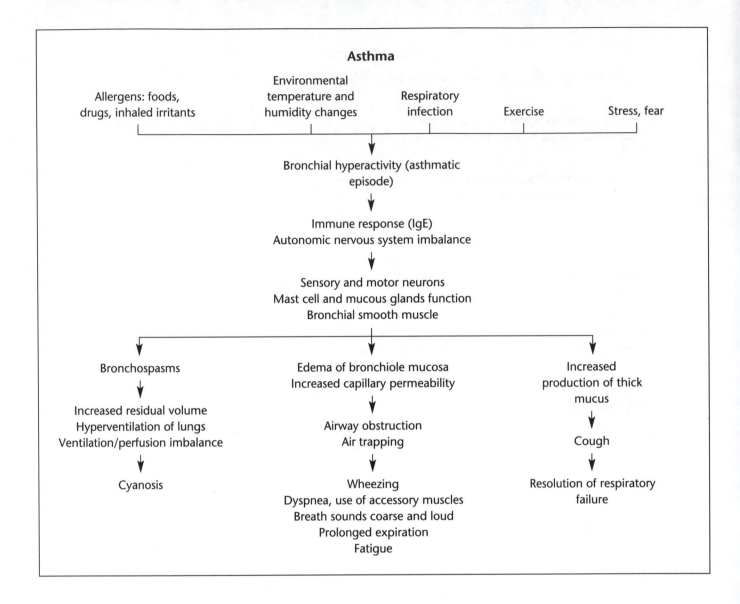

CHAPTER 2.2

INFLUENZA

Influenza is an acute inflammation of the nasopharynx, trachea, and bronchioles, with associated edema, congestion, and possible necrosis of these respiratory structures. It occurs in epidemic proportions usually in the late fall or early winter, and complications, such as hemorrhagic bronchitis, pneumonia, and death can ensue in severe cases. The highest risk group includes those over age 65, those patients with chronic cardiovascular or pulmonary diseases, and residents of long-term, chronic-care facilities.

Also known as the "flu," or the "grippe," influenza is caused by an RNA virus that has a center composed of helical nucleic acid and soluble nucleoprotein antigens. Based on testing of these antigens with specific antibodies, the virus is usually classified as one of three types, A, B, or C. Influenza A is normally the most frequent type seen, with a prevalence for the young, the aged, and the chronically ill.

Several different strains of the virus cause the disease and new strains appear, which result in yearly changes in immunization precautions for the elderly. Proliferation of the disease occurs by person-to-person contact or airborne droplet contamination, with a 2-day incubation period. Symptoms include malaise, generalized aches and pains, especially in the back and legs, headache, photophobia, sore throat, cough, and fever. As the systemic symptoms decrease, respiratory symptoms become worsened. Some symptoms may linger for days to weeks, especially in the elderly. Sometimes, a secondary bacterial infection also occurs, and should be anticipated if the patient continues with symptoms longer than 5 days, or has a relapse after a period of improvement from 5–15 days. Usually bacterial organisms that cause pneumonia include *Pneumococcus*, *Staphylococcus aureus*, *Haemophilus influenzae*, and other gram-positive and gram-negative organisms. Elderly patients, especially those with concurrent chronic medical diseases, may be responsible for at least 50% of all hospitalizations and for more than 80% of deaths attributable to influenza (Beers & Berkow, 2000).

A vaccine provides some immunity in approximately 85% of people for up to 1 year; the vaccine's content changes from year to year and is established by use of the prevailing types of strains of influenza from the former year. The vaccine is contraindicated for persons who exhibit a hypersensitivity to eggs or other components of the vaccine, people with an acute febrile illness, or patients who have thrombocytopenia. Immunity is greatest after approximately 2 weeks.

Treatment of the flu is aimed at supportive care, prevention of complications, and decreasing the duration of symptoms with the use of drugs, such as amantadine or rimantadine. Ribavirin has been used successfully in treatment of severely ill patients who have influenza A or B.

MEDICAL CARE

Laboratory: CBC used to identify secondary infection with shifts to the left on a differential; leukocyte count may be normal in an uncomplicated case; leukopenia with lymphocytosis may be present; viral testing done to isolate the specific virus from nasal, oral, mucoid, or lung tissue specimens; serologic testing may be used but is not used frequently because of the lengthy time it requires to obtain the specimen (usually at least 10 days after the onset of the disease); myoglobin in the urine may be seen with influenza B; liver profiles may be used to identify complications that may occur, such as hepatitis or liver dysfunction that may occur with use of antiviral drugs

Radiography: chest X-rays used to evaluate possible lung involvement with complications, such as pneumonia

Prophylaxis: vaccines help to provide immunity to those at risk, with the mixture made up of influenza strains from the previous year; amantadine can be used prophylactically for influenza A, but is ineffective against type B

Antipyretics and analgesics: acetaminophen (Tylenol), ibuprofen (Motrin, Advil, Genpril, Ibuprofen, Nuprin, Trendar), and acetylsalicylic acid (ASA, aspirin) used to reduce temperature by the action on the hypothalamus control center, and to treat the headache, aches, and pains normally associated with the flu

Antivirals: amantadine hydrochloride (Symmetrel), famciclovir (Famvir), oseltamivir phosphate (Tamiflu), and zanamivir (Relenza) used to inhibit viral shedding, viral replication, or for prophylaxis after exposure to the disease; newer drugs effective for both influenza types A and B but must be given within 48 hours of onset of symptoms to be effective and reduce the duration of the symptoms

COMMON NURSING DIAGNOSES

 ### INEFFECTIVE AIRWAY CLEARANCE (see COPD)

Related to: tracheobronchial and nasal secretions, pneumonia, increased peripheral airway resistance caused by drug therapy

Defining Characteristics: rhinorrhea, irritating nonproductive cough, respiratory rate and depth changes, decreased breath sounds, adventitious breath sounds, production of sputum, restlessness, orthopnea

 ### INEFFECTIVE BREATHING PATTERN (see TB)

Related to: inflammation from viral infection, pneumonia, hemorrhagic bronchitis

Defining Characteristics: cough, tachypnea, hemoptysis, cyanosis, dyspnea, pulmonary edema, fever, weakness, diaphoresis, fatigue, leukopenia, sputum, warm, flushed skin, erythema to tonsils, soft and hard palate and pharyngeal wall, abnormal chest X-rays

ADDITIONAL NURSING DIAGNOSES

 ### ACUTE PAIN

Related to: influenza virus, coughing, pneumonia

Defining Characteristics: communication of pain, fever, cough with or without production, body aches, malaise

Outcome Criteria

✔ Patient will achieve relief from aches and pain.

NOC: *Comfort Level*

INTERVENTIONS	RATIONALES
Assess patient for complaints of headache, sore throat, redness of throat, general malaise, muscle aches and pain.	Result of inflammation or elevated temperature.
Assess for herpes simplex lesions on lips or mouth.	Associated with viral infection.
Assess VS for changes from baselines (usually increased).	Result of autonomic response to pain.
Administer analgesic as ordered.	Controls aches and pains by inhibiting brain prostaglandin synthesis.
Provide restful, quiet environment.	Reduces stimuli that may increase pain.
Provide warm baths or heating pad to aching muscles.	Warmth causes vasodilation and decreases discomfort.
Provide cool compress to head prn.	Promotes comfort and treats headache.
Provide backrub prn.	Promotes relaxation and relieves aches.
Encourage gargling with warm water; provide throat lozenges prn.	Reduces throat discomfort.
Instruct patient/family in deep breathing, relaxation techniques, guided imagery, massage, and other nonpharmacologic aids.	Helps patient to focus less on pain, and may improve efficacy of analgesics by decreasing muscle tension.
Instruct patient/family regarding use of acetaminophen and to avoid use of aspirin.	Acetaminophen may relieve pain and headache, but should be used cautiously in patients with liver dysfunction because of acetaminophen's metabolism in the liver. Aspirin should be avoided because of potential for hemorrhage and ulceration.

NIC: *Analgesic Administration*

Discharge or Maintenance Evaluation

- Patient will achieve and maintain reduced pain and discomfort with use of analgesics and/or non-pharmacologic methods.
- Patient will have stable vital signs.
- Patient will exhibit no complications from medication therapy.
- Patient/family will be able to accurately verbalize instructions regarding use of medication and relaxation techniques.

HYPERTHERMIA

Related to: influenza viral infection, exposure to infection, alterations in fluid and electrolyte balance

Defining Characteristics: fever, warm, flushed skin, tachycardia, tachypnea, dry mucous membranes, dehydration, oliguria, seizures, changes in mental status, increased BUN and creatinine, electrolyte imbalances

Outcome Criteria

- ✔ Patient will achieve and maintain normal temperature.
- ✔ Patient will achieve and maintain balanced intake and output with adequate hydration.

NOC: *Thermoregulation*

INTERVENTIONS	RATIONALES
Monitor vital signs, especially temperature, every 2–4 hours and prn. Utilize same methods of temperature reading with each measurement.	Helps to evaluate efficacy of treatment and monitors for complications that may occur as a result of increased temperature. Consistency in methods allows for accurate data collection and correlation. Increased temperature is a response to the inflammatory process associated with the disease.
Administer antipyretics as ordered.	This type of drugs affects the hypothalamic control center to reduce elevated temperature.
Provide tepid sponge baths prn.	Increases heat loss by evaporation. Tepid baths help prevent chilling that may aggravate and increase temperature.

INTERVENTIONS	RATIONALES
Utilize cooling blanket if temperature will not decrease with use of other methods, and if temperature is above 103° F (39.4° C) as ordered. Ensure that blanket is covered with linens/blanket, that temperature is taken at least every 15 minutes, if not constantly with rectal probe, and that blanket is turned off when temperature drops to set parameters or if shivering occurs.	Hypothermia blankets remove heat by conduction via the cool solution that is circulated in the mattress placed above and/or below the patient. The cooling blanket must be covered to prevent skin tissue injury and burns. Cooling blankets may lower temperature quickly and should be monitored to ensure that a hypothermic condition does not occur. Shivering actually increases the patient's metabolic rate and temperature. Some facilities may utilize pharmacologic agents, such as thorazine, to reduce shivering if the cooling blanket is the only method of reducing temperature.
Decrease environmental temperature and remove extra blankets as warranted.	Helps to reduce temperature.
Encourage fluid intake up to 3–4 L/day, unless contraindicated.	Increases in body temperature multiply insensible fluid losses by 10% for every 1° C increase in body temperature, which may result in dehydration.
Monitor intake and output every 2–4 hours and prn.	Helps to identify fluid status changes and imbalances, and allows for prompt treatment.
Notify physician of temperature increases that do not respond to any measure used.	May indicate other source of temperature aberration and may cause permanent organ damage.
Monitor patient for seizures.	Seizures may occur with high temperatures because of hyperactivity within the brain, which can further impair tissue perfusion.
Instruct patient/family in use of hypothermia blanket, reasons for use, signs and symptoms of complications, etc.	Provides knowledge and helps to involve patient and family in care.
Instruct patient/family on medications, side effects, effects, and symptoms to report to nurse.	Involves patient and family in care and provide knowledge that facilitates compliance.

NIC: *Temperature Regulation*

Discharge or Maintenance Evaluation

- Patient will be afebrile, with stable vital signs.

- Patient will have moist mucous membranes and exhibit adequate hydration status.
- Patient will have good skin turgor and balanced intake and output.
- Patient/family will be able to accurately verbalize understanding of need for use of hypothermia blanket and medications.
- Patient will suffer no complications, such as skin trauma or burns, from the use of hypothermia blanket.

DEFICIENT KNOWLEDGE

Related to: lack of knowledge about influenza, inability to avoid complications, recurrence of disease

Defining Characteristics: verbalization of misconceptions, verbalization of questions about disease, request for information, presence of avoidable complications

Outcome Criteria

✔ Patient will be able to understand and verbalize appropriate treatment and care for influenza.

NOC: *Knowledge: Disease Process*

INTERVENTIONS	RATIONALES
Assess patient's understanding of disease process.	Patient may have seen many epidemics in which numerous people perished because of the viral illness, and may have misconceptions that should be corrected. Identification of baseline knowledge helps to facilitate and establish plan of care for patient and family education.
Ensure that patient is willing and able to listen to information about disease.	Patient may be too ill to understand and comprehend information. If patient is unwilling to listen to information, accept decision, which will help to facilitate acceptance of rights as a patient to choose level of self-participation in care.
Use limited amounts of time for teaching, with the provision of a quiet environment.	Helps the elderly patient to remember information being discussed without distracting stimuli. Limiting sessions of instruction helps to avoid over-stimulation and overload.

INTERVENTIONS	RATIONALES
Use appropriate teaching aids for patient's abilities, such as large written instructions for visually impaired patients, and so forth.	Helps to provide information in a manner that will be more easily understood by patient and remembered. Normal aging changes may cause memory loss, sensory deficits, and the need for slower, more repetitive teaching.
Instruct patient/family about influenza types, when typical outbreaks occur, and methods to avoid infection.	Influenza occurs every year, normally from November through April, and virus is spread through direct contact or by aerosol droplets. Elderly patients, who usually have other disease processes, are especially prone to infection and should avoid others who have upper respiratory symptoms when possible.
Instruct patient/family that the elderly patient should always be immunized with the flu vaccine, especially if there are other concurrent disease processes.	The vaccination should be given in October prior to the start of the outbreak of influenza season, but can be given throughout this time until late winter. Prevention of influenza is considered optimal in order to prevent complications, such as pneumonia.
Instruct patient/family about newer antiviral drugs, their effects, when to seek medical attention, and side effects.	Tamiflu (oseltamivir phosphate) and Relenza (zanamivir) are effective for influenza types A and B. Rimantadine and amantadine are effective for influenza A. These drugs should be given within 48 hours of the onset of symptoms for maximum efficacy. Caution should be used if patients have other respiratory diseases or renal insufficiency. Patients should also be advised these drugs are not a replacement for their annual vaccination.

NIC: *Teaching: Disease Process*

Discharge or Maintenance Evaluation

- Patient/family will be able to accurately verbalize understanding of the influenza disease and methods to use to avoid contracting illness.
- Patient/family will be able to notify physician immediately during flu season if patient begins to

have symptoms of influenza in order to be treated appropriately with antivirals.

■ Patient will suffer no complications, such as pneumonia, requiring hospitalization.

■ Patient will be compliant with obtaining annual influenza vaccination.

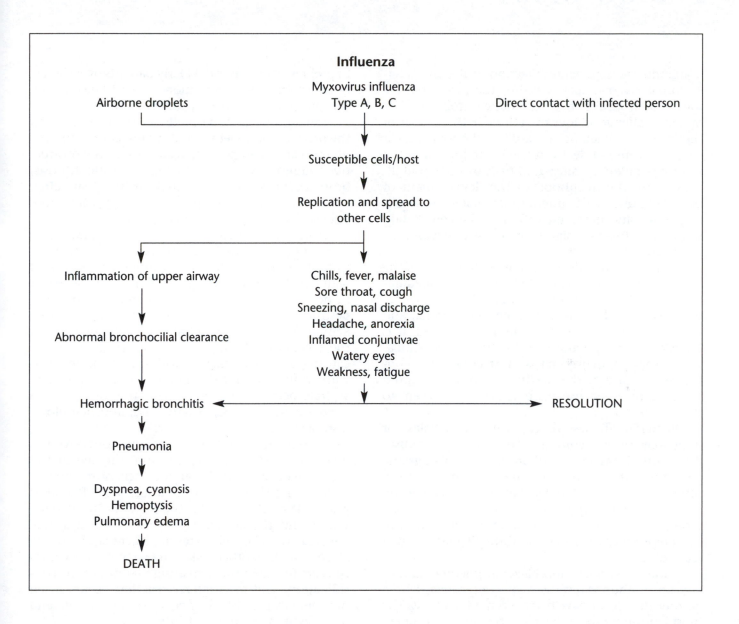

CHAPTER 2.3

PNEUMONIA

Pneumonia is an acute infection of the lung's terminal alveolar spaces and/or the interstitial tissues, which results in gas exchange problems. The major challenge is identification of the source of the infection. Pneumonia ranks as the fourth most common cause of death in the United States in the elderly population, caused, in part, by comorbid illnesses and the likelihood of the development of complications from pneumonia, such as sepsis, empyema, and meningitis (Beers & Berkow, 2000). Influenza is the most significant cause of pneumonia in the elderly.

When the infection is limited to a portion of the lung, it is known as segmental, or lobular, pneumonia; when the alveoli adjacent to the bronchioles are involved, it is known as bronchopneumonia, and when the entire lobe of the lung is involved, it is known as lobar pneumonia. In the elderly population, bronchopneumonia is most commonly contracted because of the decline in immunity and a presence of other diseases that predispose them to this condition.

Bacteria, viruses, mycoplasma, rickettsias, or fungi may cause pneumonia. The causative organism gains entry by aspiration of oropharyngeal or gastric contents, inhalation of respiratory droplets, from others who are infected, by way of the bloodstream, or directly with surgery or trauma. Viral types are more common in some areas, but identification of causative organisms may be difficult with limited technology.

Patients who develop bacterial pneumonia usually are immunosuppressed or compromised by a chronic disease, or have had a recent viral illness. The most common type of bacterial pneumonia is pneumococcal pneumonia, in which the *Streptococcus pneumoniae* organism reaches the lungs via the respiratory passageways and results in the collapse of alveoli. The inflammatory response that this generates causes protein-rich fluid to migrate into the alveolar spaces and provides culture media for the organisms

to proliferate and spread. Elderly patients over the age of 65 are from 3–5 times more prone to death from this pneumonia than are younger patients.

Pneumonia may be predisposed to occur with the presence of upper respiratory infections, chronic illness, cancer, surgery, atelectasis, chronic obstructive pulmonary disease, asthma, cystic fibrosis, bronchiectasis, influenza, malnutrition, smoking, alcoholism, immunosuppressive therapy, aspiration, sickle cell disease, head injury, or coma.

Aspiration pneumonia occurs after aspiration of gastric or oropharyngeal contents, or other chemical irritants, into the trachea and lungs. Stomach acid damages the respiratory endothelium and may result in noncardiogenic pulmonary edema, hemorrhage, destruction of surfactant-producing cells, and hypoxemia. The pH of the aspirated material determines the severity of the injury, with a pH less than 2.5 causing severe damage. Morbidity is high even with treatment, and the elderly are more prone to aspirate because of age-related conditions, such as altered consciousness, sedative use, and neurologic disorders.

In pneumonia's early stages, pulmonary vessels dilate and erythrocytes spread into the alveoli and cause a reddish, liver-like appearance, or red hepatization, in the lung consolidation area. Polymorphonuclear (PMNs) cells then enter the alveolar spaces and the consolidation increases to a gray hepatization. The leukocytes trap bacteria against the alveolar walls or other leukocytes so that more organisms are found in the increasing margins of the consolidation. The macrophage reaction occurs when mononuclear cells advance into the alveoli and phagocytize the exudate debris.

Diagnosis may be assisted with the observation of sputum characteristics, with bacterial pneumonia having mucopurulent sputum, viral and mycoplasmic pneumonias having more watery secretions, pneumococcal pneumonia having rust-colored sputum, and *Klebsiella* noted to have dark red mucoid secretions. A diagnosis should not be made based on sputum characteristics alone because expectorated sputum does not differentiate colonization from distinct pulmonary infection.

The initial signs and symptoms include: a sudden onset of shaking chills, fever, purulent sputum, pleuritic chest pain that is worsened with respiration or coughing, tachycardia, tachypnea, and use of accessory muscles for breathing. In the elderly, however, the usual clinical features of pneumonia may be understated and subtle, with an initial presentation of acute confusion, deterioration of baseline function, tachypnea, and/or tachycardia.

Staphylococcal pneumonia is frequently noted after influenza or in hospitalized patients with a nosocomial superinfection following surgery, trauma, or immunosuppression. Pleural pain, dyspnea, cyanosis, and productive coughing with copious pink secretions are common symptoms. Streptococcal pneumonia occurs as a complication after influenza, and is the most common bacterial cause of community-acquired pneumonia in the elderly. Klebsiellal pneumonia is virulent and necrotizing, and is usually seen with alcoholic or severely debilitated patients. Pneumonia that is caused by *Haemophilus influenzae* occurs after viral upper respiratory infections, or concurrently with bronchopneumonia, bronchitis, and bronchiolitis. Sputum is usually yellow or green, and patients have fever, cough, cyanosis, and arthralgias. Viral pneumonia may be caused by influenza, adenoviruses, respiratory syncytial virus (RSV), rhinoviruses, cytomegalovirus, herpes simplex virus, and childhood diseases, and is usually milder. Symptoms include headache, anorexia, and occasionally mucopurulent sputum that is bloody.

Pneumonia can be prevented, or minimized, in two types—influenza and pneumococcal—by obtaining a yearly influenza vaccine. The pneumococcal vaccine is suggested for high-risk elderly patients with reimmunization every 6–10 years.

Treatment of pneumonia is aimed at supportive care, drainage of empyemas and pleural effusions, drug therapy to eradicate the causative organism, pulmonary hygiene, and reduction of complications. Pneumonia in the elderly may be a terminal event with comorbid illnesses, and sometimes supportive comfort measures are more suitable than antimicrobial therapy. An advanced directive should be obtained and can assist the family and physician in making appropriate choices for the patient based on the patient's condition and wishes concerning quality of life.

MEDICAL CARE

Laboratory: CBC used to identify presence of infection, as well as identification of improvement or worsening of condition; WBC may be normal or low, but usually elevated with polymorphonuclear neutrophils; cultures of sputum, blood, and CSF obtained to identify the causative organism and appropriate antimicrobial agent needed for eradication; electrolyte profiles used to show imbalances, with a prevalence normally of decreases in sodium and chloride levels; serology and cold agglutinins used for identification of viral titers; sedimentation rate usually elevated; liver profiles used to identify elevations in alkaline phosphatase, LDH, and AST; renal profiles used to identify renal dysfunction

Radiography: chest X-rays used to reveal areas affected by consolidation of lungs; progression with multilobular association frequently noted in the elderly; with staphylococcal pneumonia, early X-rays may show numerous small rounded densities that shortly enlarge and group together to form abscesses; presence of a large pleural effusion is normally seen with streptococcal pneumonia; in pneumonias caused by gram-negative bacilli and *Klebsiella*, an enlarged lobe and a downward curve of the horizontal lobar fissure may be seen, as well as cavitation; X-ray may be clear with mycoplasmal pneumonia

Oxygen: used to supplement room air, and to treat hypoxemia that may occur

Pulmonary function studies: used to evaluate ventilation/perfusion problems; volumes may be decreased because of alveolar collapse; airway pressures may be increased; lung compliance may be decreased

Arterial blood gases: used to evaluate adequacy of oxygen and respiratory therapies, as well as to identify acid–base imbalances and acidotic/alkalotic states

Chest physiotherapy: percussion and pulmonary hygiene used to assist with patients who have a poor cough reflex and effort to assist with removing the thick secretions

Antimicrobials: used to treat causative organism once culture results obtained; method of action may vary but usually involves inhibition of cell wall synthesis or preventing protein biosynthesis; for *Streptococcus pneumoniae*, penicillin, macrolides (azithromycin [Zithromax], clarithromycin [Biaxin], dirithromycin [Dynabac], erythromycin base, estolate, ethylsuccinate, lactobionate, or stearate [E-Mycin, Eryc, Erythromycin, Ilosone, EES, EryPed, Erythrocin]), fluoroquinolones (ciprofloxacin [Cipro], enoxacin [Penetrex], gatifloxacin [Tequin], levofloxacin [Levaquin], lomefloxacin hydrochloride [Maxaquin], moxifloxacin hydrochloride [Avelox], nalidixic acid [NegGram], norfloxacin [Noroxin], ofloxacin [Floxin], sparfloxacin [Zagam], or trovafloxacin mesylate [Trovan]), or first-generation cephalosporins (cefadroxil [Duricef], cefazolin sodium [Ancef, Kefzol, Zolicef], cephalexin hydrochloride [Keftab, Biocef, Keflex], or cephradine [Velosef]) are generally used; for *Haemophilus influenzae*, cefuroxime (Ceftin, Kefurox, Zinacef), trimethoprim-sulfamethoxazole (Bactrim, Bethaprim, Comoxol, Septra, Sulfatrim), levofloxacin (Levaquin), and third-generation cephalosporins (cefdinir [Omnicef], cefixime [Suprax], cefoperazone sodium [Cefobid], cefotaxime sodium [Claforan], cefpodoxime proxetil [Vantin], ceftazidime [Ceptaz, Fortaz, Tazicef, Tazidime], ceftibuten [Cedax], ceftizoxime sodium [Cefizox] or ceftriaxone sodium [Rocephin]) are used; for *Pseudomonas aeruginosa*, ceftazidime (Ceptaz, Fortaz, Tazicef, Tazidime) in addition with an aminoglycoside, such as tobramycin (Nebcin, Tobrax) or amikacin (Amikin), or an antipseudomonal penicillin (mezlocillin sodium [Mezlin], piperacillin sodium [Pipracil], or ticarcillin disodium [Ticar]) is used; for *Staphylococcus aureus*, cephalothin (Keflin, Cephalothin), cefamandole (Mandol), vancomycin (Vancocin, Vancoled, Lyphocin), or an antistaphylococcal penicillin (cloxacillin sodium [Cloxapen, Tegopen], dicloxacillin sodium [Dycill, Dynapen, Pathocil], nafcillin sodium [Nallpen, Unipen], oxacillin sodium [Bactocill], or piperacillin sodium/taxzobacam sodium [Zosyn]) is used; for gram-negative bacilli, imipenem (Primaxin), aztreonam (Azactam), or third-generation cephalosporins (cefdinir [Omnicef], cefixime [Suprax], cefoperazone sodium [Cefobid], cefotaxime sodium [Claforan], cefpodoxime proxetil [Vantin], ceftazidime [Ceptaz, Fortaz, Tazicef, Tazidime], ceftibuten [Cedax], ceftizoxime sodium [Cefizox] or ceftriaxone sodium [Rocephin]) are used; for anaerobic bacilli, clindamycin (Cleocin) or penicillin is used; for *Legionella*, a fluoroquinolone (ciprofloxacin [Cipro], enoxacin [Penetrex], gatifloxacin [Tequin], levofloxacin [Levaquin],

lomefloxacin hydrochloride [Maxaquin], moxifloxacin hydrochloride [Avelox], nalidixic acid [NegGram], norfloxacin [Noroxin], ofloxacin [Floxin], sparfloxacin [Zagam], or trovafloxacin mesylate [Trovan]), a macrolide (azithromycin [Zithromax], clarithromycin [Biaxin], dirithromycin [Dynabac], erythromycin base, estolate, ethylsuccinate, lactobionate, or stearate [E-Mycin, Eryc, Erythromycin, Ilosone, EES, EryPed, Erythrocin]), or erythromycin with the addition of rifampin (Rifadin, Rifampicin, Rimactane) may be used; for influenza A viruses, rimantadine (Flumadine), amantadine (Symmetrel), and some other antibiotic may be used in cases where a superimposed bacterial infection is present

Vaccines: influenza and pneumonia vaccines are recommended for the elderly patient; influenza vaccine should be taken yearly, and the pneumonia vaccine should be administered approximately every 5–7 years

Expectorants: guaifenesin (Anti-Tuss, Hytuss, Naldecon, Robitussin, Uni-tussin) used to stimulate bronchial secretory cells to increase the production of respiratory tract secretions and to irritate the gastric mucosa to stimulate gastric reflex and production of respiratory secretions

Mucolytics: acetylcysteine (Mucomyst, Mucosil) used to liquefy thick, tenacious mucus for easier removal and mobilization by coughing

Antipyretics and analgesics: acetaminophen (Tylenol), ibuprofen (Motrin, Advil, Genpril, Ibuprofen, Nuprin, Trendar), and acetylsalicylic acid (ASA, aspirin) are used to reduce temperature by the action on the hypothalamus control center, and to treat the headache, aches, and pains normally associated with the flu

Thoracentesis: used to remove fluid if pleural fluid is present; assists in the diagnosis of pleural empyema

Surgery: may be required for open lung biopsy or treatment of effusions and empyema; bronchoscopy with bronchial brushings may be indicated for progressive pneumonias that are unresponsive to medical treatment; insertion of thoracotomy tubes for re-expansion of a lung collapse caused by mucus obstruction

Nerve blocks: intercostal nerve blocks may be required to control pleuritic pain

COMMON NURSING DIAGNOSES

 ### INEFFECTIVE AIRWAY CLEARANCE (see COPD)

Related to: bronchospasm, increased work of breathing, increased mucus production, infection, decreased energy

Defining Characteristics: dyspnea, tachypnea, bradypnea, bronchospasms, increased work of breathing, use of accessory muscles, increased mucus production, cough with or without productivity, thick secretions, airway obstruction, fatigue, adventitious breath sounds, abnormal arterial blood gases

 ### INEFFECTIVE BREATHING PATTERN (see TB)

Related to: decreased lung volume, decreased lung capacity, increased metabolic needs, pneumothorax

Defining Characteristics: cough with or without production, hemoptysis, increased respiratory rate, tachycardia, use of accessory muscles, nasal flaring, pursed-lip breathing, orthopnea, dyspnea, sternal retractions, diaphoresis, abnormal arterial blood gases, fever, pain, decreased oxygen saturation, adventitious breath sounds

 ### IMBALANCED NUTRITION: LESS THAN BODY REQUIREMENTS (see COPD)

Related to: inability to take in enough food, increased metabolism resulting from disease process, decreased level of consciousness, inability to absorb nutrients because of biologic or psychological factors

Defining Characteristics: actual inadequate food intake, altered taste, altered smell sensation, weight loss, body weight 20% or more under ideal for height and frame, anorexia, absent bowel sounds, decreased peristalsis, muscle mass loss, decreased muscle tone, changes in bowel habits, nausea, vomiting, abdominal distention, lack of interest in food, satiety immediately after ingesting food, abdominal pain or discomfort, sore, inflamed buccal cavity, depression, anxiety, social isolation, difficulty in feeding self, changes in mental status, fatigue from work of breathing

 ### IMPAIRED PHYSICAL MOBILITY (see PACEMAKERS)

Related to: pain, immobilization, intolerance of activity

Defining Characteristics: inability to move as desired, imposed restrictions on activity, decreased muscle strength, decreased muscle coordination, pain, limited range of motion, pain, decreased endurance

 ### ACUTE PAIN (see INFLUENZA)

Related to: pneumonia, coughing, rib fractures

Defining Characteristics: communication of pain, fever, cough with or without production, body aches, malaise, fractures

 ### HYPERTHERMIA (see INFLUENZA)

Related to: infection, exposure to infection, alterations in fluid and electrolyte balance

Defining Characteristics: fever, warm, flushed skin, tachycardia, tachypnea, dry mucous membranes, dehydration, oliguria, seizures, changes in mental status, increased BUN and creatinine, electrolyte imbalances

 ### DEFICIENT KNOWLEDGE (see TB)

Related to: lack of knowledge about pneumonia, difficulty understanding about disease process, lack of coping skills, cognitive impairment

Defining Characteristics: verbalization of questions, verbalization of incorrect information, noncompliant behavior, presence of preventable complications, inability to follow instructions, inappropriate behaviors, agitation, restlessness, apathy, depression, withdrawal

ADDITIONAL NURSING DIAGNOSES

IMPAIRED GAS EXCHANGE

Related to: inflammation, infection, ventilation/perfusion mismatching, fever, changes in oxyhemoglobin dissociation curve, bronchospasm

Defining Characteristics: dyspnea, tachycardia, cyanosis, hypoxia, hypoxemia, abnormal arterial blood gases, confusion, restlessness, inability to move secretions, dysrhythmias, decreased oxygen saturation by oximetry, fever, airway obstruction, tenacious secretions, cough, elevated WBC with shift to the left on differential

Outcome Criteria

✔ Patient will have arterial blood gases within normal range for patient, with no signs of ventilation/perfusion mismatching.

NOC: *Respiratory Status: Gas Exchange*

INTERVENTIONS	RATIONALES
Monitor pulse oximetry for oxygen saturation and notify physician if <90%.	Oximetry readings of 90 correlate with PaO$_2$ of 60 mm Hg. Levels below 60 mm Hg do not allow for adequate perfusion to tissues and vital organs. Oximetry uses light waves to identify differences between saturation and reduced hemoglobin of the tissues and may be inaccurate in low blood flow states.
Monitor transcutaneous oxygen tension if available.	Measures the oxygen concentration of the skin, but may cause burns if monitor site is not rotated frequently. Skin, blood flow, and temperature may affect these readings.
Administer oxygen as ordered.	Provides supplemental oxygen to benefit patient. Low-flow oxygen delivery systems use some room air and may be inadequate for patient's needs if their tidal volume is low, respiratory rate is high, or if ventilation status is unstable. High levels of oxygen may cause severe damage to tissues, oxygen toxicity, increases in A-a gradients, microatelectasis, and ARDS.
Observe patient for changes in mental status, restlessness, anxiety, confusion, dysrhythmias, hypotension, tachycardia, and/or cyanosis.	May indicate impending or present hypoxia and hypoxemia.

INTERVENTIONS	RATIONALES
Monitor ABGs for changes and/or trends, and notify physician for specific parameters set for patient.	Provides information on measured levels of oxygen and carbon dioxide as well as acid–base balance. Promotes prompt intervention for deteriorating airway status. PaO$_2$ alone does not reflect tissue oxygenation; ventilation must be adequate to provide gas exchange. In the elderly patient, what may be considered a "normal" value for ABGs may not reflect the normal range for the patient because of normal physiologic changes related to aging, such as respiratory muscle inelasticity and vascular changes.
Monitor patient for signs/symptoms of oxygen toxicity: nausea, vomiting, dyspnea, coughing, retrosternal pain, extremity paresthesias, pronounced fatigue, or restlessness.	Oxygen toxicity may result when oxygen concentrations are greater than 40% for lengthy durations of time, usually 8 to 24 hours, and may cause actual physiologic changes in the lungs. Progressive respiratory distress, cyanosis, and asphyxia are late signs of toxicity. Oxygen concentrations should be maintained as low as possible in order to maintain adequate PaO$_2$.
Instruct patient regarding need for measurements of oxygen saturation via ABGs.	Provides information to facilitate early detection of hypoxia, hypoxemia, or oxygen toxicity, and also provides patient with knowledge to facilitate compliance.
Instruct patient/family in signs/symptoms of oxygen toxicity (see above), and to notify nurse or physician if family notices changes in sensorium.	May be indicative of oxygen toxicity or hypoxia.

NIC: *Acid–Base Management*

Discharge or Maintenance Evaluation

■ Patient will have ABGs within normal limits for patient and his disease process.

■ Patient will be eupneic with adequate oxygenation and no signs/symptoms of oxygen toxicity.

■ Patient and family will be compliant with instructions given.

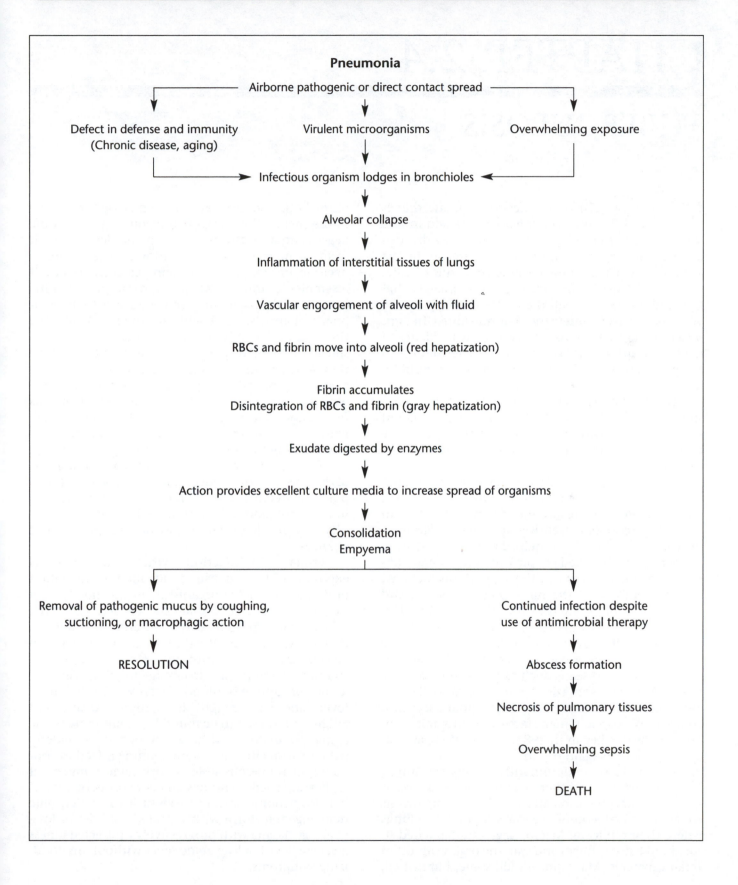

Pneumonia

Airborne pathogenic or direct contact spread

Defect in defense and immunity
(Chronic disease, aging)

Virulent microorganisms

Overwhelming exposure

Infectious organism lodges in bronchioles

Alveolar collapse

Inflammation of interstitial tissues of lungs

Vascular engorgement of alveoli with fluid

RBCs and fibrin move into alveoli (red hepatization)

Fibrin accumulates
Disintegration of RBCs and fibrin (gray hepatization)

Exudate digested by enzymes

Action provides excellent culture media to increase spread of organisms

Consolidation
Empyema

Removal of pathogenic mucus by coughing,
suctioning, or macrophagic action

RESOLUTION

Continued infection despite
use of antimicrobial therapy

Abscess formation

Necrosis of pulmonary tissues

Overwhelming sepsis

DEATH

CHAPTER 2.4

TUBERCULOSIS

Tuberculosis (TB) is an infectious disease that is caused by *Mycobacterium tuberculosis*, and in rare instances, by *Mycobacterium bovis*. TB, once a dreaded disease, had previously nearly disappeared in the last decades, but with a new resurgence of this disease, the World Health Organization now predicts that four million people will die of TB annually by the year 2004. This re-emergence has transpired, in part, by a lack of attention to the disease, the incidence of new strains of the disease that are drug-resistant, and the prevalence of HIV which increases susceptibility to TB.

TB, also known as the "white plague" and "consumption," has produced acute, chronic, and latent forms of the disease that involve every organ of the body, although most people assume it involves only the lungs.

Historically, TB patients have been refused admission to this country since 1906, and in 1912 laws were endorsed restricting anyone with TB from attending schools or renting apartments. Sanitariums were developed and helped to limit the disease by segregating infected people from the general public. Forms of treatment in the sanitariums included surgical removal of the lung, pneumothorax, and insertion of ping-pong balls into the chest. In 1944, streptomycin was discovered and was found to be effective in the treatment of TB. As the disease mutated, other drugs had to be added to the regimen to eradicate the disease, such as para-aminosalicylic acid (PAS) and isoniazid hydrochloride (INH). By 1980, sanatariums were closed, and pharmaceutical companies stopped manufacturing streptomycin. The resurgence began in 1985, and by 1990, an epidemic had once again begun.

Tuberculosis predominantly affects the lungs, but may extend to other organs. The organism is spread by droplet inhalation and these organisms collect in the alveoli of the lower lobes of the lungs where they replicate. Macrophages are launched to surround the organism and wall the organisms off in small tubercles. Macrophages kill some, but not all, of the bacilli, so more and more macrophages come to the site. As the macrophages join together, some degenerate and others clean up the debris, which forms a mass called a granuloma. The center is necrotic and referred to as being caseous because it resembles crumbly cheese. A focal pneumonitis occurs and the bacilli may achieve access to the lymphatic channels; the bacilli are then disseminated throughout the body via the bloodstream. They may spread to the hilar lymph nodes leading to calcification. A patient may remain asymptomatic except for a positive tuberculin skin test or positive chest X-ray. New TB cases are really reactivation of organisms from a dormant stage and are called reactivation TB, which occurs when the immune system is compromised and cell-mediated immunity is impaired.

The elderly are at high risk for contracting this disease because of the decrease in mucociliary transport, ineffective cough reflex, immune system impairment, and reduction in cell-mediated immunity as a result of aging and normal physiologic changes.

Primary TB infection, without any previous exposure to the organism, is acquired by inhalation of droplets of viable organisms. In the elderly, it is frequently difficult to diagnose TB because of the nonspecific symptoms exhibited and presentations that are remote from the disease site. Pulmonary TB creates respiratory symptoms of coughing, excess sputum, hemoptysis from necrotizing cavitary lesions or rupture of blood vessels within the lungs, fever, anorexia, weight loss, night sweats, and fatigue, but these can be found less commonly in the aging population. Miliary TB occurs in elderly patients with either an overwhelming infection consisting of numerous lesions with large numbers of replicating bacilli, and has an acute onset of a fever, hepatosplenomegaly, and weight loss, or a chronic hematogenous form with repeated episodes of low-grade bacillemia with progressively protracted illness associated with a low-grade fever without any localizing symptoms.

Other sites that are affected by TB are the brain, spine, joints, kidneys, bladder, prostate, lymph nodes, liver, gallbladder, intestine, pericardium, middle ear, and carpal tunnel. Some extrapulmonary types of TB used to be caused by ingesting milk that was contaminated by *Mycobacterium bovis* bacilli, but with the process of pasteurizing milk, what frequently occurs is the seed of a TB organism is planted in a distant organ and lies dormant for years until the health of the patient fails and allows the old site to reactivate.

Treatment is normally based on drug utilization, with first-line drugs being isoniazid, rifampicin, streptomycin, ethambutol and pyrazinamide. Second-line drugs, used when the first-line drugs fail, are ethionamide, para-aminosalicylic acid, kanamycin, amikacin, cycloserine, capreomycin, thiacetazone, and the bacille Calmette–Guerin (BCG) vaccine. Other drug therapies are continually being discovered, with the initial therapy aimed at rapidly reducing the large number of organisms, followed by a second phase of maintenance that lasts long enough to eradicate the dormant bacilli. Currently therapy is given for at least 6 months to ensure a cure. Surgical treatment of TB is much less common and is only utilized when drug therapy has failed, for removal of necrotic lung tissue, for persistent bronchopleural fistulas, for intractable hemorrhaging, and for repair of postsurgical complications.

MEDICAL CARE

Laboratory: CBC used to identify infection, anemia, or thrombocytosis; liver profiles used to identify increases seen in military TB; coagulation profiles used to identify DIC; electrolyte profiles used to identify imbalances, especially hyponatremia that may result from SIADH, and hypercalcemia; urinalysis used to identify pyuria without bacteriuria with renal TB; acid-fast cultures/stains used as the traditional way to identify tubercule bacilli; cultures of sputum or urine used to identify mycobacteriologic invasion; DNA probes in combination with radiometric cultures can be used to confirm identification of tuberculosis-specific RNA sequences, but is only in the early testing phase; immunoassay is another new test for mycobacterial antigens in CSF of patients with tuberculosis meningitis; CSF levels of tubercule bacilli are usually too sparse to be identified and may not be helpful; serum uric acid levels used to identify problems when pyrazinamide is used; hepatitis pro-

files done to evaluate for symptoms that are commonly an adverse effect of INH; BUN and creatinine levels may be monitored to evaluate for renal impairment

Radiography: chest X-rays used to identify pulmonary TB, pleural effusions, hilar and mediastinal adenopathy, infiltrates, consolidations, and calcifications; used to identify pericardial effusions; IVP used to show cavitary lesions of the renal parenchyma in renal TB

Electrocardiography: used to identify baseline cardiac rhythm, alterations in conduction associated with pericardial effusion or pericarditis, dysrhythmias occurring from electrolyte imbalances, or cardiac involvement

Echocardiography: used to identify presence of pericardial effusions, tamponade, and pretamponade states

Periocardiocentesis: may be required to drain fluid out of the pericardial sac with tuberculous pericarditis

Surgery: may be required to remove an abscess in the brain resulting from TB; laparotomy or laparoscopy may be required to diagnose genitourinary TB in women; synovial biopsy may be required in tuberculosis of the joints and articular capsule to ensure diagnosis; bone marrow and liver biopsies are required to assist with diagnosis in military tuberculosis; bronchoscopy may be done to identify pleural and mediastinal lesions and to assist with diagnosis; may be required for removal of damaged lung tissue, persistent bronchopleural fistula, repair of postsurgical complications, and for intractable hemorrhage; chest tube insertion may be required for pneumothorax

Skin testing: Mantoux skin testing with purified protein derivative (PPD) antigen is the standard testing procedure and replicates the delayed test hypersensitivity response to *Mycobacterium tuberculosis*

Drug therapy: currently the first-line antituberculous chemotherapy drugs are ethambutol hydrochloride (Myambutol), isoniazid (INH, Laniazid, Nydrazid, Tubizid), rifampin (Rifadin, Rifampicin, Rimactane), rifapentine (Priftin), and streptomycin; these bactericidals penetrate into the cells wall and interfere with nucleic acid biosynthesis; the second-line drugs used when first-line pharmaceuticals prove not effective are currently ethionamide (Trecator-SC), para-aminosalicylic acid (PAS), kanamycin (Kantrex,

Kanamycin), amikacin (Amikin), cycloserine (Seromycin), capreomycin (Capastat Sulfate), thiacetazone (not approved for use in the U.S.), and Bacille Calmette–Guerin (BCG) vaccine (usually not used in the U.S.); rifaburin (Mycobutin) is used to block protein synthesis of bacteria usually with patients who have advanced HIV infection, and should not be used in patients with active TB because single-drug use of this increases the potential for resistance of TB bacteria to rifabutin and rifampin

NURSING DIAGNOSES

 ## INEFFECTIVE BREATHING PATTERN

Related to: tuberculosis, decreased lung volume, decreased lung capacity, increased metabolic needs, pneumothorax

Defining Characteristics: cough with or without production, hemoptysis, increased respiratory rate, tachycardia, use of accessory muscles, nasal flaring, pursed-lip breathing, orthopnea, dyspnea, sternal retractions, diaphoresis, abnormal arterial blood gases, fever, adventitious breath sounds, lung cavitation, lung collapse

Outcome Criteria

✔ Patient will achieve and maintain normal respiratory pattern and rate, with no adventitious breath sounds to auscultation.

NOC: *Respiratory Status: Ventilation*

INTERVENTIONS	RATIONALES
Assess vital signs, especially respiratory status for baseline rate, rhythm, and character, and notify physician of significant changes.	Changes may reflect early signs of respiratory compromise and insufficiency.
Monitor pulse oximetry readings and notify physician if <90%.	Oximetry approximates arterial blood gas oxygen saturation, and helps to identify oxygenation dysfunction and respiratory status changes.
Auscultate breath sounds every 2–4 hours and prn. Notify physician of changes.	Assists with identification of changes in respiratory status, presence of adventitious breath sounds or decreased breath sounds. The elderly patient may

INTERVENTIONS	RATIONALES
	have infiltrates in the interstitium, bilateral lobes, and anterior and lower lung fields.
Administer oxygen as ordered.	Provides supplemental oxygen and helps alleviate respiratory distress caused by hypoxemia.
Assess patient for complaints of pain and medicate as needed.	Pain decreases respiratory effort and chest excursion, which decreases ventilation and perfusion. Analgesia relieves pain and promotes improved respiratory effort.
Encourage patient to maintain semi-Fowler's or high Fowler's position as tolerated.	Promotes chest expansion and enhances respiratory effort.
Encourage patient and assist with use of incentive spirometry, nebulizers, etc., as ordered.	Assists to prevent atelectasis and ensures proper use of equipment.
Perform chest physiotherapy, chest percussion and postural drainage, as ordered.	Helps to improve airway clearance and respiratory effort. Promotes clearing of secretions.
Encourage patient to change position every 2 hours and prn, and assist as needed.	Facilitates comfort and mobilizes pulmonary secretions.
Provide and encourage fluid intake of at least 2 L/day unless contraindicated.	Maintains hydration and helps to liquefy secretions to enable patient to expectorate sputum.
Maintain ordered isolation techniques.	Prevents cross contamination and exposure to pathogens.
Instruct patient/family regarding isolation requirements, and ensure that they adhere to proper techniques.	Provides knowledge, decreases fear, and helps to prevent further tuberculosis spread.
Instruct patient in use of pillow to splint chest with cough efforts.	Assists to reduce pain associated with cough.
Instruct patient in relaxation techniques, guided imagery, muscle relaxation, and breathing exercises.	Assists in pain reduction and alleviates anxiety which may improve respiratory effort and oxygenation.

NIC: *Respiratory Monitoring*

Discharge or Maintenance Evaluation

■ Patient will achieve and maintain a normal respiratory rate and rhythm with no adventitious breath sounds to auscultation.

■ Patient will be able to expectorate secretions.

- Patient will maintain and adhere to isolation precautions.
- Patient will be able to utilize relaxation techniques to improve pain and facilitate breathing.

RISK FOR INFECTION

Related to: risk factors that threaten physical well-being, such as crowded living conditions, unsanitary living conditions, presence of HIV infection, presence of chronic illnesses, history of exposure to TB, poor nutritional status, history of substance abuse, increased instance of tuberculosis, immigration from Africa, Asia, or South America, immunosuppression

Defining Characteristics: positive TB cultures, fever, cough, hemoptysis, lung consolidation, cavitation, abscesses, positive skin testing, sputum production, anorexia, weight loss, night sweats, fatigue, dementia, confusion, neurologic deficits, flank pain, dysuria, hematuria, abnormal urinary sediment, abnormal chest X-rays, pleural effusions, pericardial effusions, pleural or chest wall pain, dyspnea, decreased pulmonary function, pneumothorax, gastrointestinal obstruction, diarrhea with bleeding, abdominal tenderness, jaundice, hepatomegaly, bone and joint pain, loss of bowel and/or bladder control, multiple perforations of the tympanic membrane, hoarseness, dysphagia, inadequate ingestion of proper nutritional elements, use of recreational substances, HIV infection

Outcome Criteria

✔ Patient will be able to achieve and remain free of infection and complications from tuberculosis.

✔ Patient/family will be compliant with anti-infective regimen and will maintain safety precautions.

✔ Patient will not have infection spread to other people with whom patient has contact.

NOC: *Risk Control*

INTERVENTIONS	RATIONALES
Assess patient for exposure to tuberculosis or for physical signs/symptoms of exposure.	Concurrent diagnoses of HIV or other immunocompromised disease processes place patient at higher risk for TB. Knowledge of exposure and potential for disease allows for proper and

INTERVENTIONS	RATIONALES
	timely intervention to prevent spread of disease.
Administer PPD testing and read results in 48–72 hours.	Provides screening test, but frequently the skin test reaction decreases with time, and in the elderly patient, the test should be repeated later to detect the booster phenomenon. Most elderly patients with TB disease have a positive test result. The amount of induration links to the probability of TB. A chest X-ray should be done to confirm diagnosis.
Assess vital signs every 2–4 hours and notify physician of significant changes, such as increased work of breathing, tachypnea, increased blood pressure, increased heart rate initially, then may decrease to bradycardia.	May indicate impending respiratory insufficiency and failure with progression of disease.
Observe characteristics of sputum, and obtain cultures as ordered.	Purulent sputum may indicate a secondary infection is also present. Sputum will frequently be bloody because of irritation in the pleural areas.
Maintain appropriate isolation techniques. Standard Precautions should be utilized with all patients, but if TB is suspected, respiratory precautions may be added.	Prevents the spread of tuberculosis, which may be transmitted through aerosolized droplet method.
If patient is to be transported to another department, ensure that the patient has mask applied.	Prevents the potential spread of TB.
Ensure patient has easy access for disposal of tissues with secretions, and is able to perform good handwashing frequently.	Helps to avoid spreading pathogens.
Monitor lab work for electrolytes, hepatic profiles, renal profiles, and thyroid function tests.	INH and rifampicin can cause hepatotoxicity and hepatitis, streptomycin can cause nephrotoxicity and hypokalemia, pyrazinamide can cause hepatotoxicity and hyperuricemia, ethionamide can cause hypothyroidism, para-amino salicylic acid can cause hypernatremia and hepatotoxicity, and kanamycin, amikacin, and careomycin can cause renal toxicity.

(continues)

(continued)

INTERVENTIONS	RATIONALES
Assess patient for peripheral neuropathy, ototoxicity, optic neuritis, decreased visual acuity, color blindness, metallic taste, vestibular toxicity, and impaired coordination.	INH can cause peripheral neuropathy, ethambutol can cause optic neuritis, decreased visual acuity, and color blindness, ethionamide can cause metallic taste sensations, kanamycin, amikacin, and capreomycin can cause vestibular toxicity and auditory toxicity, and ethambutol, pyrazinamide, and cycloserine can cause skin rashes.
Administer vitamin B₆ as ordered.	Pyridoxine is usually given to help prevent any peripheral neuropathy that might ensue from the use of INH.
Instruct patient/family in all medications, effects, side effects, and signs and symptoms to report to physician.	Promotes knowledge, facilitates compliance, and allows for prompt identification of complications that may require changes in treatment plan and drug therapy.
Instruct patient/family in isolation techniques, need for precautions, especially in handling respiratory secretions, and ensure that they comply.	Isolation rooms, or rooms with high efficiency particulate air (HEPA) filters should be used. Acid-fast bacillus isolation prevents patients with pulmonary or laryngeal tuberculosis from transmitting disease to others by use of a special ventilation system and private room with the door closed. Caregivers and visitors entering the room should use a mask and wear a gown if handling soiled linens or clothing. Although gloves are not mandatory for this isolation type, it is recommended for use with Standard Precautions. Masks should be worn to prevent aerosolized transmission of disease.
Instruct patient to take medications precisely as instructed to do so.	Omitting doses and other mistakes in self-administering medications results in a prolonged length of treatment. Currently, a patient is usually on chemotherapy drugs for TB for at least 6–9 months before they are deemed to be cured.
Instruct patient/family about signs and symptoms that require medical attention, such as increasing cough, hemoptysis, weight loss, fevers, and night sweats.	Early identification allows for prompt treatment to control the spread of disease.

INTERVENTIONS	RATIONALES
Instruct patient to keep all appointments with physician as well as lab exams.	Promotes compliance with treatment regimen. Sputum is normally cultured on a monthly basis while receiving drug therapy, until cultures are negative; then cultures are done every 3 months for the duration of drug therapy.
Provide consultation with community resources, support groups, and so forth.	Assists patient to obtain assistance in receiving financial assistance for drugs, foods, and other medical supplies patient may need but cannot afford. Helps to increase patient's sense of independence.
Instruct patient that soft contact lenses may become discolored by drug therapy.	Rifampin turns body secretions red orange and may permanently discolor contact lenses. Knowledge of this helps patient to prepare for adverse effect.

NIC: *Infection Control*

Discharge or Maintenance Evaluation

- Patient will be compliant with drug regimen to eradicate infection.
- Patient will be able to avoid contaminating others with tuberculosis bacterium.
- Patient/family will be able to practice adequate safety measures/isolation techniques.
- Patient will achieve and maintain negative cultures and have no complications with any body system.
- Patient will be able to access community resources for assistance postdischarge.

DEFICIENT KNOWLEDGE

Related to: lack of knowledge about tuberculosis, stigma of disease, difficulty understanding about disease process, lack of coping skills, cognitive impairment

Defining Characteristics: verbalization of questions, verbalization of incorrect information, noncompliant behavior, presence of preventable complications, inability to follow instructions, inappropriate behaviors, agitation, restlessness, apathy, depression, withdrawal

Outcome Criteria

✔ Patient will be able to exhibit understanding of disease process, medication regimen, and treatment plan of care.

NOC: *Knowledge: Disease Process*

INTERVENTIONS	RATIONALES
Assess patient's understanding of disease process. Consider the older patient's life experiences.	Provides baseline of understanding from which to establish a plan of care. New information can be based upon the patient's existing knowledge base and life experience. The patient may have known others who had tuberculosis during the time of epidemics, when people were sent away to sanatoriums and had various treatments for the disease, and may believe this is the same treatment he or she must face.
Instruct patient/family about tuberculosis, detection, methods of transmission, signs and symptoms of relapse, treatments, and prevention of complications. Limit length of teaching sessions and provide quiet environment for each session.	Elderly patients may only be aware of old information and the stigma that was attached to tuberculosis, and may require re-education regarding current treatments. Reduction of extraneous stimuli assists with learning and the ability to process new information without distraction. Short sessions allow patient to learn at own speed and prevent information overload.
Instruct patient/family in tuberculosis disease process, including other sites of tuberculosis, such as kidneys, GI system, and so forth.	Patient and family may be only familiar with pulmonary TB and will not be alert to signs or symptoms of problems or relapses at different sites.
Instruct patient/family regarding medications and need for compliance with dosages, scheduling, and physician follow-up.	Provides knowledge and facilitates compliance with treatment regimen.

INTERVENTIONS	RATIONALES
Provide time for questions and concerns to be voiced, and answer questions honestly. If possible, give patient/family written materials to refer back to later.	Provides for correction of misinformation and written materials allow for documentation to assist with care once patient is discharged.
Instruct patient/family regarding the need to continue medication therapy for the entire length prescribed, and to be compliant with medical follow up.	Patients who are in the active phase of tuberculosis usually are given several medications for at least 2 months. Some patients may require therapy for up to 9 months, or until sensitivity tests indicate that bacillus has been eradicated. Frequent monitoring and lab tests should be performed during the course of therapy for the potential side effect of hepatitis as a result from INH, and to see if toxic levels in the liver occur that may require discontinuation of INH therapy. Sputum cultures are usually done monthly until negative results are noted, and q 3 months thereafter.

NIC: *Teaching: Disease Process*

Discharge or Maintenance Evaluation

■ Patient will be able to accurately verbalize understanding of tuberculosis and its treatment.

■ Patient will be able to comply with medication regimen and to notify physician if he or she experiences untoward side effects.

■ Patient/family will be able to identify and demonstrate safety precautions to prevent spread of the disease.

■ Patient will exhibit no signs or symptoms of adverse medication reactions.

■ Patient will have negative sputum cultures.

Tuberculosis

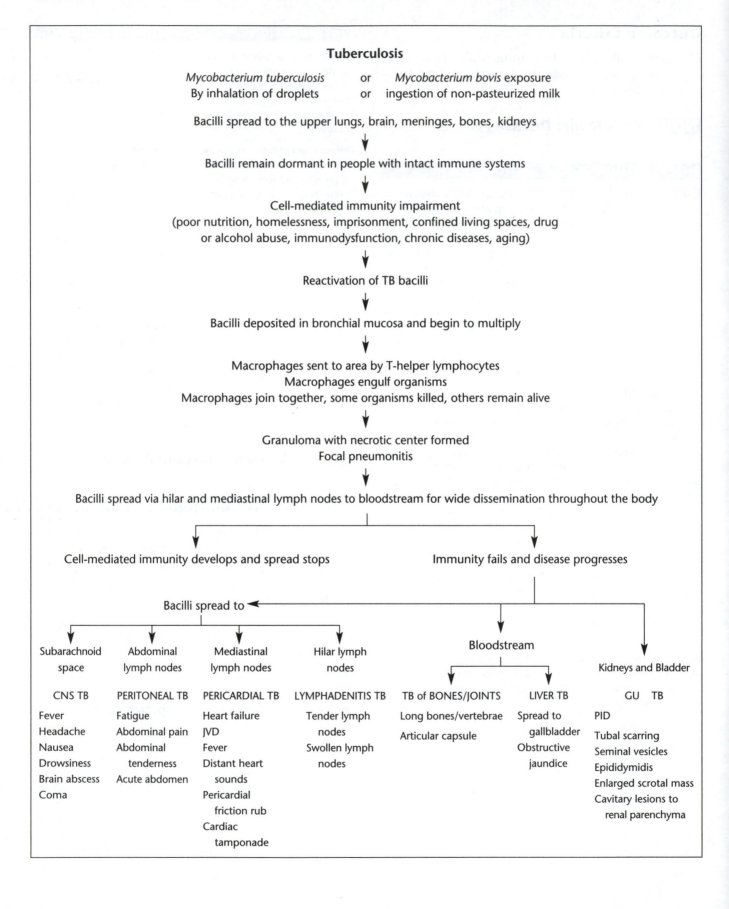

Mycobacterium tuberculosis   or   *Mycobacterium bovis* exposure
By inhalation of droplets   or   ingestion of non-pasteurized milk

Bacilli spread to the upper lungs, brain, meninges, bones, kidneys

Bacilli remain dormant in people with intact immune systems

Cell-mediated immunity impairment
(poor nutrition, homelessness, imprisonment, confined living spaces, drug
or alcohol abuse, immunodysfunction, chronic diseases, aging)

Reactivation of TB bacilli

Bacilli deposited in bronchial mucosa and begin to multiply

Macrophages sent to area by T-helper lymphocytes
Macrophages engulf organisms
Macrophages join together, some organisms killed, others remain alive

Granuloma with necrotic center formed
Focal pneumonitis

Bacilli spread via hilar and mediastinal lymph nodes to bloodstream for wide dissemination throughout the body

Cell-mediated immunity develops and spread stops   Immunity fails and disease progresses

Bacilli spread to

Subarachnoid space	Abdominal lymph nodes	Mediastinal lymph nodes	Hilar lymph nodes	Bloodstream		Kidneys and Bladder
CNS TB	PERITONEAL TB	PERICARDIAL TB	LYMPHADENITIS TB	TB of BONES/JOINTS	LIVER TB	GU TB
Fever	Fatigue	Heart failure	Tender lymph nodes	Long bones/vertebrae	Spread to gallbladder	PID
Headache	Abdominal pain	JVD	Swollen lymph nodes	Articular capsule	Obstructive jaundice	Tubal scarring
Nausea	Abdominal tenderness	Fever				Seminal vesicles
Drowsiness	Acute abdomen	Distant heart sounds				Epididymidis
Brain abscess		Pericardial friction rub				Enlarged scrotal mass
Coma		Cardiac tamponade				Cavitary lesions to renal parenchyma

UNIT 3
NEUROLOGIC SYSTEM

CHAPTER 3.1

ALZHEIMER'S DISEASE

Alzheimer's disease, or AD, is the most conventional form of dementia that affects the elderly population but it has been recognized as such for only the last decade or so when more information became known about the disease. Historically, Dr. Alois Alzheimer first recognized AD in the early 1900s after one of his patients who suffered dementia and hallucinations died and the autopsy revealed brain lesions and distortions that could not be classified into any existing diagnosis. Senility and dementia were often thought to be a disease of the aging, and patients were tended to at home. By the 1970s, scientists had established the disease as being of significance and that patients with AD had a noted neurochemical deficiency.

AD is the most common form of dementia and is a progressive and irreversible, fatal disease. Progression of the disease is done in phases, until all cognitive function is destroyed. Typically, the disease begins after the age of 65, although younger patients have been known to have the disorder. Pathologic consequences include the loss of neurons in multiple areas within the brain, atrophy with wide sulci and dilated ventricles of the brain, the presence of plaques composed of neurites, astrocytes, and glial cells that surround an amyloid center, and neurofibrillary tangles. Apolipoprotein E is a protein that is connected with Alzheimer's disease. Because the diagnosis of AD can only be actually made postmortem, the identification of AD is established based upon the clinical presentation, and only after all other types of dementia are ruled out. Pick's disease and frontal lobe dementias are very similar to Alzheimer's disease, but they generally are more quickly progressive, and have more neurologic and behavioral changes earlier in the disease.

Every type of dementia can be classified as being associated with one of two types of brain deterioration: cortical or subcortical. The cortex of the brain is responsible for the complex functions of the brain and these types of dementia are noted by memory disturbances. Alzheimer's disease is a result of cortical interruption and all lobes of the brain are involved to some extent.

Subcortical dementias, such as Parkinson's disease and Huntington's disease, affect the basal ganglia, thalamus, and the brain stem, which control motor coordination, vital functions, central nervous system arousal, timing, and sequential activity. Tremors and rigidity are early manifestations in this type of dementia, whereas in AD, these symptoms occur late in the course of the disease.

Symptoms seen in AD are the result of the destruction of numerous neurons in the hippocampus and the cerebral cortex. The enzyme, choline acetyl transferase, has a decreased action with AD patients, which results in impaired conduction of impulses between the nerve cells caused by lack of acetylcholine production.

Potential and theoretical causes of AD include genetic predisposition, declining glucose metabolism, hypercalcemia, extended exposure to glucocorticoids, aluminum and zinc exposure, food-borne poisons, and viruses.

There are four stages of AD, and clinical symptoms may be present for an extended time prior to identification by the family. The first stage, or early stage, involves memory loss that may be variable initially. Family and others may credit the symptoms to "old age." As memory loss progresses, it is apparent that the changes are not normal, and the patient is extremely depressed because he or she realizes something is wrong, but is unable to do anything about it. This stage can persist for up to two years.

Stage 2, or the middle stage, involves intensifying memory loss that interferes with daily living and the ability to cope in unfamiliar surroundings. This stage may last from two to five years, and during this period, the patient becomes unable to identify time and place, gets lost in familiar areas, is unable to express his or her thoughts in a comprehensible manner, and either is unable to make decisions or spends a lengthy time to make a simple choice. Inhibitions are lost, errors in judgment, inability to concentrate, and hoarding become commonplace. Wandering and pacing begin during this stage.

Stage 3, or the late stage, entails all the symptoms of stage 2, but with much more progressive failure. It is during this time that the patient fails to recognize family and friends, hyperorality and perseveration occur. Agnosia and apraxia are present. This stage may last from two to five years.

Stage 4, or the terminal phase, continues the progressive deterioration. If the patient has diligent caregivers, the patient can remain physically healthy and only rarely will have complications that are known to be associated with chronic illness. The patient is no longer able to make any decisions and is totally dependent on others, and ultimately, the disease will result in death.

MEDICAL CARE

Laboratory: CBC used to identify anemia, infection, or other causes for confusion; electrolyte profiles used to identify imbalances; serum glucose used to identify hypoglycemia which may occur; chemistry profiles to identify dysfunction, especially hypercalcemia; aluminum and zinc levels to identify increases; liver function studies to evaluate for dysfunction; renal profiles to identify renal insufficiency; thyroid function studies to identify hypothyroidism or hyperthyroidism; ELISA test used to reveal presence of HIV; blood test for ApoE may provide data regarding genetic predisposition for AD, but is not recognized as a predictor for AD

Radiography: chest X-rays used to identify concurrent lung-related problems, evaluate cardiac silhouette, and identify hypertrophy of the heart; CT scans may be used to identify brain atrophy and enlargement of the ventricles in the latter stages of the disease; positron emission tomography (PET) may be used to identify active areas within the brain by tracking the flow of oxygen and glucose in the blood; magnetic resonance spectroscopy imaging (MRSI) may be used to identify metabolites within the brain, but as of the present time, it is unknown how metabolites that change with aging relate to AD and cognitive impairment

Mental status testing: used to assess orientation, function, judgment, memory, ability for abstract thinking, math, and reading, and thus can identify the level of cognitive impairment

Antipsychotics: chlorpromazine hydrochloride (Thorazine), clozapine (Clozaril), fluphenazine (Modecate, Prolixin, Permitil), haloperidol (Haldol, Haloperidol Intensol), loxaine (Loxitane), mesoridazine besylate (Serentil), olanzapine (Zyprexa), perphenazine (Trilafon), pimozide (Orap), quetiapine fumarate (Seroquel), risperidone (Risperdal), thioridazine hydrochloride (Mellaril), or thiothixene (Navane) may be required for severe levels of AD to improve the patient's emotional and mental well-being; act by blocking postsynaptic dopamine or serotonin receptors in the brain, but may have side effects such as sedation, extrapyramidal symptoms, tardive dyskinesia, orthostatic hypotension, and anticholinergic effects

Antidepressants: amitriptyline hydrochloride or pamoate (Elavil, Endep), amoxapine (Asendin), bupropion hydrochloride (Wellbutrin), citalopram hydrobromide (Celexa), clomipramine hydrochloride (Anafranil), desipramine hydrochloride (Norpramin), doxepin hydrochloride (Sinequan), fluoxetine hydrochloride (Prozac), imipramine hydrochloride (Norfranil, Tipramine), mirtazaprine (Remeron), nefazodone hydrochloride (Serzone), nortriptyline hydrochloride (Aventyl, Pamelor), paroxetine hydrochloride (Paxil), phenelzine sulfate (Nardil), sertraline hydrochloride (Zoloft), tranylcypromine sulfate (Parnate), trazodone hydrochloride (Desyrel, Trazon, Trialodine), trimipramine maleate (Surmontil), or venlafaxine hydrochloride (Effexor) may be used to lessen symptoms of depression by several actions; tricyclics block the reuptake of norepinephrine and serotonin in the nerve endings and increase the action of these chemicals within the nerve cells; MAOIs increase the concentration of endogenous epinephrine, norepinephrine, serotonin and dopamine

Antianxiety drugs: alprazolam (Xanax), buspirone hydrochloride (BuSpar), chlordiazepoxide hydrochloride (Libritabs, Librium), clorazepate dipotassium (Tranxene, Gen-XENE), diazepam (Valium, Diazepam), hydroxyzine embonate or hydrochloride (Atarax, Anx, Vistaril, Hydroxacen), lorazepam (Ativan, Lorazepam, Intensol), meprobamate (Equanil, Miltown, Probate, Trancot), midazolam hydrochloride (Versed), or oxazepam (Serax) may be used to inhibit the action of serotonin or to depress subcortical levels of the central nervous system to help relieve anxiety

Cholinergic replacement therapy: donepezil (Aricept), rivastigmine tartrate (Exelon), and tacrine (Cognex)

inhibit acetylcholinesterase which increases the available acetylcholine to temporarily improve Alzheimer's patients' function and memory; these drugs utilized in an attempt to hypothetically halt the disease process; some have proven partially successful in slowing down memory loss and impaired thinking ability temporarily if given during the early stages, but can result in liver dysfunction

Nonsteroidal anti-inflammatory drugs (NSAIDs): celecoxib (Celebrex), diclofenac potassium or sodium (Cataflam, Voltaren), etodolac (Lodine), fenoprofen calcium (Nalfon), flurbiprofen (Ansaid, Ocufen), ibuprofen (Advil, Motrin, Genpril, Nuprin, Trendar), indomethacin (Indocin, Indocid PDA), ketoprofen (Actron, Orudis, Oruvail), ketorolac tromethamine (Toradol), meloxicam (Mobic), nabumetone (Relafen), naproxen (Naprosyn, Aleve, Naprelan, Anaprox), oxaprozin (Daypro), piroxicam (Feldene), rofecoxib (Vioxx), or sulindac (Clinoril) used experimentally to slow the progression of Alzheimer's symptoms

Estrogen: use is being clinically studied as a treatment for early stage AD; initial data show that increased estrogen dosages and longer duration of use decreased the risk of AD; it has been proposed that estrogen interacts with the nerve growth factor to protect the neurons from degeneration

Antioxidants: use is being clinically studied as a treatment for AD; initial theories propose that oxygen free radicals can be neutralized by antioxidants, which might slow the progression of AD by reduced damage to the brain neurons with use of antioxidants

COMMON NURSING DIAGNOSES

IMBALANCED NUTRITION: LESS THAN BODY REQUIREMENTS (see COPD)

Related to: Alzheimer's disease progression, inability to take in enough food, increased metabolism resulting from disease process, decreased level of consciousness, inability to absorb nutrients because of biologic or psychological factors, dysphagia

Defining Characteristics: actual inadequate food intake, altered taste, altered smell sensation, weight loss, body weight 20% or more under ideal for height and frame, anorexia, absent bowel sounds, decreased peristalsis, muscle mass loss, decreased muscle tone, changes in bowel habits, nausea, vomiting, abdomi-

nal distention, lack of interest in food, satiety immediately after ingesting food, abdominal pain or discomfort, sore, inflamed buccal cavity, depression, anxiety, social isolation, difficulty in feeding self, inability to feed self, changes in mental status, fatigue from work of breathing, decreased cough and gag reflexes, confusion, food left in mouth, hyperorality

ADDITIONAL NURSING DIAGNOSES

DISTURBED THOUGHT PROCESSES

Related to: Alzheimer's disease, changes in cognitive abilities, impaired memory, disorientation, chemical imbalances in the brain, neuronal destruction in the brain, dementia

Defining Characteristics: disorientation to time, place, person, and circumstance, decreased ability to reason or conceptualize, inability to reason, impaired ability to calculate, memory loss, decreased attention span, easy distractibility, inability to follow commands, deterioration in personal care and appearance, dysarthria, dysphagia, convulsions, inappropriate social behavior, paranoia, combativeness, inability to cooperate, wandering, disturbance in judgment and abstract thoughts, explosive behavior, illusions, delusions, hallucinations, deterioration in intellect, loss of sexual drive and desire, reduced control of sexual behavior, inappropriate behavior, lack of inhibitions, egocentricity, hypervigilance, hypovigilance, alteration in sleep pattern, lethargy

Outcome Criteria

✔ Patient will have maintenance of mental and psychological function as long as possible, and reversal of behaviors when possible.

✔ Family members will be able to exhibit understanding of required care and will demonstrate appropriate coping skills and ability to utilize community resources.

NOC: *Distorted Thought Control*

INTERVENTIONS	RATIONALES
Assess patient's ability for thought processing every shift. Observe for cognitive functioning, memory changes,	Changes in status may indicate progression of deterioration or improvement in condition.

INTERVENTIONS	RATIONALES
disorientation, difficulty with communication, or changes in thinking patterns.	
Assess level of confusion and disorientation.	Confusion may range from slight disorientation to agitation and may develop over a short period of time or slowly over several months. May indicate effectiveness of treatment or decline in condition.
Assess patient's ability to cope with events, interest in surroundings and activity, motivation, and changes in memory pattern.	The elderly patient may have a decrease in memory for more recent events and more active memory for past events and reminisce about the pleasant ones. Patient may exhibit assertiveness or aggressiveness to compensate for feelings of insecurity, or develop more narrowed interests and have difficulty accepting changes in lifestyle.
Orient patient to environment as needed, if patient's short term memory is intact. Use calendars, radio, television, newspapers, and so forth.	Reality orientation techniques help improve patient's awareness of self and environment only for patients with confusion related to delirium or with depression. Depending on the stage of AD, it may be reassuring for patients in the very early states who are aware that they are losing their sense of reality, but it does not work when dementia becomes irreversible because the patient can no longer understand reality. Television and radio programs may be overstimulating and increase agitation, and can be disorienting to patients who cannot make a distinction between reality and fantasy or what they may view on television.
Assess patient for sensory deprivation, concurrent use of CNS drugs, poor nutrition, dehydration, infection, or other concomitant disease processes.	May cause confusion and mental status changes.
Maintain a regular daily scheduled routine to prevent problems that may result from thirst, hunger, lack of sleep, irregular elimination, or inadequate exercise.	If needs of AD patients are not met, it may cause the patient to become agitated and anxious. Predictable behavior is less threatening to the patient and does not tax limited ability of function with ADLs.

INTERVENTIONS	RATIONALES
Allow patient the freedom to sit in chair near the window, utilize books or magazines as desired, and so forth.	Validates patient's sense of reality and assists the patient in differentiating between day and night. Respect for the patient's personal space allows patient to exert some control.
Label drawers, use written reminder notes, pictures, or color-coding for articles to assist patient.	Assists patient's memory by use of reminders of what to do and location of articles.
Allow hoarding and wandering in a controlled environment within acceptable limitations.	Increases patient's security and decreases hostility and agitation by permitting behaviors that are difficult to prevent, to be allowed within the confines of a safe, supervised environment.
Provide positive reinforcement and feedback for positive behaviors.	Promotes patient confidence and reinforces progress.
Provide opportunity for social involvement with others, but do not force interaction.	Helps to prevent isolation. Forcing interaction will usually result in confusion, agitation, and hostility.
Limit decisions that patient makes. Be supportive and convey warmth and concern when communicating with patient.	Patient may be unable to make even the simplest choice decisions and this will result in frustration and distraction. By avoiding this, the patient has an increased feeling of security. Patients frequently have feelings of loneliness, isolation, and depression, and they respond positively to a smile, friendly voice, and gentle touch.
Inform patient of care to be done, with one instruction at a time.	Patients with AD require extended time for processing information. Removal of decision making may facilitate improved compliance and feelings of security.
Instruct family in methods to use with communication with patient: to listen carefully, to listen to stories even if they've heard them many times previously, and to avoid asking questions that the patient may not be able to answer.	Comments from the patient may involve reliving experiences from previous years and may be totally appropriate within that context. In the early stages of AD, questions may cause embarrassment and frustration when the patient is presented with another reminder that abilities are decreasing.
Instruct family members in the disease process, what can be expected, and assist with providing a list of community resources for support.	Once a diagnosis is made, the family should be prepared to make long-term plans in order to discuss problems before they arise. Choices for resuscitation,

(continues)

(continued)

INTERVENTIONS	RATIONALES
	legal competency and guardianship, and financial responsibility need to be addressed. The care of a person with AD is expensive, time-consuming, as well as energy-draining and emotionally devastating for the family. Community resources can help delay the need for placement in a long-term care facility and may help defray some of the costs.

NIC: *Dementia Management*

Discharge or Maintenance Evaluation

■ Patient will achieve functional ability at his optimum level with modifications and alterations within his environment to compensate for deficits.

■ Patient will have improved thought processing or will be maintained at a baseline level.

■ Patient will be aware and oriented if possible, and reality will be maintained at an optimal level.

■ Patient will have behavioral problems identified and controlled.

■ Patient's family will be able to access community resources and make informed choices regarding patient's care, both currently and for future care.

CHRONIC CONFUSION

Related to: Alzheimer's disease, dementia

Defining Characteristics: decreased ability to interpret one's environment, decreased capacity for thought, memory impairment, disorientation, behavioral changes, personality changes, altered interpretation and response to stimuli

Outcome Criteria

✔ Patient will have minimal confusion, cognitive impairment, and other dementia manifestations.

NOC: *Cognitive Orientation*

INTERVENTIONS	RATIONALES
Assess patient for reversible or irreversible dementia, causes, ability to interpret the environ-	Determines type and extent of dementia to establish a plan of care to enhance cognition and
ment, intellectual thought processes, disturbances with orientation, memory loss, behavior, and socialization.	emotional functioning at optimal levels.
Utilize cognitive function testing.	Identifies current level of dementia.
Maintain consistent scheduling, with allowances for patient's specific needs, and avoid frustrating situations and overstimulation.	Prevents patient agitation, erratic behaviors, and combative reactions. Scheduling may need revision to show respect for the patient's sense of worth and to facilitate completion of tasks.
Avoid or terminate emotionally charged situations or conversations. Avoid anger and expectation of patient to remember or follow instructions. Do not expect more than the patient is capable of doing.	Catastrophic emotional responses are prompted by task failure when the patient feels expected to perform beyond ability and becomes frustrated and angry. Responding calmly to the patient validates feelings and causes less stress.
Provide time for reminiscing if patient so desires.	Allows for memory of past pleasant events. Patient may be reliving events in the past and the caregiver should identify this behavior and respect it.
Limit sensory stimuli and independent decision-making.	Decreases frustration and distractions from environment. Decreasing stress of making a choice helps to promote security.
Assist with establishing cues and reminders for patient's assistance.	Assists patients with early AD to remember location of articles, and facilitates some orientation.
Identify family members and/or support systems for patient.	Helps to determine appropriate person to notify for changes, to assist with care, and someone familiar to patient to help deal with his confusion.
Ask family members about their ability to provide care for patient.	Identifies family's need for assistance.
Instruct family and provide them with information regarding community services and long-term health care facilities.	Patient may require ongoing skilled nursing care that the patient's family is unable or unwilling to provide.
Instruct family regarding avoidance of arguing with patient about what he thinks, sees, or hears.	Patient may have delusions and hallucinations, that are real to patient, and no amount of persuasion will convince him or her otherwise. The patient may become agitated or violent if contradicted.

INTERVENTIONS	RATIONALES
Instruct family to consider if what patient believes has some basis in reality.	Sometimes portions of conversations can be heard and misinterpreted by the patient, or environment may have noises or lighting that may cause misinterpretation.
Instruct family to consider if what patient believes has some basis in reality from previous years ago.	Patient may be reliving times in the past and the reality may be decades ago.
Instruct family to avoid having patient watch violent television shows.	Patients cannot make a distinction of reality from fiction, and witnessing violent acts on the screen may be frightening to the patient.
Instruct family to utilize distraction techniques, such as music, going for a walk, or looking at picture albums if patient has delusions.	Distraction may be effective to calm patient if stressful situations occur.

NIC: *Behavior Management: Overactivity/Inattention*

Discharge or Maintenance Evaluation

- Patient will have stable, safe environment with routine scheduling of activities to decrease anxiety and confusion.
- Patient will exhibit minimal or reduced confusion, memory loss, and cognitive disturbances, depending upon stage of AD.
- Patient will be able to tolerate stimuli when introduced slowly in a nonthreatening manner, with one item at a time.
- Patient will be able to be distracted or use other techniques to avoid stressful situations that may cause aggressive, hostile behaviors or frustration.
- Family will be able to utilize information effectively in dealing with patient with confusion with regard to limitations of stimulation and validation of patient's thoughts.
- Family will be able to utilize information to begin making decisions for long-term plans for patient.

IMPAIRED VERBAL COMMUNICATION

Related to: Alzheimer's disease dementia, psychological barriers, psychosis, decreased circulation to brain, age-related factors, lack of stimuli

Defining Characteristics: confusion, anxiety, restlessness, disorientation to person, place, time, and circumstance, repetitive speech, agitation, flight of ideas, inability to speak, stuttering, slurring, impaired articulation, difficulty with phonation, inability to name words, inability to identify objects, difficulty comprehending communication, difficulty forming words or sentences, aphonia, dyslalia, dysarthria, inappropriate verbalizations, aphasia, dysphasia, apraxia, dyslexia

Outcome Criteria

✔ Patient will be able to have effective speech and understanding of communication, or will be able to use another method to communicate and make needs known.

NOC: *Communication Ability*

INTERVENTIONS	RATIONALES
Assess patient's ability to speak, language deficit, cognitive or sensory impairment, presence of aphasia, dysarthria, aphonia, dyslalia, or apraxia, presence of psychosis, and/or other neurologic disorders affecting speech.	Identifies problem areas and speech patterns to help establish a plan of care.
Assess effects of communication deficit.	Communication becomes progressively impaired as AD advances. The left side cerebral functions consisting of language, reasoning, and calculation are decreased. Receptive and expressive aphasia are major symptoms of Alzheimer's disease and affect speaking, reading, writing, and math. The mechanics of speech production is usually intact until the last stages of AD but the patient has difficulty concentrating on what has been said, understanding and processing what was said, and then preparing a response. In the first stage of AD, vocabulary skill decreases and the patient has trouble finding the correct word to use, resulting in word substitution. The patient can usually understand most messages but forgets them because of memory deficits. As the disease evolves,

(continues)

(continued)

INTERVENTIONS	RATIONALES
	the ability to comprehend written and spoken language is decreased. False details about past events may be invented to try to camouflage the inability to remember. Ultimately the patient will become mute.
Monitor patient for nonverbal communication, such as facial grimacing, smiling, pointing, crying, and so forth, and encourage the use of speech when possible.	Indicates that feelings or needs are being expressed when speech is impaired. Excessive mumbling, striking out, or nonverbalization clues may be the only method left for the patient to express discomfort.
Attempt to anticipate patient's needs.	Helps to prevent frustration and anxiety.
When communicating with patient, face patient and maintain eye contact, speaking slowly and enunciating clearly in a moderate or low-pitched tone.	Clarity, brevity, and time provided for responses promotes the opportunity for successful speech by allowing patient time to receive and process the information.
Remove competing stimuli, and provide a calm, unhurried atmosphere for communication.	Reduces unnecessary noise and distractions and allows patient time to decrease frustration.
Use simple, direct questions requiring one-word answers. Repeat and reword questions if misunderstanding occurs.	Promotes self-confidence of the patient who is able to achieve some degree of speech or communication.
Utilize pencil and paper or magic slate to write messages.	Provides an alternative method of communication if fine motor function is not impaired.
Assess patient for hearing deficits, and use appropriate adaptive devices if needed. Minimize glare in room, speak normally, but distinctly, and use short phrases with speech attempts.	If patient is deaf or requires hearing aids, make sure battery is working and that aid is correctly placed to enhance hearing ability. Shouting usually increases the pitch of the voice and does not help with hearing. Glare makes it more difficult for patient to read your lips.
Encourage patient to breathe prior to speaking, pause between words, and use tongue, lips, and jaw to speak.	Promotes coordinated speech and breathing.
Encourage patient to control the length and rate of phrases, over-articulate words, and separate syllables, emphasizing consonants.	Helps to promote speech in the presence of dysarthria.

INTERVENTIONS	RATIONALES
Avoid rushing patient when struggling to express feelings and thoughts. If you cannot understand, let the patient know you accept his or her efforts to speak and you empathize with patient's frustration.	Impaired verbal communication results in patient's feelings of isolation, despair, depression, and frustration. Compassion helps to foster a therapeutic relationship and sense of trust and is important for continuing communication.
Encourage patient to take part in social activities.	Helps to reduce feelings of isolation, which then result in further depression and unwillingness to communicate, even if patient is physically able to do so.
Instruct patient/family regarding need to use glasses, hearing aids, dentures, and so forth.	Helps to promote communication with sensory or other deficits.
Provide consultation with speech therapist as warranted.	Helps to facilitate speech ability and provides potential alternatives for communication needs.
Instruct patient/family in the performance of facial muscle exercises, such as smiling, frowning, sticking tongue out, moving tongue from side to side and up and down.	Promotes facial expressions used to communicate by increasing muscle coordination and tone.

NIC: *Communication Enhancement: Speech Deficit*

Discharge or Maintenance Evaluation

- Patient will be able to use assistive devices and techniques to improve ability to communicate.
- Patient will be able to speak in an understandable way when possible.
- Patient will be able to understand communication.
- Patient will exhibit minimal frustration and anxiety with speech attempts.
- Patient will be able to make needs known utilizing nonverbal methods if required.
- Family will be compliant and supportive of patient's attempts at communication.

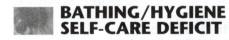

BATHING/HYGIENE SELF-CARE DEFICIT

Related to: Alzheimer's disease, dementia, memory loss, cognitive impairment, neuromuscular impairment

Defining Characteristics: inability to wash body or body parts, inability to obtain bath supplies, inability to obtain water source, inability to get into and out of bathroom, inability to dry body, inability to take off necessary clothing, inability to maintain appearance at satisfactory level, inability to brush teeth, inability to comb/brush hair, inability to shave

Outcome Criteria

✔ Patient will have self-care needs met and have few, if any, complications.

✔ Patient's family will be able to carry out self-care program on a daily basis.

NOC: *Self-Care: Bathing, Hygiene*

INTERVENTIONS	RATIONALES
Assess patient's appearance, body odors, ability to recognize and use articles for washing and grooming, and any other self-care deficits.	Identifies specific needs and the amount of assistance that the patient will require in order to establish a plan of care.
Assess and identify patient's previous history of grooming and bathing, and attempt to maintain similar care.	Promotes familiarity with routine bathing time and type of bath/shower, and lessens further confusion and agitation.
Ensure all needed items are present in bathroom prior to the patient's arrival. Ensure that water temperature in tub is appropriate.	Prevents the need to leave the patient unattended, which may result in injury. Elderly patients are easily chilled, and have fragile skin that is susceptible to scalding.
Allow patient to perform as much of the task as able.	Fosters independence and promotes self-care as long as possible. Once the skill is lost, it is lost forever with AD.
Assist with as much of activity as needed. Give patient a wash-cloth or hand towel to hold on to.	Promotes independence and self-esteem when patient is allowed to control situation. Patients with AD frequently will grasp the nurse's hands during a bath, and use of a washcloth helps them to have something to hold on to.
Inspect the patient's skin during the bath.	Provides the opportunity to observe for the presence of rashes, pressure areas, lesions, bruises, growths, or unclean skin areas, which may require more

INTERVENTIONS	RATIONALES
	assistance with hygiene to prevent further skin deterioration.
Instruct patient in activity with short step-by-step method without rushing.	Promotes self-esteem and feelings of accomplishment.
Instruct family members in bathing techniques and what to observe for during bath.	Provides knowledge and decreases anxiety.
Instruct family to reassure patient with simple statements such as, "You're in the tub," "I'm right here," and so forth.	Reduces panic that may be caused by fear of drowning.

NIC: *Self-Care Assistance: Bathing/Hygiene*

Discharge or Maintenance Evaluation

■ Patient will be able to maintain an acceptable appearance.

■ Patient will be able to perform a portion of self-care within the limitations of the disease.

■ Patient will accept assistance with self-care when needed.

■ Patient and family will be able to use assistive devices to perform self-care.

■ Family will be able to competently provide bathing and hygiene care for patient.

DRESSING/GROOMING SELF-CARE DEFICIT

Related to: Alzheimer's disease, dementia, musculoskeletal impairment, cognitive impairment

Defining Characteristics: inability to put on or take off clothing, inability to choose clothing, inability to maintain appropriate appearance, inability to fasten clothing, inability to obtain clothing, inability to pick up clothing, inability to brush/comb hair, inability to shave, inability to brush teeth

Outcome Criteria

✔ Patient will be appropriately groomed and dressed independently or with assistance.

NOC: *Self-Care: Dressing, Grooming*

INTERVENTIONS	RATIONALES
Assess patient's functional and cognitive ability to provide self-care.	Identifies functional level and helps to establish plan of care to meet patient's needs.
Provide assistive devices as needed.	Facilitates independence in some tasks.
Allow patient to perform as much care as able, giving simple instructions, step-by-step.	Fosters self-confidence and self-esteem.
Assist patient with dressing and grooming as needed.	Patients with AD have difficulty with dressing because of the need to have fine and gross motor skills, balance, sequencing ability, and the ability to tell right from left, and top from bottom. Dressing is less difficult if patient's clothes are large enough and made of material that is soft, slick, and stretchy. As the patient becomes more dependent, the clothing choices will require adaptation for patient needs. Elastic waistbands and Velcro closures are easier for the patient and caregiver to handle.
Provide oral care after meals and at bedtime. Use adaptive devices as required.	Patient requires oral care to remove any leftover food particles, to prevent decay, and promote dental hygiene. Patients may be unable to understand directions for spitting out toothpaste or rinsing with water, and may be unable to open mouth for flossing. Adaptive devices may be used to facilitate proper dental hygiene.
Instruct family regarding removal of clothing that is out of season or no longer fits, to lay out clothes in the order they are to be put on, and to use larger sized clothing with fasteners that are easier to handle.	Assists patient in self-care while still able to do part of care, and will assist the caregivers when they assume this duty.
Instruct family in the use of electric razors for men and cream depilatory products for women.	May facilitate ease in grooming process.
Instruct family that patient will require oral care at least twice daily, and in the use of artificial saliva.	Daily oral care will help lower the risk of needing extensive dental care later. Oral care may be difficult especially in the latter stages of AD because the patient

INTERVENTIONS	RATIONALES
	may not be able to spit the toothpaste out or rinse the mouth. Artificial saliva may be required if patient suffers from dry mouth caused by medications or lack of fluid intake.
Instruct family regarding the possibility of cutting the patient's hair and keeping it in a short, simple style.	Helps to keep patient's appearance neat and tidy. Long hair requires more intensive care and pain caused by combing/brushing hair, shampooing, or curling hair; may cause aggressive behavior and frustration in the AD patient.

NIC: *Self-Care Assistance: Dressing/Grooming*

Discharge or Maintenance Evaluation

- Patient will have self-care needs met.
- Patient will have a satisfactory appearance.
- Patient will not exhibit any signs of symptoms of infection or lack of skin integrity.
- Family will be able to provide adequate self-care for patient on a daily basis.
- Patient will exhibit no signs of complications, such as dental abscesses.

TOILETING SELF-CARE DEFICIT

Related to: Alzheimer's disease, dementia, cognitive impairment, neurologic impairment, physiologic impairment, psychological dysfunction, environmental impairment

Defining Characteristics: inability to carry out toileting routine, inability to flush toilet, inability to get to bathroom, inability to manipulate clothing for toileting, inability to sit on or rise from toilet or commode, incontinence of stool or urine

Outcome Criteria

✔ Patient will have self-care needs met without any complications.
✔ Patient's family will be able to carry out toileting routine program.

NOC: *Self-Care: Toileting*

INTERVENTIONS	RATIONALES
Assess patient for functional, perceptual, or cognitive ability for self-care.	Identifies problems to help establish a plan of care.
Allow patient to perform toileting routine, as able, and provide sufficient time so as to avoid rushing patient.	Facilitates patient's independence as much as condition will allow. Rushing promotes excessive stress and leads to failure.
Assist patient with toileting as needed.	Allows patient to perform independently for as long as possible.
Establish urinary and bowel care program if patient is unable to complete self-care.	Monitoring success or failure of the plan of care helps to identify and resolve areas of failure.
Monitor patient for sudden changes in urinary status.	Incontinence usually does not occur until the latter stages of AD, so sudden urinary incontinence may indicate the presence of infection, prostatic hyperplasia, urethral sphincter failure, bladder irritation, or certain medication effects.
Observe patient and monitor for wandering, rubbing the genital area, or irritability.	May indicate signs of a full bladder.
Encourage fluid intake of at least 2–3 L/day unless contraindicated, and ensure that patient actually drinks the fluid.	Provides hydration and enhances renal function. The patient may not drink fluids just because they are available.
Establish a scheduled toileting and habit training program for the patient. Take the patient to the bathroom every 2 hours, run the water, place the patient's hands in warm water, or pour warm water over the genitalia. Administer stool softeners/laxatives/suppositories and take patient to bathroom at same time each day to promote stool evacuation.	Helps to establish toileting routines.
Instruct family regarding toileting program, times to take patient to bathroom, and need to maintain consistent schedule.	Promotes knowledge, and facilitates continuity of care to promote toileting routines.
Instruct family in procedure for administration of suppositories or enemas, and the potential for manual removal of stool.	Provides knowledge and helps to instill confidence in family members who provide care. This may also induce family members to realistically decide if they can personally care for patient or will need a long-term care facility for the patient.

INTERVENTIONS	RATIONALES
Provide information to family regarding community resources, support groups, long-term facilities, respite care, and so forth.	Assists to reinforce activities and planned care once patient is discharged, and to plan for care needs in the future.

NIC: *Self-Care Toileting*

Discharge or Maintenance Evaluation

- Patient will have self-care needs met without complications.
- Family will be able to provide self-care for patient.
- Family will be able to access community resources for support as needed.
- Family will have adequate information to decide if long-term care is required for patient's needs.

IMPAIRED PHYSICAL MOBILITY

Related to: Alzheimer's disease progression, dementia, inability to bear weight, poor nutrition, perceptual impairment, cognitive impairment

Defining Characteristics: inability to move at will, weakness, inability to bear weight, immobility, gait disturbances, balance and coordination deficits, difficulty turning, decreased fine and gross motor movement, decreased range of motion, tremors, instability while standing, dyspnea, decreased reaction time, incoordination, jerky movement, shuffling, swaying

Outcome Criteria

✔ Patient will maintain functional mobility as long as possible within limitations of disease process.
✔ Patient will have few, if any, complications related to immobility as disease condition progresses.

NOC: *Mobility Level*

INTERVENTIONS	RATIONALES
Assess patient's functional ability for mobility and note changes.	Identifies problems and helps to establish a plan of care. Mobility deteriorates as AD progresses, but most patients are ambulatory until the latter stages.
Assess patient's degree of cognitive impairment and ability to follow commands, and adapt interventions as needed.	Helps to determine the presence of deficits.

(continues)

(continued)

INTERVENTIONS	RATIONALES
Provide patient with enough time to perform a mobility-related assignment. Use simple instructions.	Patient may need repetitive instruction and comprehensive assistance to perform the task.
Provide range of motion exercises every shift. Encourage active range of motion exercises.	Helps to prevent joint contractures and muscle atrophy.
Reposition patient every 2 hours and prn.	Turning at regular intervals prevents skin breakdown from pressure injury.
Apply trochanter rolls and/or pillows to maintain joint alignment.	Prevents musculoskeletal deformities.
Assist patient with walking if at all possible, utilizing sufficient help. A one- or two-person pivot transfer utilizing a transfer belt can be used if the patient has weight-bearing ability.	Preserves patient's muscle tone and helps prevent complications of immobility.
Use mechanical lift for patients who cannot bear weight, and get them out of bed at least daily.	Provides a change of scenery, movement, and encourages participation in activities.
Avoid restraints if possible.	Inactivity created by the use of restraints may increase muscle weakness and poor balance.
Avoid the use of walkers and canes.	Most Alzheimer's patients cannot use them properly because of their cognitive impairment, and they may actually increase potential for injury.
Instruct family regarding ROM exercises, methods of transferring patient from bed to wheelchair, and turning at routine intervals.	Prevents complications of immobility and knowledge assists family members to be better prepared for home care.
Instruct family in community resources, support groups, and other resources as needed.	Provides alternative approaches for care and for support postdischarge.

NIC: *Teaching: Prescribed Activity/Exercise*

Discharge or Maintenance Evaluation

- Patient will maintain functional mobility within limitations of disease process.
- Patient will exhibit no evidence of skin breakdown or contractures.
- Family will be able to accurately perform exercises and repositioning techniques.

- Family will be able to access community resources as needed.

RISK FOR INJURY

Related to: Alzheimer's disease, dementia, lack of awareness of environmental hazards, poor judgment, medications, hallucinations, choking, hyperorality

Defining Characteristics: confusion, disorientation, malnutrition, altered mobility, skin breakdown, agitation, physical discomfort, choking, wounds, falls, wandering, shadowing, sundowning, pillaging, hoarding, aggression, overstated emotional response, delusions, hallucinations

Outcome Criteria

✔ Patient will remain safe from environmental hazards resulting from cognitive impairment.

✔ Family will ensure safety precautions are instituted and followed.

NOC: *Safety Status: Physical Injury*

INTERVENTIONS	RATIONALES
Assess patient's surroundings for hazards and remove them.	Alzheimer's disease decreases awareness of potential dangers, and disease progression coupled with hazardous environment could lead to accidents.
Maintain adequate lighting and clear pathways.	Allows patient to be able to see and find the way around room without danger of tripping or falling.
Assess patient for hyperorality.	AD patients frequently have this syndrome of unexplained movements of the mouth and tongue. The patient may chew on the fingers or put other items in the mouth. This can be dangerous and lead to medication overdose or the ingestion of poisonous substances.
During the middle and later stages of Alzheimer's disease, the patient must not be left unattended.	Patients with AD have impaired thinking and cannot rationalize cause and effect. This can result in the patient wandering outside without clothes on, become dehydrated or ill from exposure. Thermal injuries may occur with careless use of smoking materials or incorrect use of the stove.

INTERVENTIONS	RATIONALES
Instruct family regarding removal or locking up knives and sharp objects, cleaning supplies, insecticides, other household chemicals, all medications, aerosol sprays, weapons, power tools, small appliances, smoking materials, and breakable items.	Prevents physical injury from ingestion, burns, overdoses, or accidents.
Instruct family to apply protective guards over electrical outlets, thermostats, and stove knobs.	Prevents accidental injury.
Instruct family to keep pathways clear, move furniture against the wall, remove throw rugs, remove wheels on beds and chairs, and keep rooms and hallways well lighted.	Prevents risk of falls.
Instruct family to double lock doors and windows, swimming pool areas, and install warning buzzers on doors.	Helps to reduce risks to AD patients who wander.
Instruct family to ensure that patient has hearing aids, glasses, and so forth if they have a sensory deficit.	Reduces the risk for patients who need supplemental assistance with sensory status.
Instruct family to provide nonslip shoes, and shoes without laces when possible.	Helps to prevent tripping and falls.

NIC: *Risk Identification*

Discharge or Maintenance Evaluation

- Patient will remain safe in environment with no complications or injuries obtained.
- Family will identify and eliminate hazards in the patient's environment.

DISTURBED SLEEP PATTERN

Related to: internal factors of Alzheimer's disease, depression, confusion, boredom, environmental stimuli, obstructive sleep apnea

Defining Characteristics: interrupted sleep, difficulty falling asleep, awakening early, fatigue, lethargy, irritability, disorientation, complaints of not feeling rested, insomnia, sleeplessness, naps during the day, expressionless face, snoring, long periods of silence, apnea, sleepiness during the day, yawning, morning headache, loss of libido

Outcome Criteria

- ✔ Patient will achieve and maintain restorative, restful sleep.
- ✔ Patient will exhibit no behavioral symptoms, such as restlessness, irritability, or lethargy.

NOC: *Sleep*

INTERVENTIONS	RATIONALES
Assess patient's sleep patterns and changes, naps and frequency, amount of activity, sedentary status, number and time of awakenings during night, and patient's complaints of fatigue, apathy, lethargy, and impotence.	Provide information on which to establish a plan of care for correction of sleep deprivation. If patient is sleeping during the day, Sundowner's syndrome may be the problem, with the patient's day and night mixed up. By keeping the patient up during the day, sleeping at night may return.
Assess patient for complaints or signs of pain, dyspnea, nocturia, or leg cramps.	May be causes of frequent awakenings and interruptions of sleep cycle.
Monitor patient's medications, use of alcohol, and caffeine ingestion.	These drugs can alter REM sleep, which may cause irritability and lethargy. Drug action, absorption, and excretion may be delayed in the elderly patient, and toxicity may place the patient at risk.
Ensure environment is quiet, well-ventilated, absent of odor, and has a comfortable temperature.	External stimuli interferes with going to sleep and increases awakenings.
Provide ritualistic procedures of warm drink, extra covers, clean linens, and/or a warm bath prior to bedtime.	Prevents disruption of established pattern and promotes comfort and relaxation before sleep.
Provide backrubs, music, and other relaxation techniques.	Promotes relaxation before sleep and reduces anxiety and tension. AD patients respond well to therapeutic touch.
Provide sleep apnea apparatus if required.	Provides for completion of all stages of sleep resulting in restorative rest.
If all efforts fail, allow patient to remain awake in a recliner by the nurse's station.	Provides for surveillance of the patient, and the patient may willingly return to bed later.
Instruct family regarding Sundowner's syndrome, methods of coping with this, and possibility	The patient may not be able to be reverted back to a "normal" day/night cycle, and either the

(continues)

(continued)

INTERVENTIONS	RATIONALES
of changing their sleeping cycle to match that of the patient's once discharged.	caregiver will have to change his or her own sleeping pattern, hire a sitter during the night, or placement in a long-term facility may be required. Persistent Sundowner's is a frequent reason for admission to a long-term care facility because the caregiver becomes stressed from sleep deprivation, and is afraid that the patient may wander outside or become injured.
Instruct family to avoid putting out patient's clothes for the next day if the patient exhibits a sleep disorder.	The patient may believe he or she is supposed to get dressed and go somewhere.
Instruct family regarding need for patient to obtain exercise.	May promote sleep.
Provide information regarding community resources, respite care, and long-term care facilities.	Family may choose these options in order to cope with patient and the illness.

NIC: *Sleep Enhancement*

Discharge or Maintenance Evaluation

- Patient will achieve and maintain a normalized sleeping cycle with all sleeping phases obtained.
- Patient will have no sleep disruptions.
- Patient will not exhibit any signs or symptoms of sleep deprivation.
- Family will be able to utilize techniques to care for patient with Sundowner's syndrome.
- Family will be able to utilize community resources or choose to place patient in a long-term care facility.

DISTURBED SENSORY PERCEPTION: VISUAL, AUDITORY, KINESTHETIC, GUSTATORY, TACTILE, OLFACTORY

Related to: Alzheimer's disease, dementia, altered sensory reception, transmission and/or integration of neurologic disease or deficit, altered status of sensory organs, inability to communicate, understand, speak, or respond, sleep deprivation, CNS stimulants or depressants, environmental factor of socially restricted institutionalization, aging, chronic illness

Defining Characteristics: disorientation to time, place, person, or circumstance, change in sensory acuity, altered abstraction or conceptualization, change in problem solving abilities, apathy, complaints of fatigue, altered communication patterns, lack of concentration, noncompliance, disordered thought sequencing, visual and auditory distortions, motor incoordination, posture alterations, changes in behavior, changes in response to stimuli, restlessness, rapid mood swings, exaggerated emotional responses, anger, irritability, depression, bizarre thinking

Outcome Criteria

✔ Patient will have preservation of sensory/perceptual function and controlled effects of deficits within limits of disease process.

NOC: *Cognitive Orientation*

INTERVENTIONS	RATIONALES
Assess for confusion state, disorientation, difficulty and slowing of mental ability, changes in behavior and emotional responses.	Cognitive dysfunction behavior change may result from sensory deficits/deprivation caused by physiologic, psychological, and/or environmental factors.
Assess visual acuity, visual difficulties and loss and effects from these changes (withdrawal, isolation), presence of cataract, glaucoma, macular degeneration and status of remaining vision.	Presbyopia is common in the elderly; other visual changes caused by physiologic changes require correction by surgery or with eye glasses. Visual deficits create mobility and socialization changes.
Assess auditory acuity, cerumen in ears, responses to noises and effect on hearing, ability to communicate, amount of loss and effect, and difficulty in locating and identifying sounds.	Presbycusis is common in the elderly. Conductive loss results in a false interpretation of the world and creates poor communication, isolation, depression, and impaired thought processes as interactions are not heard.
Assess olfactory/gustatory loss, changes in appetite and eating, and amount of loss and effect on nutritional status.	Deterioration results from physiologic changes of aging and creates loss of interest and pleasure of eating.
Assess tactile changes, tingling or numbness in the extremities, loss of sensation, pain, or pressure.	Tactile perception is reduced in the aged and discriminating different sensations is decreased and creates risk of injury.
Assess kinesthetic perception, expression or behavior indicating	Cognitive deficits or aging neurologic changes may prevent

INTERVENTIONS	RATIONALES	INTERVENTIONS	RATIONALES
awareness, extent and direction of movement.	awareness, control of muscles, muscle movements and create risk of falls.	with proper pitch, use short sentences and gestures, maintain position even with patient to allow view of lips, and use touch to hold attention.	
Administer eye drops as ordered.	Mydriatics act to improve vision with cataracts; miotics facilitate flow of aqueous humor through canal of Schlemm.	Allow time for answers, rephrase message using different words if patient is confused, puzzled or gives inappropriate response.	May need time to sort out and identify sounds or may not understand certain frequency sounds.
Administer softening agent to ear and irrigate with bulb syringe or low-pulsating water pic.	Softens cerumen and emulsifies it for easier removal to facilitate hearing.	Use hand-held device if appropriate.	Hearing horns and speaking tubes enhance communication.
Promote use of assistive devices: hearing aid, corrective glasses, or contact lenses.	Provides for correction of deficit.	Offer sweet and salt substitutes.	Satisfies desire for these tastes as taste buds decrease with aging without compromising special dietary regimens.
Provide reading materials with large print, recorded material, telephone with large numbers, and posters with contrasting colors.	Provides for visual aids that allow for more control and independence.	Allow for interaction during mealtime.	Promotes interest in eating.
Provide magnifying glass, reading stand with magnifier attached, or brighter lighting.	Promotes visual acuity.	Provide alarm and flashing light type smoke detector, and safety alarms for stoves and heating units.	Reduces risk of injury if olfactory perception is reduced.
Suggest sunglasses or visor.	Reduces glare that is a common complaint in the elderly.	Prevent any exposure to extreme temperatures, and pressure to skin.	Reduces risk of burns or injury if tactile perception is impaired.
Arrange articles in familiar fashion and maintain same location. Follow through with food on table, personal hygiene articles, clothing, and furniture.	Provides alteration in environment that facilitates independence with limited vision and promotes safety.	Provide assistance when ambulating or performing ADLs as appropriate.	Reduces risk of falls or injury if visual acuity is reduced or if kinesthetic perception is impaired.
Suggest to use colors that are bright and contrasting; avoid blues and greens.	Minimizes problem of distinguishing items from one another as colors tend to blend.	Encourage participation in physical/social interactions.	Prevents isolation and sensory deficit.
Provide for adequate lighting at night; avoid abrupt movement from bright light to dim light.	Prevents confusion and accidents as ability to adjust to differences in lighting is decreased.	Instruct patient/family in the application of eye and/or ear medications. Stress the importance of drug compliance.	Preserves visual acuity and prevents vision loss, and otic solutions promote auditory acuity.
Provide telephone amplifier on receiver and bell tone, flashing light on phone, loud speakers for TV, radio, tape and CD players.	Promotes auditory perception and acuity.	Instruct patient/family in cleansing of glasses with mild soap and water, and drying with lint free cloth.	Promotes vision through clean glasses.
Determine type of hearing loss if head turned to hear, asks for repeat of conversations frequently, or has inability to follow verbal conversation.	The elderly with conductive loss experiences loss of hearing of all frequencies and will hear any loudly spoken words. Sensorineural loss experiences loss of hearing even when speech is loud enough to be heard.	Instruct patient/family regarding application of hearing aids, removal of them 2 times per week, and cleaning ear and device. Instruct about troubleshooting device according to manufacturer's recommendations.	Prevents cerumen accumulation and enhances hearing. Cleansing of hearing aid prevents buildup of cerumen and dirt, which can result in dysfunction.
Eliminate background noise.	Interferes with hearing.	Instruct family that patient requires screening exams for vision and hearing at least yearly.	Provides for adjustments in corrective devices.
Face the patient, use eye contact and speak loud enough to be heard, speak slowly and clearly	Enhances communication if hearing is impaired and promotes feelings of warmth and caring.	Instruct family in environmental modifications to enhance vision, hearing, taste, smell, and touch as appropriate.	Provides for patient safety by preventing injury in the presence of sensory impairment.

(continues)

(continued)

INTERVENTIONS	RATIONALES
Instruct family regarding the use of pet therapy.	Small pets provide sensory stimulation, encourage movement, as well as facilitating social interaction and non-verbal communication. Even in advanced stages of AD, patients respond favorably to kittens and puppies.
Instruct family regarding horticulture activities and their healing and therapeutic properties.	Plants grow and provide patients with the prospect of caring and nurturing, as well as sensory stimulation when working with the soil.

NIC: *Peripheral Sensation Management*

Discharge or Maintenance Evaluation

- Patient will be able to identify sounds and objects correctly.
- Patient will be able to use assistive devices to minimize deficits.
- Family will be compliant with making adjustments in the patient's environment for prevention of accidents or injuries.
- Family will be compliant with medication administration, and intraocular pressure increases will be prevented.

SOCIAL ISOLATION

Related to: Alzheimer's disease progression, alterations in mental status, confusion, memory loss, agitation, combativeness, unacceptable social behavior

Defining Characteristics: uncommunicative, withdrawn, cognitive impairment, impaired sleep pattern, hostile behavior, feelings of rejection, indifference of others, inability to meet expectations of others, isolation from others

Outcome Criteria

✔ Patient will be able to maintain social interaction with others within limitations of disease process.

NOC: *Social Involvement*

INTERVENTIONS	RATIONALES
Assess patient's feelings about his behavioral problems, negative feelings about self, ability to communicate, anxiety, depression, and feeling of powerlessness.	Determines extent of loneliness and isolation and reasons for it.
Identify possible support systems and ability to participate in social activities.	Community resources are available for clients and families dealing with stages of Alzheimer's disease that provide information and assistance.
Provide diversional activities as appropriate for functional ability.	Provides stimuli and promotes psychosocial functioning.
Provide rest and sleep periods; avoid situations that cause frustration, agitation, or sensory overload.	Permits coping with stimuli and prevents violent reactions.
Instruct patient/family regarding plan for periods of rest and activities during the day.	Promotes social interaction and activity.
Instruct family regarding establishing a consistent bedtime routine.	Promotes sleep and helps to avoid frustration and confusion from sleep deprivation.
Instruct family regarding resources in community that can be accessed for assistance.	Provides social outlets, financial assistance, and psychological counseling assistance.

NIC: *Socialization Enhancement*

Discharge or Maintenance Evaluation

- Patient will have increased participation in social activities within limitations of disease stage.
- Patient will exhibit a reduction in isolation from others.
- Family will be able to access support sources for assistance and counseling.

COMPROMISED FAMILY COPING

Related to: Alzheimer's disease, dementia, chronic illness, progression of disease that exhausts the supportive capacity of the family unit, progressive dependence of the patient on the family

Defining Characteristics: fatigue, anxiety, stress, social isolation, financial insecurity, expression of inadequate understanding of crisis and patient's responses to his health problem and necessary supportive behaviors, unsatisfactory results of attempts to assist patient, need for autonomy, preoccupation with reaction to patient's health problem, withdrawal from patient at his time of need

Outcome Criteria

✔ Family members will achieve increased coping ability concerning patient's dementia and care needs.

NOC: *Family Coping*

INTERVENTIONS	RATIONALES
Assess family's knowledge of patient's disease and erratic behaviors, and possible violent reactions.	Knowledge will enhance the family's understanding of the dementia associated with the disease and development of coping skills and strategies.
Assess for level of family's fatigue, reduced social exposure of family, feelings about role reversal in caring for patient and increasing demands of patient.	Long-term needs of the patient may affect the physical and psychosocial health of the caregiver, their economic status, and prevent the family from achieving their own goals in life.
Provide for opportunity for family to express concerns and lack of control of situation.	Promotes venting of feelings and reduces anxiety.
Assist in defining problem and use of techniques to cope and solve problems.	Provides support for problem-solving and management of family's fatigue and chronic stress.
Assist family to identify patient's reactions and behaviors and reasons for them.	May indicate onset of agitation and allow for interventions to prevent or reduce frustration.
Instruct family and demonstrate time-saving, energy-conserving techniques to be used to assist patient.	Assists family to provide personal care while conserving their energy.
Instruct family and demonstrate the use of assistive devices for walking, lift belts, equipment to be used in the care of the patient, and removal of environmental hazards.	Assists family to prevent injury or accident to patient or themselves.
Instruct family regarding the need to maintain their own health and social contacts.	Fatigue, isolation, and anxiety will affect the physical health and care capabilities of the caregiver.

INTERVENTIONS	RATIONALES
Instruct family regarding community resources available for Alzheimer's disease patients/ families, as well as utilization of respite care.	Provides information and support from those people that understand and empathize with these families. Respite care may facilitate caregiver's sense of well-being. Some families may feel that asking for help indicates a lack of caring for the patient.
Consult with social worker as appropriate.	May be helpful for providing assistance for financial help and respite services, as well as identifying need for long-term care facility need.
Instruct family regarding the use of the Alzheimer's Disease and Related Disorders Association.	Provides information for association that offers support for the safety, legal, financial, ethical issues, and needs of patients as the disease causes disruption within all aspects of family life.

NIC: *Support System Enhancement*

Discharge or Maintenance Evaluation

- Family will maintain their own optimal health.
- Family will be able to access support groups, counseling, and ADRDA for assistance as needed.
- Family will increase their knowledge about the disease and the care of the patient to enable them to feel more in control of their situation.
- Family will have reduced anxiety and be able to cope and use problem-solving techniques.
- Family will be able to adjust to role reversal status and resolve conflicts regarding the care of the patient.

WANDERING

Related to: Alzheimer's disease, dementia, age, previous use of wandering as a coping mechanism, mental illness, continuous ambulation or pacing

Defining Characteristics: aimless ambulation, frequent or continuous movement, persistent searching for people or objects, movement without planned destination, shadowing, pacing, inability to locate familiar landmarks, inability to be persuaded to remain in present location, pain, neurosensory deficits, attraction to random stimuli

Outcome Criteria

✔ Patient will have minimized wandering behavior.

✔ Patient will be able to ambulate safely, and will not have unplanned outings.

NOC: *Cognitive Orientation*

INTERVENTIONS	RATIONALES
Assess patient for presence of wandering behavior, noting times, places, and people with whom he ambulates.	Helps to identify gravity of the problem and to establish a plan of care. Purposeful wandering occurs when the patient has some intent for his movement, such as to escape boredom or for exercise. Aimless wandering is usually purposeless and involves disoriented patients who may enter other patients' rooms and take their belongings. The escapist wanderer usually has a destination in mind and is able to leave the premises undetected even though closely supervised.
Assess specific reasons for wandering, if patient is able to verbalize motivation.	Helps to identify possible causes for wandering and the needs that this behavior may be meeting.
Inquire how family handles the patient's wandering behavior.	Helps to identify potential appropriate methods of management of patient's behavior by using consistent methods.
Maintain safe environment and structured routine for patient.	Allows patient to wander within boundaries in a safe environment. Structure in the patient's routine may decrease wandering tendencies.
Encourage patient to participate in activities if able to do so.	Exercise helps to decrease restlessness and may decrease potential for wandering.

INTERVENTIONS	RATIONALES
Install bed alarms or pressure-sensitive doormats.	Provides alarm to alert nurses of movement and to help prevent injury to patient.
Avoid using restraints if at all possible.	Restraints increase agitation, anxiety, and cause complications of immobility, feelings of powerlessness, and actually increase tendency for wandering.
Assess patient for thirst, hunger, pain, discomfort, or need for toileting.	Patient may wander about looking for these needs to be fulfilled.
Instruct family regarding installing dead-bolt locks, fences, locks on gates, and locks on doors and windows.	Helps to prevent unsafe exits from home and for the protection of the patient.
Instruct family to notify neighbors and local police regarding patient's condition and penchant for wandering.	Provides awareness of others to prevent patient from becoming lost or injured.
Instruct family regarding community resources and support groups.	Assists caregivers to cope with patient's wandering behavior.
Instruct family to be prepared for possible escape and to keep up-to-date picture, and other information available.	Provides for information that may be used by police or other authorities to find a lost person.

NIC: *Seclusion*

Discharge or Maintenance Evaluation

■ Patient will be able to participate in activities.

■ Patient will have minimal wandering behaviors, and will experience no injuries.

■ Family will be able to identify hazards within home and neighborhood, and to provide safety measures to prevent patient escape and potential injury.

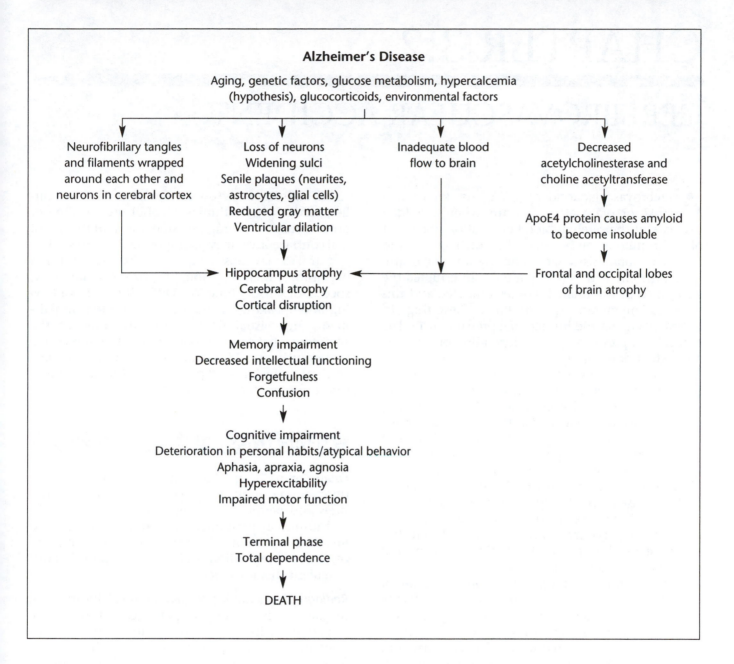

Alzheimer's Disease

Aging, genetic factors, glucose metabolism, hypercalcemia
(hypothesis), glucocorticoids, environmental factors

Neurofibrillary tangles and filaments wrapped around each other and neurons in cerebral cortex

Loss of neurons
Widening sulci
Senile plaques (neurites, astrocytes, glial cells)
Reduced gray matter
Ventricular dilation

Inadequate blood flow to brain

Decreased acetylcholinesterase and choline acetyltransferase

ApoE4 protein causes amyloid to become insoluble

Frontal and occipital lobes of brain atrophy

Hippocampus atrophy
Cerebral atrophy
Cortical disruption

Memory impairment
Decreased intellectual functioning
Forgetfulness
Confusion

Cognitive impairment
Deterioration in personal habits/atypical behavior
Aphasia, apraxia, agnosia
Hyperexcitability
Impaired motor function

Terminal phase
Total dependence

DEATH

CHAPTER 3.2

CEREBROVASCULAR ACCIDENT

A cerebrovascular accident (CVA), also known as a stroke or brain attack, occurs when a sudden decrease in the cerebral blood circulation as a result of a thrombosis, embolus, or hemorrhage leads to hypoxia of brain tissues, causing swelling and death. When the circulation is impaired or interrupted the small area of the brain becomes infarcted and this changes membrane permeability, resulting in increased edema and intracranial pressure (ICP). The clinical symptoms may vary depending on the area and extent of the injury.

Thrombosis of small arteries in the white matter of the brain account for the most common cause of strokes. A history of hypertension, diabetes mellitus, cardiac disease, vascular disease, or atherosclerosis may lead to thrombosis, which causes ischemia to the part of the brain supplied by the vessel involved. Risk factors that predispose patients to stroke increase with age, resulting in the greatest incidence of the disease in the elderly population, and the aged are least likely to seek medical attention in a timely manner. People over the age of 75 have the greatest risk of stroke but are the least aware of signs and symptoms of brain attack.

Embolism is the second most common cause of CVA, and happens when a blood vessel is suddenly occluded with blood, air, tumor, fat, or septic particulate. The embolus migrates to the cerebral arteries and obstructs circulation causing edema and necrosis.

When hemorrhage occurs, it is usually the sudden result of ruptured aneurysms, tumors, or AV malformations, or involves problems with hypertension or bleeding dyscrasias. The cerebral bleeding decreases the blood supply and compresses neuronal tissue.

Patients who have strokes frequently have had prior events, such as TIAs (transient ischemic attacks) with reversible focal neurologic deficits lasting less than 24 hours, or RINDs (reversible ischemic neurologic deficits) lasting more than 24 hours but leaving little, if any, residual neurologic impairment.

In addition to the disease processes discussed earlier, cardiac dysrhythmias, alcohol use, cocaine or other recreational drug use, smoking, and the use of oral contraceptives may predispose patients to strokes.

Strokes may cause temporary or permanent losses of motor function, thought processes, memory, speech, or sensory function. Difficulty with swallowing and speaking, hemiplegia, intellectual impairment, and visual field defects are some of the symptoms that can be produced. Treatment is aimed at supporting vital functions and ensuring adequate cerebral perfusion, and prevention of major complications or permanent disability.

MEDICAL CARE

Laboratory: CBC used to identify blood loss or infection; serum osmolality used to evaluate oncotic pressures and permeability; electrolytes, glucose levels, and urinalysis performed to identify problems and imbalances that may be responsible for changes in condition; coagulation studies used to monitor anticoagulant therapy efficacy

Radiography: skull X-rays may show calcifications of the carotids in the presence of cerebral thrombosis, or partial calcification of an aneurysm in subarachnoid hemorrhage; pineal gland may shift to the opposite side if mass is expanding; may reveal evidence of shift if hematoma or cerebral edema is present

CT scans: used to identify thrombosis or hemorrhagic stroke, tumors, cerebral edema, or hydrocephalus; may not reveal changes immediately

Brain scans: used to identify ischemic areas caused by CVA but usually are not discernible until up to 2 weeks postinjury; brain nuclear scans may reveal the disruption in the blood-brain barrier, area of infarction, size and location of hematoma

Magnetic resonance imaging: used to identify areas of infarction, hemorrhage, ischemia, edema, and AV malformations

Angiography: used to identify site and degree of occlusion or rupture of vessel and to assess collateral blood circulation and presence of AV malformations

Ultrasonography: may be used to gather information regarding flow velocity in the major circulation

Lumbar puncture: performed to evaluate ICP and to identify infection; bloody CSF may indicate a hemorrhagic stroke, and clear fluid with normal pressures may be noted in cerebral thrombosis, embolism, and with TIAs; protein may be elevated if thrombosis results from inflammation

Electroencephalogram: may be used to help localize area of injury based on brain wave pattern and electrical activity

Surgery: endarterectomy may be required to remove the occlusive atherosclerotic plaque from the intima of the carotid artery, or microvascular bypass may be performed to bypass the occluded area, such as the carotid artery, aneurysm, or AV malformation

Corticosteroids: betamethasone (Celestone), cortisone acetate (Cortone), dexamethasone acetate or sodium phosphate (Decadron, Dexone, Hexadrol, Solurex LA, Cortastat, Dalalone, Dexasone), hydrocortisone acetate , sodium phosphate, or sodium succinate (Cortef, Cortenema, Hydrocortone, Solu-Cortef), methylprednisolone acetate or sodium succinate (Medrol, Depo-Medrol, Duralone, Medralone, Solu-Medrol), prednisolone acetate, sodium phosphate, or terbutate (Delta-Cortef, Prelone, Cotolone, Predalone, Predate, Prenisol), prednisone (Deltasone, Meticorten, Orasone, Prednisone Intensol, Sterapred), or triamcinolone (Aristocort, Atolone, Kenacort, Azmacort, Trilog, Amcort, Trilone) used to decrease cerebral inflammation and edema

Anticonvulsants: carbamazepine (Atretol, Epitol, Tegretol), clonazepam (Klonopin), ethosuximide (Zarontin), gabapentin (Neurontin), lamotrigine (Lamictal), levatiracetam (Keppra), magnesium sulfate, oxcarbazepine (Trileptal), Phenobarbital (Barbita, Solfoton, Luminal), phenytoin sodium (Dilantin, Phenytex), primidone (Mysoline, PMS), tiagabine hydrochloride (Gabitril), topiramate (Topamax), valproate sodium or acid (Depacon, Depakene, Depakote), or zonisamide (Zonegran) are believed to

stabilize the neuronal membrane and suppress neuronal hypersynchronization; used in the treatment and prophylaxis of seizure activity

Analgesics: acetaminophen (Tylenol) or ibuprofen (Motrin, Advil, Genpril, Ibuprofen, Nuprin, Trendar) used for discomfort and pain; aspirin and aspirin-containing products are contraindicated with hemorrhage

t-PA (tissue plasminogen activator): the only drug currently approved by the FDA for the treatment of ischemic stroke; used to help dissolve blood clots, but is contraindicated for hemorrhagic stroke

Neuroprotective agents: drugs such as glutamate antagonists, calcium antagonists, and antioxidants being investigated for helping to reduce injury to neurons, and may help stop or lessen damaging biochemical changes that result in secondary brain impairment after a stroke

Anticoagulants: enoxaparin sodium (Lovenox), heparin calcium and sodium (Calciparin, Heparin), and warfarin (Coumadin) are used to reduce risk of further thrombus accumulation and to prevent recurrent clot formation by inhibiting prothrombin synthesis and reducing vitamin K dependent clotting factors

Platelet aggregation inhibitors: acetylsalicylic acid (ASA, aspirin) prevents platelet aggregation; cilostazol (Pletal) decreases platelet aggregation by inhibiting phosphodiesterase III; clopidogrel bisulfate (Plavix) inhibits platelet aggregation by binding to and changing the platelet ADP receptor to inhibit ADP-mediated platelet activation and platelet aggregation; dipyridamole (Persantine) increases adenosine and inhibits platelet aggregation; eptifibatide (Integrilin) and tirofiban hydrochloride (Aggrastat) binds to the glycoprotein IIb/IIIa receptor to inhibit aggregation of platelets; these drugs are used to prevent clot formation and subsequent occlusion

Antihypertensives: vasodilators (hydralazine [Apresoline], minoxidil [Loniten], and nitroprusside sodium [Nitropress]) are used to relax smooth muscle in the arterioles that help to reduce peripheral resistance; beta-adrenergic blockers: ([Sectral], atenolol [Tenormin], betaxolol [Kerlone], bisoprolol fumarate [Zebeta], carteolol hydrochloride [Cartrol], carvedilol [Coreg], metoprolol [Lopressor], nadolol [Corgard], penbutolol [Levatol], pindolol [Visken], propranolol [Inderal], and timolol maleate [Blocadren]) used to decrease blood pressure by inhibiting the impulse through the sympathetic pathways and to decrease cardiac output, sympathetic stimulation, and renin secretion by the kidneys; alpha-adrenergic blockers: (doxazosin mesylate [Cardura], fenoldopam mesylate [Corlopam], labetalol hydrochloride [Normodyne, Trandate], phentolamine mesylate [Regitine], prazosin hydrochloride [Minipress], and terazosin hydrochloride [Hytrin]) used to reduce blood pressure by acting on the peripheral vasculature to generate vasodilatory action and to decrease peripheral vascular resistance; calcium channel blockers: (diltiazem [Cardizem], felodipine [Plendil], isradipine [DynaCirc], nicardipine [Cardene], nifedipine [Procardia], nisoldipine [Sular], and verapamil [Calan, Isoptin]) used to reduce blood pressure by the inhibition of calcium ion influx across the smooth muscle and cardiac cells which reduces arteriolar resistance; angiotensin-converting enzyme (ACE) inhibitors: (benazepril hydrochloride [Lotensin], candesartan cilexetil [Atacand], captopril [Capoten], enalapril maleate [Vasotec], eprosartan mesylate [Teveten], fosinopril sodium [Monopril], moexipril hydrochloride [Univasc], perindopril erbumine [Aceon], quinapril hydrochloride [Accupril], ramipril [Altace], telmisartan [Micardis], and trandolapril [Mavik]) used to lower blood pressure by inhibiting ACE which prevents the conversion of angiotensin I to angiotensin II, which is a strong vasoconstrictor; the reduction in angiotensin II helps to reduce the peripheral arterial resistance and decreases aldosterone secretion, which effectively reduces the water and sodium retention to lower blood pressure; angiotensin II receptor blockers: (irbesartan [Avapro], losartan potassium [Cozaar], and valsartan [Diovan]) used to reduce blood pressure by blocking the binding of angiotensin II to the receptor sites in the vascular smooth muscle to help inhibit the pressor effect of the renin-angiotensin-aldosterone system; central-acting adrenergics: (clonidine hydrochloride [Catapres], guanabenz acetate [Wytensin], guanfacine hydrochloride [Tenex], hydralazine hydrochloride [Apresoline], lisinopril [Prinivil, Zestril], and methyldopa hydrochloride [Aldomet]) used to help decrease sympathetic outflow to the heart, kidneys, and peripheral vessels in order to decrease peripheral vascular resistance, heart rate, and blood pressure

Hyperosmotics: mannitol (Osmitrol) and urea carbamide (Ureaphil) used to reduce intracranial pressure caused by cerebral edema

COMMON NURSING DIAGNOSES

INEFFECTIVE AIRWAY CLEARANCE (see COPD)

Related to: decreased level of consciousness, tracheobronchial obstruction, potential for aspiration

Defining Characteristics: ineffective cough, tachypnea, dyspnea, abnormal breath sounds, respiratory rate and depth changes, decreased response to stimuli, choking, ineffective swallowing, abnormal arterial blood gases, decreased oxygen saturation, paralysis, obstruction, ECG changes, hemorrhage

IMPAIRED PHYSICAL MOBILITY (see ALZHEIMER'S DISEASE)

Related to: CVA effects, paralysis, paresthesias, neuromuscular impairment, impaired cognition, weakness

Defining Characteristics: inability to move at will, muscle incoordination, decreased range of motion, decreased muscle strength, paralysis, muscle atrophy, flaccidity, deformity, contracture of limb(s), tremors, alteration in gait, shuffling, swaying, difficulty with turning, weakness, paresthesias

DISTURBED SENSORY PERCEPTION: VISUAL, KINESTHETIC, GUSTATORY, TACTILE, OLFACTORY (see ALZHEIMER'S DISEASE)

Related to: stroke, neurologic trauma/deficit, stress, altered reception of stimuli, altered integration from neurologic disease

Defining Characteristics: behavior changes, disorientation to time, place, self, and circumstance, diminished concentration, inability to focus, alteration in thought processes, decreased sensation, paresthesias, paralysis, altered ability to taste and smell, inability to recognize objects, muscle incoordination, muscle weakness, inappropriate communication, changes in visual acuity

IMBALANCED NUTRITION: LESS THAN BODY REQUIREMENTS (see COPD)

Related to: stroke, inability to ingest food, dysphagia, absent gag reflex

Defining Characteristics: anorexia, choking, aspiration, inability to feed self, food remaining in mouth, weight loss, coma, weakness of muscles involved with eating, altered taste sensation, lack of interest in eating, abdominal pain, diarrhea, inadequate food intake, loss of weight despite adequate food intake, paralysis, paralysis of muscles involved with eating

BATHING/HYGIENE SELF-CARE DEFICIT (see ALZHEIMER'S DISEASE)

Related to: stroke, weakness, decreased muscle strength, muscle incoordination, paralysis, paresthesia, pain, functional impairment

Defining Characteristics: inability to wash body or body parts, inability to obtain bath supplies, inability to obtain water source, inability to get into and out of bathroom, inability to dry body, inability to take off necessary clothing, inability to maintain appearance at satisfactory level, inability to brush teeth, inability to comb/brush hair, inability to shave

DRESSING/GROOMING SELF-CARE DEFICIT (see ALZHEIMER'S DISEASE)

Related to: stroke, musculoskeletal impairment, cognitive impairment

Defining Characteristics: inability to put on or take off clothing, inability to choose clothing, inability to maintain appropriate appearance, inability to fasten clothing, inability to obtain clothing, inability to pick up clothing, inability to brush/comb hair, inability to shave, inability to brush teeth

TOILETING SELF-CARE DEFICIT (see ALZHEIMER'S DISEASE)

Related to: stroke, cognitive impairment, neurologic impairment, physiologic impairment, psychological dysfunction, environmental impairment

Defining Characteristics: inability to carry out toileting routine, inability to flush toilet, inability to get to bathroom, inability to manipulate clothing for toileting, inability to sit on or rise from toilet or commode, incontinence of stool or urine, gastric paresis

CONSTIPATION (see HEART FAILURE)

Related to: immobility, less than adequate physical activity, lack of dietary bulk, neuromuscular impairment, dysphagia, paralysis

Defining Characteristics: passage of hard, formed stool, decreased bowel sounds, inability to evacuate stool, abdominal pain, abdominal distention, ileus, absent bowel sounds, nausea, vomiting

RISK FOR IMPAIRED SKIN INTEGRITY (see PERIPHERAL VASCULAR DISEASE)

Related to: stroke, skin changes associated with the aging process, pressure on skin surfaces, bed rest, immobility, intermittent claudication, alteration in arterial and venous circulation, alterations in tissue perfusion, presence of shearing forces on skin, paralysis

Defining Characteristics: thin, dry skin on extremities, redness to pressure areas, edema, ulcerations or lesions to extremities, dermatitis, pigmentation to legs, mottling, cyanosis, pallor, decreased or absent pulses, warmth to area, disruption of skin surface, excoriation of skin, decreased tactile sensation, open wounds, decreased temperature to extremities, paralysis, paresthesias

INEFFECTIVE SEXUALITY PATTERNS (see CAD)

Related to: stroke, functional impairment, physiologic changes related to aging, medications, paralysis, paresthesia

Defining Characteristics: verbalization of difficulties with sexual activity, verbalization of limitations or change in sexual activity imposed by illness, impotence, inability to achieve sexual satisfaction

INEFFECTIVE COPING (see DEPRESSION)

Related to: stroke, life changes, limitations imposed by disease process, inadequate coping methods

Defining Characteristics: inability to meet role expectations, inability to meet basic needs, fatigue, changes in social participation, inability to problem-solve, inappropriate use of defense mechanisms, inappropriate use of coping strategies, risk-taking behaviors, sleep disturbances, verbalization of inability to cope with situation, changes in communication

DEFICIENT KNOWLEDGE (see CAD)

Related to: lack of information about strokes, cognitive limitations, medications, neurological impairment

Defining Characteristics: request for information, anxiety regarding potential errors, presence of preventable complications, noncompliance with instructions, misperceptions about illness

ADDITIONAL NURSING DIAGNOSES

INEFFECTIVE TISSUE PERFUSION: CEREBRAL

Related to: occlusion, hemorrhage, interruption of cerebral blood flow, vasospasm, edema

Defining Characteristics: changes in level of consciousness, mental changes, personality changes, memory loss, restlessness, combativeness, vital sign changes, motor function impairment, sensory impairment, lethargy, stupor, coma, increased intracranial pressure, headache, cognitive dysfunction

Outcome Criteria

✔ Patient will have improved or normal cerebral perfusion with no mental status changes or complications.

NOC: *Tissue Perfusion: Cerebral*

INTERVENTIONS	RATIONALES
Measure blood pressure in both arms with each vital sign check.	Cerebral injury may cause variations in blood pressure readings. Hypotension may result from circulatory collapse, and increased ICP may result from edema or clot formation. Differences in readings between arms may indicate a subclavian artery blockage.
Maintain head of bed in elevated position with head in a neutral position.	Helps to improve venous drainage, reduce arterial pressure, and may improve cerebral perfusion.

INTERVENTIONS	RATIONALES
Provide calm, quiet environment with adequate rest periods between activities.	Bed rest may be required to prevent rebleeding after initial hemorrhage. Activity may increase ICP.
Administer t-PA as ordered.	Tissue plasminogen activator must be administered only to patients with ischemic type strokes, and must be done within 3 hours of symptom onset to be effective. t-PA helps to dissolve blood clots and allow reperfusion of cerebral arteries, but if it is administered after an extended time, the drug may result in cerebral edema and actually increase morbidity.
Administer anticoagulants as ordered.	May be warranted to improve blood flow to cerebral tissues and to prevent further clotting and embolus formation. These are contraindicated in hypertension because of the potential for hemorrhage.
Administer antihypertensives as ordered.	Hypertension may be transient when occurring during the CVA, but chronic hypertension will require judicious treatment to prevent further tissue ischemia and damage.
Administer vasodilators as ordered.	Helps to improve collateral circulation and to reduce the incidence of vasospasm.
Administer neuroprotective agents as ordered.	Numerous drugs are being investigated for their capacity to shield neurons from damaging effects of ischemia. Glutamate antagonists, calcium antagonists, and antioxidants may help halt or decrease the harmful biochemical changes that result in secondary brain injury after a stroke. Brain regenerative drugs are being investigated to see if they can restrict the amount of damage caused by a stroke and assist in repairing damaged brain tissues.
Instruct patient on the use of stool softeners and avoidance of straining at stool evacuation.	Valsalva's maneuvers increase ICP and may result in rebleeding. Stool softeners help to prevent straining.

INTERVENTIONS	RATIONALES
Prepare patient for surgery as warranted.	May be required to treat problem and prevent further complications.
Instruct patient/family regarding signs and symptoms of stroke, importance of seeking medical attention promptly, and modifying lifestyle risk factors.	Promotes knowledge and enhances likelihood of patients seeking help in a timely manner. It has been shown in studies that most stroke patients do not seek help for 24 hours after the onset of symptoms. Controllable risk factors include elevated blood pressure, atrial fibrillation, smoking, alcohol consumption, use of cocaine, and an elevated red blood cell count.

NIC: *Cerebral Perfusion Promotion*

Discharge or Maintenance Evaluation

- Patient will achieve reperfusion of cerebral arteries and experience no lasting adverse side effects.
- Patient will experience no complications from treatment.
- Patient will maintain cerebral perfusion and suffer no lasting neurologic deficits.
- Patient/family will be able to accurately verbalize signs and symptoms of CVA and will seek medical help in a timely manner if these signs are present.

IMPAIRED VERBAL COMMUNICATION

Related to: CVA, weakness, loss of muscle control, cerebral circulation impairment, neuromuscular impairment

Defining Characteristics: inability to speak, inability to identify objects, inability to comprehend language, inability to write, inability to choose and use appropriate words, dysarthria

Outcome Criteria

✔ Patient will be able to communicate normally or will be able to make needs known by some form of communication.

NOC: *Communication Ability*

INTERVENTIONS	RATIONALES
Evaluate patient's ability to speak or understand language.	Provides a baseline from which to begin planning interventions. Determination of specific areas of brain injury involvement will preclude what type of assistance will be required.
Assess whether patient suffers from aphasia or dysarthria.	Aphasic patients have difficulty using and interpreting language, comprehending words, and inability to speak or make signs. Dysarthric patients can understand language, but have problems forming or pronouncing words as a result of weakness or paralysis of the oral muscles.
Evaluate patient's response to simple commands.	Inability to follow simple commands may indicate receptive aphasia.
Evaluate patient's ability to name objects.	Inability to do so indicates expressive aphasia.
Evaluate patient's ability to write simple sentences or own name.	May indicate patient's disability with receptive and expressive aphasia.
Avoid talking down to patient or making patronizing comments.	Intellect frequently remains unimpaired after injury.
When asking questions, use yes or no type questions initially, and progress as patient is able to answer more specific questions.	Provides for method of communication without necessity of response to large volumes of information. As patient progresses, the intricacy of questions may increase.
Provide a method of communication for patient, such as a writing board, magic slate, or communication board, to which patient may point.	Allows for communication of needs and allays anxiety.
Consult with speech therapy.	May be required to identify cognition, function, and plan interventions for recovery of speech.
Instruct patient/family on methods to use for communication.	Provides method for patient to communicate his needs.

NIC: *Communication Enhancement: Speech Deficit*

Discharge or Maintenance Evaluation

- Patient will be able to communicate effectively.
- Patient will be able to understand communication problem and access resources to meet needs.

IMPAIRED SWALLOWING

Related to: stroke, neuromuscular impairment

Defining Characteristics: inability to swallow effectively, choking, aspiration

Outcome Criteria

✔ Patient will be able to swallow effectively with no incidence of aspiration.

NOC: *Swallowing Status*

INTERVENTIONS	RATIONALES
Evaluate patient's ability to swallow, extent of any paralysis, and ability to maintain airway.	Provides baseline information from which to plan interventions for care.
Maintain head position and support, with head of bed elevated at least 30 degrees or more during and immediately after feeding.	Helps to prevent aspiration and facilitates ability to swallow.
Place food in the unaffected side of patient's mouth.	Allows for sensory stimulation and taste, and may assist to trigger swallowing reflexes.
Provide foods that are soft and require little, if any, chewing, or provide thickened liquids.	These types of foods are easier to control and decrease potential for choking or aspiration.
Assist with stimulation of tongue, cheeks, or lips as warranted.	May help to retrain oral muscles and facilitate adequate tongue movement and swallowing.
Administer tube feedings or enteral alimentation as warranted/ordered.	May be required if oral intake is not sufficient.
Instruct patient/family to use straw for drinking liquids. Maintain swallowing precautions identified by speech therapist.	Helps to strengthen facial and oral muscles to decrease potential for choking.
Encourage family to bring patient's favorite foods, within limitations of dietary restrictions.	May be helpful to have familiar foods and may increase oral intake.
Instruct family to maintain rehabilitation with speech therapist.	Provides for continued instruction and guidance postdischarge. Speech therapist may be able to identify interventions that enable patient to avoid risk of aspiration.

NIC: *Swallowing Therapy*

Discharge or Maintenance Evaluation

- Patient will be able to eat and swallow normally.
- Patient will be able to ingest an adequate amount of nutrients without danger of aspiration.
- Patient will be able to follow instructions and strengthen muscles used for eating and swallowing.
- Patient/family will be able to access resources for continued therapy as needed.

UNILATERAL NEGLECT

Related to: stroke, effects of disturbed perceptual abilities, neurologic trauma/illness, neurological impairment

Defining Characteristics: consistent inattention to stimuli on affected side, does not look at affected side, leaves food on plate on affected side, inability to protect affected side, inability to perform self-care

Outcome Criteria

✔ Patient will exhibit no injury to the affected side and will have an absence of safety hazards in environment.

NOC: *Body Image*

INTERVENTIONS	RATIONALES
Assess for safety hazards for patient that ignores affected side.	Removes potential for injury when unaware of injury threat.
Utilize siderails, soft restraints or surveillance of positioning of affected side.	Protects affected side from injury.
Arrange articles in the environment for daily needs within perceptual field; follow by placing on affected side and encouraging to attend to affected side.	Compensates for deficit.
Assist patient to judge position and distance and assist with activities.	Prepares for independence.
Provide clear pathways, good lighting, and eliminate small rugs.	Prevents accidental falls.
Continue reminding patient to turn head to affected and unaffected sides, and to rub and touch affected side frequently.	Increases awareness of affected side.

INTERVENTIONS	RATIONALES
Provide instructions verbally and in small amounts. Refer to affected side frequently.	Promotes communication and understanding by patient.
Instruct patient/family to remind to care for affected side, perform daily exercises of affected side, and to utilize affected limb when possible.	Prevents neglect and deterioration of affected side.

NIC: *Unilateral Neglect Management*

Discharge or Maintenance Evaluation

- Patient will exhibit no trauma or injury to affected arm and/or leg.
- Patient will begin to include affected limb in daily care.
- Family will be compliant with reminding patient to use affected limb.

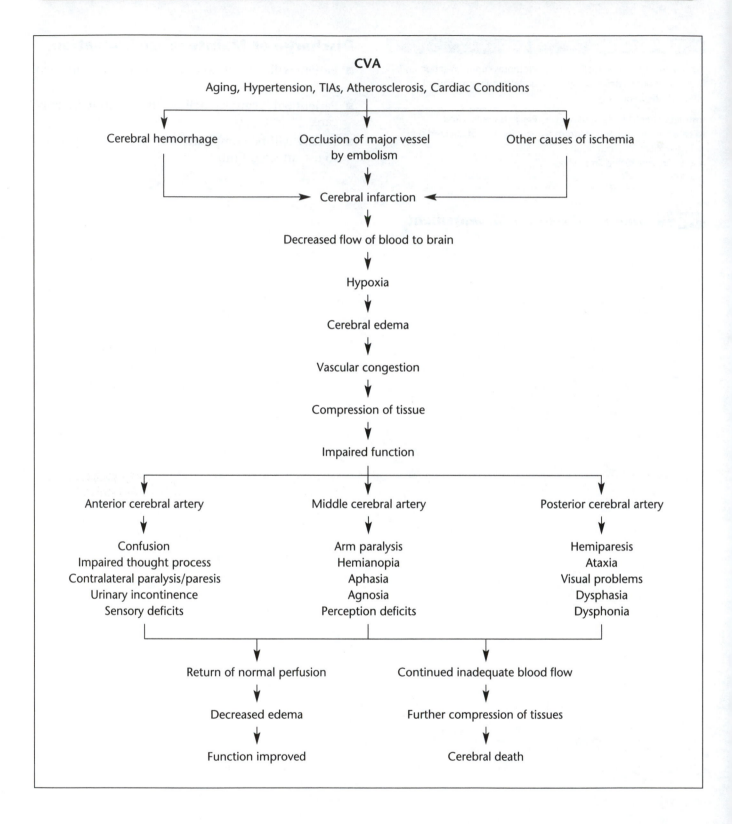

CVA

Aging, Hypertension, TIAs, Atherosclerosis, Cardiac Conditions

Cerebral hemorrhage   Occlusion of major vessel   Other causes of ischemia
                                  by embolism

Cerebral infarction

Decreased flow of blood to brain

Hypoxia

Cerebral edema

Vascular congestion

Compression of tissue

Impaired function

Anterior cerebral artery   Middle cerebral artery   Posterior cerebral artery

Confusion   Arm paralysis   Hemiparesis
Impaired thought process   Hemianopia   Ataxia
Contralateral paralysis/paresis   Aphasia   Visual problems
Urinary incontinence   Agnosia   Dysphasia
Sensory deficits   Perception deficits   Dysphonia

Return of normal perfusion   Continued inadequate blood flow

Decreased edema   Further compression of tissues

Function improved   Cerebral death

CHAPTER 3.3

DEPRESSION

Depression in the elderly is identified as a lowered mood disorder and a lack of psychic energy that is experienced by the patient and either reported or observed. The elderly frequently react with depressed moods and feelings of hopelessness when a dramatic event occurs, such as the loss of friends or a spouse, a change in home location, physical or economic changes, or a physical illness, and these major events in their lives make them more at risk for depression.

Depression can refer to deviations from normal emotional responses, be singled out as a clinical symptom, or can refer to a group of symptoms and signs that are consistent with a clinical syndrome, but it is the most prevalent psychological problem in the elderly today. One type of depression that affects the elderly is a masked depression state that is frequently missed as "depression" because the behavior does not exhibit the typical signs that a younger person might express, and is usually disregarded in older individuals as their being uncooperative or irritable. Reactive depression occurs in response to some stimulus, and depressive states that are associated with dementias are two other varieties of depression.

Depression has been mistakenly thought to be an expected outcome of the aging process. It frequently poses a challenge to diagnose because of the complexity with concomitant complications from physical illness, fatigue, and organic brain syndromes, but it can be treated effectively. Older patients also contribute to this lack of treatment because they commonly are on fixed incomes and cannot afford psychological help, or transportation may be a problem, or the stigma of having a mental illness may cause them to fear the loss of their freedom.

Some health care personnel find it difficult to distinguish the 3 D's—dementia, delirium, and depression. Dementia deals with a persistent cognitive impairment resulting from an illness, with memory loss being the first noted symptom. Delirium is a state of clouded consciousness with misperceptions and nonattention to various stimuli. It can occur because of metabolic, structural, or infectious origins. Drug toxicity, metabolic dysfunction, nutritional deficiencies, endocrine disorders, brain dysfunction, meningitis, and encephalitis are some of the causes of delirium. Depression occurs frequently in the elderly because of numerous issues, such as important life changes, losses of significant others, deterioration of physical and cognitive abilities, and the ever-present recognition of one's mortality. If depression is not recognized and treated, the illness can result in suicide in the elderly, which ranks as being three times the statistical rate of the general population.

MEDICAL CARE

Laboratory: CBC used to identify anemia or infectious processes; chemistry panel to identify deficiency states that may mimic depression; Vitamin B_{12} and folate levels used to identify deficiency and potential for anemias; thyroid profile used to identify hypothyroidism or hyperthyroidism that may have some symptoms similar to depression; urinalysis used to identify potential urinary tract dysfunction; cardiac isoenzymes may be used to identify concurrent myocardial conditions; DST (dexamethasone suppression test) used to identify endogenous depression if result is positive; electrolyte profiles used to identify imbalances and metabolic changes that may be associated with depression; drug levels used to identify therapeutic and toxic levels of medications being used in the patient's treatment

Radiography: chest X-rays used to identify the presence of any infectious process; CT scans may be used to identify lesions that may be associated with dementia

Electroencephalogram: used to identify brain waves associated with depressive states

Antidepressants: amitriptyline hydrochloride or pamoate (Elavil, Endep), amoxapine (Asendin), bupropion hydrochloride (Wellbutrin), citalopram hydrobromide (Celexa), clomipramine hydrochloride (Anafranil), desipramine hydrochloride (Norpramin), doxepin hydrochloride (Sinequan), fluoxetine hydrochloride (Prozac), imipramine hydrochloride (Norfranil, Tipramine), mirtazaprine (Remeron), nefazodone hydrochloride (Serzone), nortriptyline hydrochloride (Aventyl, Pamelor), paroxetine hydrochloride (Paxil), phenelzine sulfate (Nardil), sertraline hydrochloride (Zoloft), tranylcypromine sulfate (Parnate), trazodone hydrochloride (Desyrel, Trazon, Trialodine), trimipramine maleate (Surmontil), or venlafaxine hydrochloride (Effexor) may be used to lessen symptoms of depression by several actions; tricyclics block the reuptake of norepinephrine and serotonin in the nerve endings and increase the action of these chemicals within the nerve cells; MAOIs increase the concentration of endogenous epinephrine, norepinephrine, serotonin and dopamine; many are used in conjunction with psychotherapy

Psychotherapy: useful in the elderly to alleviate anxiety and to maintain or rehabilitate the patient's psychological ability to function

Electroconvulsive therapy (ECT): once controversial, but currently proven to be effective in treating severe depression that has not responded to medications or psychotherapy; ECT elevates mood within one week, and may provide faster and safer treatment in some patients; ECT may be contraindicated for some patients who have cardiac problems

COMMON NURSING DIAGNOSES

DECREASED CARDIAC OUTPUT (see CAD)

Related to: depression, use of antidepressants

Defining Characteristics: elevated blood pressure, decreased cardiac output <4 L/min, cardiac index <2.5 L/min/m^2, decreased stroke volume, increased peripheral vascular resistance >250 dynes/second/cm^{-5}, increased systemic vascular resistance >1400 dynes/second/cm^{-5}, decreased blood pressure, orthostatic hypotension

IMBALANCED NUTRITION: LESS THAN BODY REQUIREMENTS (see COPD)

Related to: depression, inability to take in enough food, increased metabolism caused by disease process, decreased level of consciousness, inability to absorb nutrients because of biologic or psychological factors related to aging

Defining Characteristics: actual inadequate food intake, altered taste, altered smell sensation, weight loss, body weight 20% or more under ideal for height and frame, anorexia, absent bowel sounds, decreased peristalsis, muscle mass loss, decreased muscle tone, changes in bowel habits, nausea, vomiting, abdominal distention, lack of interest in food, satiety immediately after ingesting food, abdominal pain or discomfort, sore, inflamed buccal cavity, depression, anxiety, social isolation, difficulty in feeding self, inability to feed self, changes in mental status, fatigue from work of breathing, decreased cough and gag reflexes, confusion

CONSTIPATION (see HEART FAILURE)

Related to: use of antidepressants, immobility, less than adequate physical activity because of aging process, lack of dietary bulk, depression

Defining Characteristics: passage of hard, formed stool, decreased bowel sounds, inability to evacuate stool, abdominal pain, abdominal distention, ileus, absent bowel sounds, nausea, vomiting

INEFFECTIVE SEXUALITY PATTERNS (see CAD)

Related to: depression, antidepressants, functional impairment related to aging, medications

Defining Characteristics: verbalization of difficulties with sexual activity, verbalization of limitations or change in sexual activity imposed by illness, impotence, inability to achieve sexual satisfaction

IMPAIRED VERBAL COMMUNICATION (see ALZHEIMER'S DISEASE)

Related to: depression, medications, psychological barriers, psychosis, decreased circulation to brain, age-related factors, lack of stimuli

Defining Characteristics: confusion, anxiety, restlessness, disorientation to person, place, time, and circumstance, repetitive speech, agitation, flight of ideas, inability to speak, stuttering, slurring, impaired articulation, difficulty with phonation, inability to name words, inability to identify objects, difficulty comprehending communication, difficulty forming words or sentences, aphonia, dyslalia, dysarthria, inappropriate verbalizations, aphasia, dysphasia, apraxia, dyslexia

 DISTURBED SLEEP PATTERN (see ALZHEIMER'S DISEASE)

Related to: depression, antidepressant medications, confusion, boredom, environmental stimuli, obstructive sleep apnea

Defining Characteristics: interrupted sleep, difficulty falling asleep, awakening early, fatigue, lethargy, irritability, disorientation, complaints of not feeling rested, insomnia, sleeplessness, naps during the day, expressionless face, snoring, long periods of silence, apnea, sleepiness during the day, yawning, morning headache, loss of libido

 SOCIAL ISOLATION (see ALZHEIMER'S DISEASE)

Related to: depression, withdrawal, loneliness

Defining Characteristics: sad, dull affect, uncommunicative, withdrawn, expresses feeling of loneliness and aloneness, rejection, grief, significant loss(es), absence of supportive significant other(s), inability to meet expectations of others, indifference by others, lack of support systems

ADDITIONAL NURSING DIAGNOSES

 RISK FOR SUICIDE

Related to: undiagnosed or untreated depression, significant losses, loneliness, decreased abilities, decreased ability to cope, hopelessness, terminal illness, chronic disease, chronic pain

Defining Characteristics: threats of killing oneself, previous history of suicide attempt, significant abrupt changes in behavior, loss of independence, terminal illness, debilitating disease, chronic pain, changing items in one's will, making plans, stockpiling medications, impulsively purchasing a gun, sudden euphoric mood swings after suffering from major depression

Outcome Criteria

✔ Patient will not harm himself.
✔ Patient will be able to discuss feelings that might precipitate suicidal attempts and will be able to recover from suicidal ideations.
✔ Patient will recover from a suicide attempt.

NOC: *Suicide Self-Restraint*

INTERVENTIONS	RATIONALES
Monitor patient closely and provide suicide precautions: removal of all hazardous and potentially hazardous items from room and possession, checking on patient every 15 minutes, placement of patient next to nurse's station, ensuring all pills are swallowed, and ensuring all eating utensils are accounted for.	Provides for patient safety by ensuring environment is free from hazards and that patient is protected.
Attempt to provide one-on-one supervision of patient if possible.	Provides protection to patient and assures patient of personnel's concern for his welfare.
Make short-term contract with the patient that he will not harm himself during a specific time period. Continue with negotiating with patient, lengthening time limit, until no further suicidal ideation is noted.	Contracting with the patient addresses the subject of suicide and places some responsibility for safety on the patient while continuing to accept patient and his or her feelings.
Ask patient openly if he has thought about killing self, and if patient answers positively, ask about any plans.	Suicide success increases if patient has developed a plan. Addressing the subject of suicide will not put this thought into the patient's mind—patient has most likely already thought about it.
Use nonjudgmental attitude in dealing with patient.	Assures patient of your unconditional positive regard to improve his self-worth.
Provide time to discuss situation with patient, express understanding, but do not reinforce denial of current situation.	Denial can mask the origins of suicidal feelings.
Encourage patient to participate in activities, being careful to maintain supervision.	Helps patient to build self-esteem and self-worth.

(continues)

(continued)

INTERVENTIONS	RATIONALES
Assist patient to identify inappropriate coping strategies and those that will help patient to enhance own personal well-being.	Allows patient to use own strengths and skills to prevent self-destructive behaviors.
Instruct patient/family regarding setting goals for psychiatric care.	Uncertainty and doubt about obtaining psychiatric care or refusal to see a therapist indicates that the patient is using denial and identifies lack of insight into the problem.
Instruct patient/family regarding community resources, crisis centers, hot lines, and counselors.	Alternatives may alleviate apprehension about the intimidation of long-term psychiatric care.
Refer patient to appropriate mental health provider, and instruct family regarding ensuring that patient receives proper care.	Professional help will allow the patient to work through suicidal feelings and cultivate healthier alternatives and behavior.
Instruct family that patient's threats should be taken seriously and they should contact physician immediately for help.	Mistaken beliefs that the patient is only "acting out" or being manipulative may cause the family members to avoid acting on patient's threat, leading to potential fatal consequences. If the patient has made a suicide attempt previously, patient is far more likely to repeat the behavior.

NIC: *Suicide Prevention*

Discharge or Maintenance Evaluation

- Patient will have environment that is safe and free from hazardous materials.
- Patient will be able to identify suicidal plan and contract to refrain from acting on this plan for the specified time period.
- Patient will be able to access community resources and counselors for help in dealing with suicidal feelings and ideations.
- Family members will recognize patient's threats and feelings as being valid and act upon them.

DISTURBED ENERGY FIELD

Related to: depression, anxiety, lifestyle changes, loss of significant other, helplessness, withdrawal

Defining Characteristics: disruption of patient's field of energy, movement of energy, increased sensitivity to sounds and temperature, visual changes

Outcome Criteria

✔ Patient will achieve increased relaxation, less tension and pain, and be able to increase sense of well-being.

NOC: *Well-Being*

INTERVENTIONS	RATIONALES
Provide therapeutic touch techniques to support restorative healing. Hands should be placed approximately 4–6 inches above the patient's body and moved over the patient's body.	A trained practitioner can become familiar with the patient's energy field that surrounds his body, being able to distinguish energy field disturbances, as evidenced by feelings of heat, cold, or electric sensations.
Obtain patient's collaboration as you perform therapeutic touch.	Facilitates efficacy of healing techniques and enhances patient participation in spiritual aspects of care.
Provide massage therapy to extremities, back, and face as warranted.	Helps to relax patient and reduce tension.
Continue treatments with therapeutic healing techniques.	Several treatments may be required to re-establish the patient's sense of inner well-being.
Instruct patient in self-healing modalities, such as meditation, guided imagery, yoga, and prayer.	Assists with patient's participation and contributes to improvement in wellness.
Instruct patient regarding appropriate breathing techniques and biofeedback as warranted.	Slower, deeper breathing helps to relax patient, allay anxiety, and promote a sense of well-being.

NIC: *Energy Management*

NIC: *Therapeutic Touch*

Discharge or Maintenance Evaluation

- Patient will exhibit signs of relaxation and improved sense of well-being.
- Patient will exhibit a reduction in tension and/or pain.

INEFFECTIVE COPING

Related to: depression, lack of coping skills, physical or emotional impairment, loss of significant other, lack of support systems, change in lifestyle

Defining Characteristics: verbalizations of inability to cope, sleep disturbances, inappropriate coping strategies, social withdrawal, destructive behavior, irritability, aggressiveness, hostility, changes in communication pattern, inability to ask for help, fatigue, increased illness, poor concentration, decreased problem-solving ability, risk-taking behaviors, substance abuse, suicidal ideations and/or attempts

Outcome Criteria

✔ Patient will exhibit improvement in emotional well-being.

✔ Patient will use acceptable strategies to cope with problems, and will have improved sense of self-worth.

✔ Patient will be able to access support systems, community resources, or counselors to assist in achieving adequate coping skills.

NOC: *Coping*

INTERVENTIONS	RATIONALES
Provide care for patient using same personnel whenever possible.	Provides for continuity of care and the establishment of a trusting relationship.
Provide uninterrupted time to be spent with patient, and encourage him to express feelings and concerns.	Allows patient time to express extreme and powerful emotional feelings, and with discussion, patient can begin to comprehend the personal meaning attached to recent events and develop a reasonable assessment of the situation in order to identify a plan to deal constructively with the situation.
Assist patient only when necessary. Offer positive feedback for independent behavior.	Dependency on nurse decreases self-esteem. Encouraging desired behaviors promotes effective coping.
Encourage patient to make choices about his care.	Reduces helplessness and enhances sense of self-esteem.

INTERVENTIONS	RATIONALES
Identify expectations from patient for behavior and what consequences will occur if limits are not honored.	Helps to set boundaries for manipulative behavior. Manipulation by the patient reduces sense of insecurity by increasing feeling of power.
Assist patient to identify behavior and accept responsibility for actions. Do not allow patient to place blame on others unfairly.	A sense of responsibility needs to be developed before any changes can occur.
Identify patient's positive qualities and accomplishments and assist patient to recognize these traits.	Patient will have less need for manipulative behavior if self-esteem is increased.
Congratulate patient when he or she uses effective coping strategies.	Helps to reinforce suitable behavior.
Encourage patient to utilize community resources, support systems, counselors, and family and friends.	Helps to maintain effective coping skills.
Instruct patient/family in appropriate coping strategies.	Provides knowledge and identifies alternatives to inappropriate behavior.
Instruct patient/family regarding need for support groups, counselors, and so forth.	May be required postdischarge to continue to complete appropriate care and enable patient to effectively maintain coping skills.

NIC: *Coping Enhancement*

Discharge or Maintenance Evaluation

■ Patient will be able to work with personnel and assist in planning care.

■ Patient will be able to identify emotions that are triggered by crisis and develop coping strategies to appropriately deal with these crises.

■ Patient will be able to access resources and support systems for assistance with coping skills.

 ## DISTURBED THOUGHT PROCESSES

Related to: psychological causes, depression, incorrect belief system, chronic illness, misperceptions

Defining Characteristics: inaccurate interpretation of environment, changes in lifestyle, loss of a significant other, egocentricity, distractibility, inappropriate thinking, memory impairment, sorrow, hypovigilance, hypervigilance, chronic illness, insomnia, inability to perform activities as before, abnormal lab studies, uncaring attitude, inappropriate manner of dress and physical appearance

Outcome Criteria

✔ Patient will be able to identify factors that elicit depressive reactions and use techniques that will effectively reduce the amount and frequency of these episodes.

✔ Patient will be compliant with therapeutic regimen.

NOC: *Distorted Thought Control*

INTERVENTIONS	RATIONALES
Assess patient for depressive behaviors, causative events, and orient patient to reality as warranted.	Identifies specific problems and allows for the establishment of a plan of care. Reality orientation helps patient to be aware of self and surroundings.
Use nonjudgmental attitude toward patient and actively listen to his feelings and concerns.	Establishes a trusting relationship and permits patient to discuss topics that you can then help patient deal with in appropriate ways.
Identify patient's medications currently being taken.	Assists with identification of any misuse of the drugs, or to evaluate for potential side effects from polypharmacy, which may cause depressive symptoms.
Assess patient's level of orientation.	Depressed patients will frequently give an "I don't know" answer while patients with dementia may give improper responses.
Assess patient for potential for suicide and suicidal ideation.	Patients who are depressed and who have already thought about a suicide plan are serious, and need emergency help.
Monitor vital signs every 4 hours and prn.	Antidepressants and other psychoactive medications may result in cardiovascular and cerebrovascular insufficiency in the elderly, with resultant hypotension or hypertensive episodes. Tricyclic antidepressants cause orthostatic

INTERVENTIONS	RATIONALES
	hypotension and increase cardiac conduction time. Drug interactions may increase because of multiple medications being taken for concurrent disease processes.
Observe patient for drug reactions and toxicity.	The action of the psychoactive drugs will be normally prolonged in the elderly because of decreased blood flow and motility, and decreased renal function reduces excretion. Frequently a "normal" dose may be toxic in the elderly and may interfere with the absorption of other drugs.
Administer antidepressants as ordered, being alert for drug interactions, side effects, and for efficacy of treatment.	Antidepressants incorporate four classes of drugs: tricyclic antidepressants (TCAs), heterocyclic antidepressants, monoamine oxidase inhibitors (MAOIs), and selective serotonin reuptake inhibitors (SSRIs). TCAs prevent reuptake of serotonin and norepinephrine into the nerves to prevent depression. Side effects include orthostatic hypotension, cardiac conduction time increases, dry mouth, blurred vision, constipation, increased intraocular pressures, seizures, asthma, prostate problems, glucose level changes, hematologic disorders, and Parkinson-like symptoms. Heterocyclics may inhibit serotonin uptake in the brain cells, increase the amount in the synapses, and change the method by which serotonin adheres to receptor sites. Common side effects include drowsiness and hypotension. MAOIs can interact with many other drugs and foods and are not usually the best choice for elderly patients or patients with cardiac disease because of the serious hypertensive effects they may have when combined with other drugs. These drugs are reserved for patients who have not responded to other pharmacologic agents. MAO is the enzyme that breaks down norepinephrine, epinephrine,

INTERVENTIONS	RATIONALES
	and serotonin, and MAOIs prevent this metabolizing effect. Side effects include hypotension, fluid retention, restlessness, and anticholinergic effects. SSRIs inhibit the uptake of serotonin into the CNS neurons, thereby reducing depression. Side effects are usually minor, and include nausea, insomnia, headache, and nervousness. These drugs are bound to proteins so they can increase the drug levels of other protein-bound drugs, such as coumadin.
Administer lithium as ordered.	May be effective in recurrent major depression and is used for short-term therapy.
Administer Wellbutrin as ordered.	This drug is not connected with the other antidepressants and is thought to act by inhibiting dopamine uptake, and lacks the autonomic, cardiovascular, and sedative effects that some of the other drugs have. Side effects include anxiety, insomnia, constipation, restlessness, tremor, and seizures.
Provide for psychotherapy for patient.	Helps to alleviate anxiety and improves psychological functions. May be used in conjunction with drug therapy for the most promising results.
Prepare patient and assist with ECT as warranted.	ECT has been proven to be effective when treating severe depressive states that are not responsive to other types of therapy. The patient's cardiac rhythm and vital signs are monitored, patient will receive IV sedation, and treatments will be at least 48 hours apart. Common side effects are headache, confusion, and short-term memory loss. It is thought that ECT improves depression by increasing the level of norepinephrine.
Instruct patient/family regarding disease process, that usually depression is a common illness	Provides knowledge and encourages patient that there is hope for recovery.

INTERVENTIONS	RATIONALES
	and may be related to chemical imbalances in the brain, or to environmental factors that can be corrected.
Instruct patient/family regarding the use of antidepressants, their side effects, and assure patient that medication use is not addictive and may correct the chemical imbalance.	Provides knowledge, facilitates compliance, and helps to identify side effects which need to be reported to medical personnel.
Instruct patient/family that drug therapy may be required for up to a year, and sometimes indefinitely, based upon the patient and the situation.	Provides knowledge and encourages the process of obtaining the best results and facilitating compliance postdischarge.
Instruct patient/family in ECT therapy as warranted.	Patients and families may have preconceived ideas and misperceptions of therapy based on older types of ECT. Providing information allows for concerns and fears to be allayed.
Provide information regarding community resources, counselors, psychiatrists, and so forth.	Psychotherapy will require continuation to improve skills needed in dealing with abrupt changes in the elderly, conditioning, and relaxation training.

NIC: *Reality Orientation*

Discharge or Maintenance Evaluation

- Patient will be able to identify causative factors associated with depression and utilize methods to effectively cope with situations.
- Patient will be compliant with drug therapy regimen.
- Patient will suffer no long-lasting side effects from antidepressants or ECT.
- Patient will be compliant with continuing psychotherapy postdischarge.
- Patient will be able to access community resources for care needed.
- Family will assist patient to continue with treatment.
- Patient and family will be able to accurately recall information relayed to them.

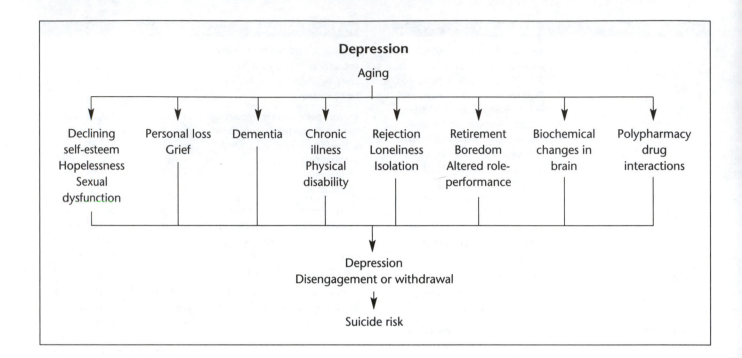

CHAPTER 3.4

PARKINSON'S DISEASE

Parkinson's disease, or paralysis agitans, is a neurologic disorder that normally occurs after the age of 50, and increases in incidence with age. Most occurrences of the disease are primary parkinsonism in which the basal ganglia of the extrapyramidal system modify the system that controls voluntary motor function. Cell loss occurs in the substantia nigra, which in turn decreases the level of striatal dopamine, and this results in illness. The disease is progressive and characterized by slowing and weakening of movements, tremors, rigidity, and continues to a state of the patient's complete dependence on others for care. Neuromuscular and motor function changes eventually result in respiratory, mobility, elimination, and nutritional impairments.

A second form of Parkinson's disease is secondary parkinsonism which occurs as a result of other causes, but frequently is initiated by the use of antipsychotic drugs. In this form of the disease, nigral cell loss can occur, the nigral striatal pathway may be damaged, or elements necessary for striatal cells may be missing. Causes of secondary parkinsonism include viral encephalitis, atherosclerosis of cerebral blood vasculature, use of antipsychotics, reserpine, metoclopramide, methyldopa, meperidine analog, carbon monoxide, manganese, hypoparathyroidism, basal ganglia brain tumors, head trauma, and dementia-type illnesses. Striatal dopamine deficiency is the classic sign in both forms of parkinsonism. The basis for nigral cell damage is unidentified completely, but researchers believe that cellular damage is a result of the process of toxic oxygen free-radicals that leads to deprivation of dopamine stores and toxic metabolic products that collect in the cells.

Shy-Drager syndrome, which is similar to Parkinson's disease, has one major distinguishing aspect that sets it apart from parkinsonism, namely, the significant autonomic dysfunction and failure. Death usually occurs from 7–10 years after the beginning of neurologic symptoms and is a result of dysrhythmias, sleep apnea, or pulmonary emboli.

Currently, there is no cure for either type of the disease, with the exception of reversible parkinsonism caused by drugs, in which removal of the drug will reverse the disease. Patients require treatment for their entire life to control the symptoms.

Symptoms of primary parkinsonism may occur in combinations of signs or as a single symptom. The hallmark manifestation is tremor of the hand, present at rest but absent during sleep, involving the fingers in a pill-rolling motion. Rigidity of the muscles during passive movement, bradykinesia, and sudden and abrupt cessation of movement are other signs noted in the disease. Eventually, a shuffling gait with short steps, rapid speech with words running together, and rapid finger tapping ensue. Patient can sometimes remain functional for several years, or may become disabled within the course of 5 years.

MEDICAL CARE

Laboratory: there are no tests to confirm diagnosis; CSF may show decreased levels of homovanilla acid but this is not conclusive

CT scan: will not show abnormalities in parkinsonism but may be helpful in diagnosis of secondary parkinsonism

Magnetic resonance imaging: will not show abnormalities in parkinsonism but may be of some help in diagnosis of secondary parkinsonism

Positron emission tomography (PET) scan: a specialized deoxyglucose PET scan of the brain may show abnormal patterns of glucose metabolism characteristic of Parkinson's disease

Antiparkinsonian drugs: benztropine mesylate (Cogentin), bromocriptine mesylate (Parlodel), carbidopa-levodopa (Sinemet), entacapone (Comton), levadopa (Dopar, Larodopa), pergolide mesylate (Permax), pramipexole dihydrochloride (Mirapex), ropinirole hydrochloride (Requip), selegiline hydrochloride (Eldepryl), tolcapone (Tasmar), or triheyphenidyl hydrochloride (Artane, Trihexane, Trihexy) are some of the drugs used to treat tremors by reducing the excess cholinergic effect associated with dopamine deficiency, but should be used cautiously in the elderly because of the side effects they produce; dopaminergics used to inhibit metabolism of dopamine and allow more of the substance to be available for transport to the brain and to activate dopamine receptors for relief of the tremor, rigidity, and kinesia; monoamine oxidase inhibitors used to augment the effect of dopamine by inhibiting the enzyme that degrades it, and may help to prevent or slow the disease progression; dopamine replacement usually done with carbidopa-levodopa which is converted to dopamine in the central nervous system

Surgery: surgical transplantation of fetal nigral cells to the patient's corpus striatum can produce and replenish the dopamine deficit in parkinsonism, but selection criteria for this procedure is very strict and the effects have not been completely evaluated; stereotactic pallidotomy reduces severe dyskinesias, improves bradykinesia, and improves rigidity; thalamotomy or implantation of a thalamic stimulator may be used to treat disabling tremors proven to be drug resistant

COMMON NURSING DIAGNOSES

 ### INEFFECTIVE AIRWAY CLEARANCE (see COPD)

Related to: parkinsonian changes in musculature, tracheobronchial obstruction, aspiration, infection, truncal rigidity, bronchospasm, fatigue, increased work of breathing, increased mucus production, thick secretions, decreased energy

Defining Characteristics: dyspnea, tachypnea, bradypnea, bronchospasms, increased work of breathing, use of accessory muscles, increased mucus production, cough with or without productivity, adventitious breath sounds, abnormal arterial blood gases

 ### DISTURBED THOUGHT PROCESSES (see DEPRESSION)

Related to: use of parkinsonian medications, psychological causes, depression, incorrect belief system, chronic illness, misperceptions

Defining Characteristics: inaccurate interpretation of environment, changes in lifestyle, loss of a significant other, egocentricity, distractibility, inappropriate thinking, memory impairment, sorrow, hypovigilance, hypervigilance, chronic illness, insomnia, inability to perform activities as before, abnormal lab studies, uncaring attitude, inappropriate manner of dress and physical appearance, memory loss, argumentative, inability to make decisions, inability to grasp ideas, toxic levels of medications, akinesia

 ### IMPAIRED VERBAL COMMUNICATION (see ALZHEIMER'S DISEASE)

Related to: physical barrier from hypertonicity from parkinsonism, rigidity of facial muscles, depression, medications, psychological barriers, psychosis, decreased circulation to brain, age-related factors, lack of stimuli

Defining Characteristics: confusion, anxiety, restlessness, agitation, flight of ideas, inability to speak, stuttering, impaired articulation, difficulty with phonation, inability to name words, inability to identify objects, difficulty comprehending communication, difficulty forming words or sentences, aphonia, dyslalia, dysarthria, inappropriate verbalizations, aphasia, dysphasia, apraxia, slurred, slow monotonous speech, drooling saliva, repetitive speech, rapid speech, high-pitched, hoarse, trembling speech, hypertonicity, facial muscle rigidity, polypharmacy

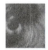 ### IMPAIRED PHYSICAL MOBILITY (see ALZHEIMER'S DISEASE)

Related to: Parkinson's disease, dementia, inability to bear weight, poor nutrition, perceptual impairment, cognitive impairment, tremors, rigidity, bradykinesia

Defining Characteristics: inability to move at will, weakness, inability to bear weight, immobility, gait disturbances, balance and coordination deficits, difficulty turning, decreased fine and gross motor movement, decreased range of motion, tremors, instability while standing, dyspnea, decreased reaction time, incoordination, jerky movement, swaying, postural disturbances, small, shuffling steps, leaning forward with head bent, akinesia, muscle rigidity, bradykinesia, dementia, cognitive decline

 IMBALANCED NUTRITION: LESS THAN BODY REQUIREMENTS (see COPD)

Related to: parkinsonian changes in musculature, facial rigidity, use of antiparkinsonian drugs, inability to take in enough food, decreased level of consciousness, inability to absorb nutrients because of biologic or psychological factors from aging process

Defining Characteristics: actual inadequate food intake, weight loss, body weight 20% or more under ideal for height and frame, anorexia, absent bowel sounds, decreased peristalsis, muscle mass loss, decreased muscle tone, changes in bowel habits, nausea, vomiting, abdominal distention, lack of interest in food, satiety immediately after ingesting food, abdominal pain or discomfort, depression, anxiety, social isolation, difficulty in feeding self, changes in mental status, fatigue from work of breathing, choking, coughing, rigidity of facial muscles

 IMPAIRED SWALLOWING (see CVA)

Related to: Parkinson's disease, neuromuscular impairment, dysphagia

Defining Characteristics: inability to swallow effectively, choking, aspiration, food remaining in oral cavity, slow eating, difficulty swallowing, chewing, stiff, masklike face, choking, drooling, weight loss, facial rigidity, muscle rigidity, tremors, aspiration

 RISK FOR INJURY (see ALZHEIMER'S DISEASE)

Related to: Parkinson's disease, dementia, lack of awareness of environmental hazards, poor judgment, medications, hallucinations, choking, bradykinesia, akinesia

Defining Characteristics: confusion, disorientation, malnutrition, altered mobility, skin breakdown, agitation, physical discomfort, choking, wounds, falls, wandering, involuntary movements, loss of postural adjustment, loss of balance, loss of arm swinging movement, difficulty initiating movement, shuffling gait, slowness of movement, orthostatic hypotension, activity intolerance, polypharmacy, hallucinations, tremors, muscle rigidity

 INEFFECTIVE COPING (see DEPRESSION)

Related to: progressive chronic disease, limitations imposed by disease, depression, lack of coping skills, physical or emotional impairment caused by normal aging changes or parkinsonism, change in lifestyle

Defining Characteristics: verbalizations of inability to cope, inappropriate coping strategies, social withdrawal, irritability, aggressiveness, hostility, changes in communication pattern, inability to ask for help, fatigue, increased illness, poor concentration, decreased problem-solving ability, risk-taking behaviors, inability to meet basic needs, poor self-esteem, insomnia, anorexia

ADDITIONAL NURSING DIAGNOSES

DEFICIENT KNOWLEDGE

Related to: lack of knowledge about Parkinson's disease, stigma of disease, difficulty understanding about disease process, lack of coping skills, cognitive impairment

Defining Characteristics: verbalization of questions, verbalization of incorrect information, noncompliant behavior, presence of preventable complications, inability to follow instructions, inappropriate behaviors, agitation, restlessness, apathy, depression, withdrawal

Outcome Criteria

✔ Patient/family will be able to exhibit understanding of disease process, medication regimen, and treatment plan of care.

NOC: *Knowledge: Disease Process*

INTERVENTIONS	RATIONALES
Assess patient's understanding of disease process. Consider the older patient's life experiences.	Provides baseline of understanding from which to establish a plan of care. New information can be based upon the patient's existing knowledge base and life experience.
Instruct patient/family about Parkinson's disease, signs and symptoms, treatments, and	Elderly patients may only be aware of old information and the stigma that was attached to

(continues)

(continued)

INTERVENTIONS	RATIONALES
prevention of complications. Limit length of teaching sessions and provide quiet environment for each session.	Parkinson's disease and dementia, and will require re-education regarding current treatments. Reduction of extraneous stimuli assists with learning and the ability to process new information without distraction. Short sessions allow patient to learn at own speed and prevent information overload.
Prepare patient for surgery as indicated.	Surgical options may be required to replenish dopamine, improve dyskinesias and rigidity, or to treat disabling drug-resistant tremors.
Instruct patient/family regarding medications and need for compliance with dosages, scheduling, and physician follow-up.	Provides knowledge and facilitates compliance with treatment regimen. Provides for timely identification of serious adverse effect from medication regimen to allow physician to be notified postdischarge from hospital.
Instruct family regarding side effects from medications and when to notify physician.	Anticholinergic drugs, such as diphenhydramine, procyclidine, and trihexyphenidyl can cause sedation, confusion, urinary retention, dry mouth, blurred vision, and hallucinations. Dopaminergic drugs, such as carbidopa-levodopa can result in nausea, anorexia, confusion, psychotic disturbances, dyskinesia, and nightmares. Dopamine agonists, such as bromocriptine, pergolide, pramiperxole, and ropinirole, can cause nausea, vomiting, confusion, hallucinations, dyskinesia, and hypotension. MAOIs, such as selegiline, can cause nausea, insomnia, and confusion. Amantadine can cause urinary retention, increased

INTERVENTIONS	RATIONALES
	intraocular pressures, and confusion. Catechol O-methyltransferase inhibitors, such as tolcapone, can result in nausea, confusion, hallucinations, diarrhea, dyskinesias, and hepatitis.
Provide time for questions and concerns to be voiced, and answer questions honestly. If possible, give patient/family written materials to refer to later.	Provides for correction of misinformation and written materials allow for documentation to assist with care once patient is discharged.
Instruct patient/family regarding need for long-term planning and potential for end-of-life care decisions.	Disease is chronic and patient will eventually become severely impaired. Drugs may lose their effectiveness, and patient may not be able to eat. Issues such as whether the patient wants resuscitation efforts, tube feedings, and so forth. should be discussed to enable patient and family to make informed choices while the patient is capable of understanding the severity of his condition.

NIC: *Teaching: Disease Process*

Discharge or Maintenance Evaluation

- Patient will be able to accurately verbalize understanding of parkinsonism and its treatment.
- Patient will be able to comply with medication regimen and to notify physician if patient experiences untoward side effects.
- Patient/family will be able to identify and demonstrate safety precautions to prevent injury.
- Patient/family will be able to identify need for long-term goals and potential for end-of-life decisions to be made.

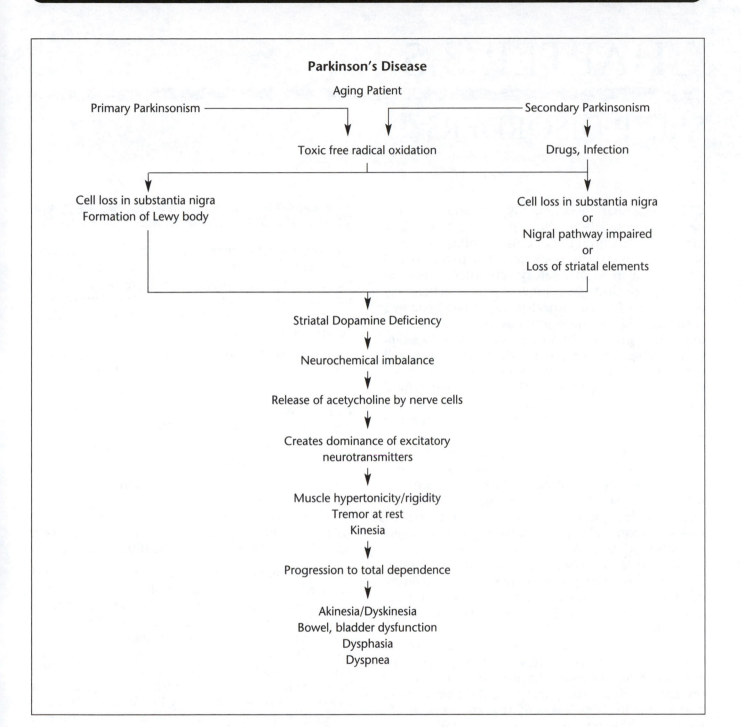

Parkinson's Disease

Aging Patient

Primary Parkinsonism ─────────────┐   ┌───────── Secondary Parkinsonism

Toxic free radical oxidation   Drugs, Infection

Cell loss in substantia nigra   Cell loss in substantia nigra
Formation of Lewy body   or
                    Nigral pathway impaired
                    or
                    Loss of striatal elements

Striatal Dopamine Deficiency

Neurochemical imbalance

Release of acetycholine by nerve cells

Creates dominance of excitatory
neurotransmitters

Muscle hypertonicity/rigidity
Tremor at rest
Kinesia

Progression to total dependence

Akinesia/Dyskinesia
Bowel, bladder dysfunction
Dysphasia
Dyspnea

CHAPTER 3.5

SLEEP DISORDERS

Sleep disorders are commonly encountered in the elderly population, with up to half of all older persons complaining about their ability to sleep. Some sleep dysfunctions are caused by psychological stressors, such as mandatory retirement, bereavement over the loss of a significant person in their life, or the loss of physical health. Age-related changes with sleeping include falling asleep earlier, awakening earlier, and less tolerance of changes in the sleep-wake cycle. Daytime naps may offset reduced nighttime sleep, but may also contribute to poor nocturnal sleeping patterns. The elderly tend to have an increase in the time it takes to fall asleep, frequency of nighttime awakenings, and a decrease in REM sleep.

The most common sleep disorders found in the elderly are insomnia and sleep apnea. Other disorders include hypersomnia or excessive sleep and nocturnal behavior. Sundowner's syndrome is manifested by disorientation and wandering during the late afternoon and evening because the patient gets days and nights confused.

Insomnia is characterized by the inability or difficulty in falling asleep, frequent awakening during sleep, awakening early in the morning, daytime fatigue, irritability, and difficulty with concentration.

Sleep apnea is characterized by cessation of breathing for periods of time during sleep, causing a decrease in oxygen concentration, which then wakes the patient before completing the REM sleep cycle. This results in sleepiness, lethargy, and exhaustion. Because of the extreme oxygen desaturations that occur, pulmonary and systemic hypertension and/or cardiac dysrhythmias may occur. Morbidity increases in obstructive sleep apnea if episodes occur more often than 10 times per hour.

MEDICAL CARE

Polysomnography: used to do overnight monitoring of patient's sleep cycles to reveal electrical activity of heart and brain, cerebral, muscle, ribcage, abdominal, and eye movements, nasal airflow, and oxygen saturation, and to diagnose the presence of sleep apnea and hypoxemia

Electroencephalogram: used to reveal sleep stages as seen by monitoring patient utilizing brain wave activity

Continuous positive airway pressure (CPAP) therapy: used in cases of severe obstructive sleep apnea to prevent oxygen desaturations by providing continuous positive pressure to keep airways open

Surgery: tracheostomy may be required for patients with severe apnea when all other measures have failed; uvulopalatopharngoplasty may be done to enlarge the pharyngeal airspace by removal of excess tissue but is effective less than half the time

Sedative-hypnotics: chloral hydrate (Aquachloral Supprettes), dexmedetomidine hydrochloride (Precedex), estazolam (ProSom), flurazepam hydrochloride (Dalmane), pentobarbital (Nembutal), secobarbital sodium (Seconal Sodium), temazepam (Restoril), triazolam (Halcion), zalepion (Sonata), or zolpidem tartrate (Ambien) used for short-term relief of insomnia; drugs act upon the limbic system and thalamus of the CNS, usually by binding to certain receptors to produce a hypnotic or sedative effect

Respiratory stimulants: methylphenidate hydrochloride (Ritalin, Ritalin-SR) used to reduce apneic episodes by increasing the respiratory drive in central apnea

COMMON NURSING DIAGNOSES

INEFFECTIVE BREATHING PATTERN (see TB)

Related to: tracheobronchial obstruction of sleep apnea, decreased lung volume, decreased lung capacity, increased metabolic needs

Defining Characteristics: snoring, apnea, hypoxia, cough with or without production, increased respiratory rate, tachycardia, use of accessory muscles, nasal flaring, pursed-lip breathing, orthopnea, dyspnea, sternal retractions, diaphoresis, abnormal arterial blood gases, fatigue, yawning, lethargy, oxygen desaturation

DISTURBED THOUGHT PROCESSES (see DEPRESSION)

Related to: sleep deprivation, sleep apnea, insomnia, psychological causes, depression, hypoxia

Defining Characteristics: inaccurate interpretation of environment, egocentricity, distractibility, inappropriate thinking, memory impairment, confusion, disorientation, lethargy, insomnia, inability to perform activities as before, toxic levels of medications, oxygen desaturation, decreased mental acuity, depression, fatigue, insomnia

DISTURBED SLEEP PATTERNS (see ALZHEIMER'S DISEASE)

Related to: internal factors of disease processes, depression, confusion, boredom, environmental stimuli, obstructive sleep apnea

Defining Characteristics: interrupted sleep, difficulty falling asleep, awakening early, fatigue, lethargy, irritability, disorientation, complaints of not feeling rested, insomnia, sleeplessness, naps during the day, expressionless face, snoring, long periods of silence, apnea, sleepiness during the day, yawning, morning headache, loss of libido, oxygen desaturations, lack of REM sleep

ANXIETY (see CAD)

Related to: sleep apnea, sleep deprivation, threat of change in health status, life-threatening crises, chronic nature of disease and effect on lifestyle, change in role functioning, decreased energy, exhaustion, sexual dysfunction

Defining Characteristics: fear, restlessness, muscle tension, helplessness, communication of uncertainty and apprehension, feeling of suffocation, feelings of inadequacy, feelings of exhaustion, insomnia, sleep apnea, verbalizations of fear of consequences of sleep apnea, impotence

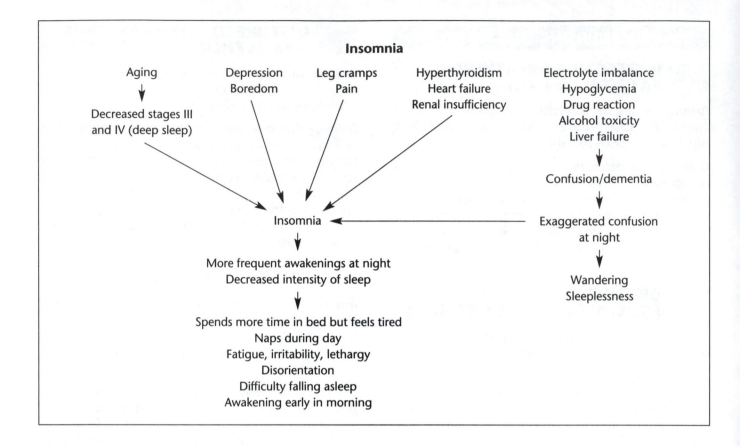

Insomnia

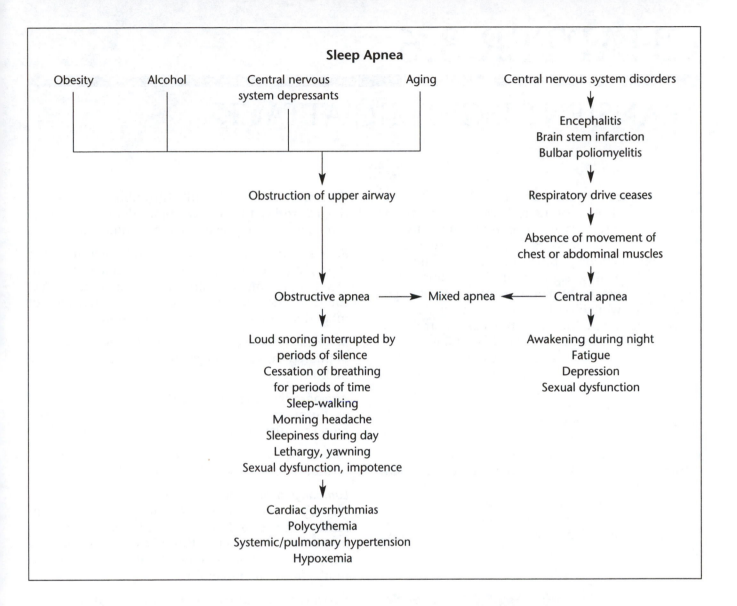

CHAPTER 3.6

TRANSIENT ISCHEMIC ATTACK

Transient ischemic attacks, or TIAs, are brief, temporary episodes of neurologic loss of vision, motor, and/or sensory function that can last from a few minutes up to 24 hours. They are caused by temporary obstructions of blood flow to the brain, and can be a warning sign of an impending CVA. Approximately one-third of those patients who experience a TIA will go on to have a completed stroke, but having a TIA increases the risk of stroke by approximately 10% (Beers & Berkow, 2000).

Symptoms of TIAs mirror those of a stroke but are temporary in nature and do not cause any irreversible damage. Signs and symptoms include a sudden weakness or paresthesia on one side of the body, abrupt dimness or loss of vision, especially in one eye, sudden slurring of speech, loss of speech, or difficulty understanding communication, dizziness, difficulty walking, loss of coordination, sudden, severe headache without any apparent cause, dysphagia, confusion, and nausea and vomiting.

Risk factors associated with TIAs include hypertension, hyperlipidemia, atherosclerosis, and polycythemia in the elderly population.

MEDICAL CARE

Laboratory: CBC used to identify blood loss or infection; serum osmolality used to evaluate oncotic pressures and permeability; electrolytes, glucose levels, and urinalysis performed to identify problems and imbalances that may be responsible for changes in condition; coagulation studies used to monitor anticoagulant therapy efficacy

Radiography: skull X-rays may show calcifications of the carotids in the presence of cerebral thrombosis, or partial calcification of an aneurysm in subarachnoid hemorrhage; pineal gland may shift to the opposite side if mass is expanding; may reveal evidence of shift if hematoma or cerebral edema present

CT scans: used to identify thrombosis or hemorrhagic stroke, tumors, cerebral edema, or hydrocephalus; may not reveal changes immediately

Brain scans: used to identify ischemic areas resulting from CVA but usually are not discernible until up to 2 weeks postinjury; brain nuclear scans may reveal the disruption in the blood-brain barrier, area of infarction, size and location of hematoma

Magnetic resonance imaging: used to identify areas of infarction, hemorrhage, ischemia, edema, and AV malformations

Angiography: used to identify site and degree of occlusion or rupture of vessel and to assess collateral blood circulation and presence of AV malformations

Ultrasonography: may be used to gather information regarding flow velocity in the major circulation

Lumbar puncture: performed to evaluate ICP and to identify infection; bloody CSF may indicate a hemorrhagic stroke, and clear fluid with normal pressures may be noted in cerebral thrombosis, embolism, and with TIAs; protein may be elevated if thrombosis results from inflammation

Electroencephalogram: used to help localize area of injury based on brain wave pattern and electrical activity

Surgery: endarterectomy may be required to remove the occlusive atherosclerotic plaque from the intima of the carotid artery, or microvascular bypass may be performed to bypass the occluded area, such as the carotid artery, aneurysm, or AV malformation

Corticosteroids: betamethasone (Celestone), cortisone acetate (Cortone), dexamethasone acetate or sodium phosphate (Decadron, Dexone, Hexadrol, Solurex LA, Cortastat, Dalalone, Dexasone), hydrocortisone acetate , sodium phosphate, or sodium succinate (Cortef, Cortenema, Hydrocortone, Solu-Cortef), methylprednisolone acetate or sodium succinate

(Medrol, Depo-Medrol, Duralone, Medralone, Solu-Medrol), prednisolone acetate, sodium phosphate, or tebutate (Delta-Cortef, Prelone, Cotolone, Predalone, Predate, Prenisol), prednisone (Deltasone, Meticorten, Orasone, Prednisone Intensol, Sterapred), or triamcinolone (Aristocort, Atolone, Kenacort, Azmacort, Trilog, Amcort, Trilone) used to decrease cerebral inflammation and edema

Anticonvulsants: carbamazepine (Atretol, Epitol, Tegretol), clonazepam (Klonopin), ethosuximide (Zarontin), gabapentin (Neurontin), lamotrigine (Lamictal), levatiracetam (Keppra), magnesium sulfate, oxcarbazepine (Trileptal), Phenobarbital (Barbita, Solfoton, Luminal), phenytoin sodium (Dilantin, Phenytex), primidone (Mysoline, PMS), tiagabine hydrochloride (Gabitril), topiramate (Topamax), valproate sodium or acid (Depacon, Depakene, Depakote), or zonisamide (Zonegran) believed to stabilize neuronal membrane and suppress neuronal hypersynchronization; used in treatment and prophylaxis of seizure activity

Analgesics: acetaminophen (Tylenol), ibuprofen (Motrin, Advil, Genpril, Ibuprofen, Nuprin, Trendar), and acetylsalicylic acid (ASA, aspirin) used to reduce discomfort and pain

t-PA (tissue plasminogen activator): only drug currently approved by the FDA for the treatment of ischemic stroke; used to help dissolve blood clots, but contraindicated for hemorrhagic stroke

Neuroprotective agents: drugs such as glutamate antagonists, calcium antagonists, and antioxidants being investigated for helping to reduce injury to neurons, and may help stop or lessen damaging biochemical changes that result in secondary brain impairment after a stroke

Anticoagulants: enoxaparin sodium (Lovenox), heparin calcium and sodium (Calciparin, Heparin), and warfarin (Coumadin) used to reduce risk of further thrombus accumulation and to prevent recurrent clot formation by inhibiting prothrombin synthesis and reducing vitamin K dependent clotting factors

Platelet aggregation inhibitors: acetylsalicylic acid (ASA, aspirin) prevents platelet aggregation; cilostazol (Pletal) decreases platelet aggregation by inhibiting phosphodiesterase III; clopidogrel bisulfate (Plavix) inhibits platelet aggregation by binding to and changing the platelet ADP receptor to inhibit ADP-mediated platelet activation and platelet aggregation; dipyridamole (Persantine) increases adenosine and inhibits platelet aggregation; eptifibatide (Integrilin) and tirofiban hydrochloride (Aggrastat) bind to the glycoprotein IIb/IIIa receptor to inhibit aggregation of platelets; these drugs used to prevent clot formation and subsequent occlusion

Antihypertensives: vasodilators (hydralazine [Apresoline], minoxidil [Loniten], and nitroprusside sodium [Nitropress]) used to relax smooth muscle in the arterioles that help to reduce peripheral resistance; beta-adrenergic blockers: ([Sectral], atenolol [Tenormin], betaxolol [Kerlone], bisoprolol fumarate [Zebeta], carteolol hydrochloride [Cartrol], carvedilol [Coreg], metoprolol [Lopressor], nadolol [Corgard], penbutolol [Levatol], pindolol [Visken], propranolol [Inderal], and timolol maleate [Blocadren]) used to decrease blood pressure by inhibiting impulse through the sympathetic pathways, and to decrease cardiac output, sympathetic stimulation, and renin secretion by the kidneys; alpha-adrenergic blockers: (doxazosin mesylate [Cardura], fenoldopam mesylate [Corlopam], labetalol hydrochloride [Normodyne, Trandate], phentolamine mesylate [Regitine], prazosin hydrochloride [Minipress], and terazosin hydrochloride [Hytrin]) used to reduce blood pressure by acting on the peripheral vasculature to generate vasodilatory action and to decrease peripheral vascular resistance; calcium channel blockers: (diltiazem [Cardizem], felodipine [Plendil], isradipine [DynaCirc], nicardipine [Cardene], nifedipine [Procardia], nisoldipine [Sular], and verapamil [Calan, Isoptin]) used to reduce blood pressure by the inhibition of calcium ion influx across the smooth muscle and cardiac cells which reduces arteriolar resistance; angiotensin-converting enzyme (ACE) inhibitors: (benazepril hydrochloride [Lotensin], candesartan cilexetil [Atacand], captopril [Capoten], enalapril maleate [Vasotec], eprosartan mesylate [Teveten], fosinopril sodium [Monopril], moexipril hydrochloride [Univasc], perindopril erbumine [Aceon], quinapril hydrochloride [Accupril], ramipril [Altace], telmisartan [Micardis], and trandolapril [Mavik]) used to lower blood pressure by inhibiting ACE which prevents the conversion of angiotensin I to angiotensin II, which is a strong vasoconstrictor; the reduction in angiotensin II helps to reduce the peripheral arterial resistance and decreases aldosterone secretion, which effectively reduces the water and sodium retention to lower blood pressure;

angiotensin II receptor blockers: (irbesartan [Avapro], losartan potassium [Cozaar], and valsartan [Diovan]) used to reduce blood pressure by blocking the binding of angiotensin II to the receptor sites in the vascular smooth muscle to help inhibit the pressor effect of the renin-angiotensin-aldosterone system; central-acting adrenergics: (clonidine hydrochloride [Catapres], guanabenz acetate [Wytensin], guanfacine hydrochloride [Tenex], hydralazine hydrochloride [Apresoline], lisinopril [Prinivil, Zestril], and methyldopa hydrochloride [Aldomet]) used to help decrease sympathetic outflow to the heart, kidneys, and peripheral vessels in order to decrease peripheral vascular resistance, heart rate, and blood pressure

Hyperosmotics: mannitol (Osmitrol) and urea carbamide (Ureaphil) used to reduce intracranial pressure caused by cerebral edema

COMMON NURSING DIAGNOSES

INEFFECTIVE TISSUE PERFUSION: CEREBRAL (see CVA)

Related to: occlusion, hemorrhage, interruption of cerebral blood flow, vasospasm, edema

Defining Characteristics: changes in level of consciousness, mental changes, personality changes, memory loss, restlessness, combativeness, vital sign changes, motor function impairment, sensory impairment, lethargy, stupor, coma, increased intracranial pressure, headache, cognitive dysfunction

INEFFECTIVE AIRWAY CLEARANCE (see COPD)

Related to: decreased level of consciousness, tracheobronchial obstruction, potential for aspiration

Defining Characteristics: ineffective cough, tachypnea, dyspnea, abnormal breath sounds, respiratory rate and depth changes, decreased response to stimuli, choking, ineffective swallowing, abnormal arterial blood gases, decreased oxygen saturation

IMPAIRED VERBAL COMMUNICATION (see CVA)

Related to: weakness, loss of muscle control, cerebral circulation impairment, neuromuscular impairment, stroke

Defining Characteristics: inability to speak, inability to identify objects, inability to comprehend language, inability to write, inability to choose and use appropriate words, dysarthria

IMPAIRED PHYSICAL MOBILITY (see ALZHEIMER'S DISEASE)

Related to: paralysis, paresthesias, effects of stroke, neuromuscular impairment, impaired cognition, weakness

Defining Characteristics: inability to move at will, muscle incoordination, decreased range of motion, decreased muscle strength, paralysis, muscle atrophy, flaccidity, deformity, contracture of limb(s), tremors, alteration in gait, shuffling, swaying, difficulty with turning

DISTURBED SENSORY PERCEPTION: VISUAL, KINESTHETIC, GUSTATORY, TACTILE, OLFACTORY (see ALZHEIMER'S DISEASE)

Related to: TIA, stroke, neurologic trauma/deficit, stress, altered reception of stimuli, altered integration from neurological disease

Defining Characteristics: behavior changes, disorientation to time, place, self, and circumstance, diminished concentration, inability to focus, alteration in thought processes, decreased sensation, paresthesias, paralysis, altered ability to taste and smell, inability to recognize objects, muscle incoordination, muscle weakness, inappropriate communication, changes in visual acuity

IMBALANCED NUTRITION: LESS THAN BODY REQUIREMENTS (see COPD)

Related to: TIA, stroke, inability to ingest food, dysphagia, absent gag reflex

Defining Characteristics: anorexia, choking, aspiration, inability to feed self, food remaining in mouth, weight loss, coma, weakness of muscles involved with eating, altered taste sensation, lack of interest in eating, abdominal pain, diarrhea, inadequate food intake, loss of weight despite adequate food intake, swallowing difficulty, paralysis, gastric paresis

IMPAIRED SWALLOWING (see CVA)

Related to: TIA, stroke, neuromuscular impairment

Defining Characteristics: inability to swallow effectively, choking, aspiration

ADDITIONAL NURSING DIAGNOSES

DEFICIENT KNOWLEDGE

Related to: lack of information about strokes and TIAs, cognitive limitations, medications, neurologic impairment

Defining Characteristics: request for information, anxiety regarding potential errors, presence of preventable complications, noncompliance with instructions, misperceptions about illness

Outcome Criteria

✔ Patient will be able to understand and comply with treatment plan and medication regimen, without progression of condition to CVA.

NOC: *Knowledge: Disease Process*

INTERVENTIONS	RATIONALES
Assess patient for knowledge of the disease process, treatment regimen, medications, and signs of impending CVA.	Provides baseline knowledge from which to identify needs and establish plan of care for teaching.
Apply cervical collar, as ordered, to avoid hyperextension, lateral movement of the neck, or any quick movement involving the head and neck.	Compression on neck vasculature resulting from cervical vertebral changes may lead to symptoms of TIA or bradycardias.

INTERVENTIONS	RATIONALES
Discuss need for proper administration of medications, including fibrinolytics, and potential outcomes.	Provides information regarding severity of condition and need to prevent further complications, such as stroke. Knowledge helps facilitate compliance.
Instruct patient/family in signs and symptoms of TIA activity, and to report these signs to physician if they continue longer than 15 minutes.	Most elderly patients do not notify their physician of what may be impending CVA symptomatology. Notification of physician allows the opportunity for early intervention, prevention of complications, and opportunity for medication adjustment.
Instruct patient in methods to use to maintain stability, holding onto furniture, use of walking aids, looking straight ahead while walking, and so forth.	Helps to prevent falls during TIA.
Instruct patient to rise from lying position slowly, sitting on side of bed for few minutes prior to rising.	Helps to allow body fluids time to equilibrate and prevents orthostatic hypotension.

NIC: *Teaching: Disease Process*

Discharge or Maintenance Evaluation

- Patient will be able to identify signs and symptoms of TIA that should be reported to physician.
- Patient will be compliant with notifying physician of any neurologic symptoms that may relate to TIA or CVA.
- Patient will be compliant with drug regimen, and be able to identify adverse side effects and report those to his physician.
- Patient will be able to avoid falls by modifying environment to minimize hazards.
- Patient will have no adverse reactions to medications administered for TIA.

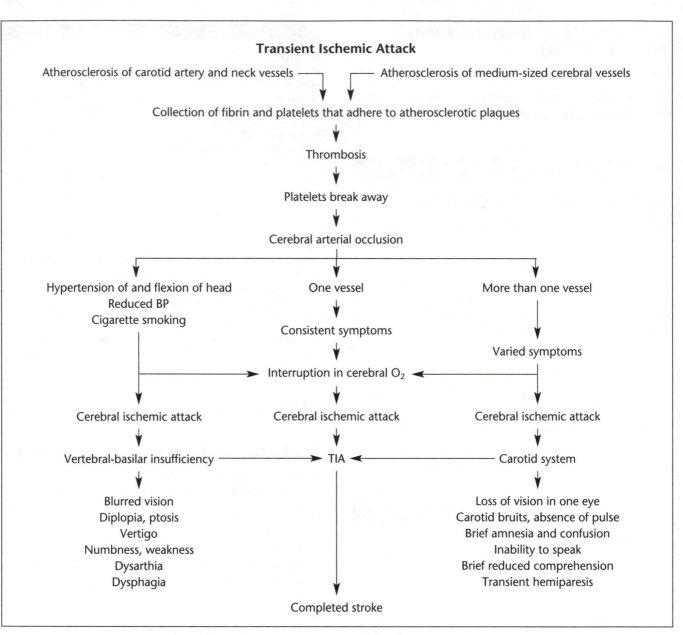

UNIT 4
GASTROINTESTINAL/ HEPATIC SYSTEMS

CHAPTER 4.1

BOWEL DISORDERS

The elderly patient is frequently preoccupied with bowel elimination. Bowel motility, the effects of medications, and changes in the physiology of defecation in the elderly contribute to the problems experienced. Autonomic nervous system control of intestinal motility may cause constipation while cortical inhibition may cause diarrhea.

Constipation is technically defined as a decrease in stool frequency, but patients frequently consider constipation to be difficult passage of hard, formed stool or a feeling of incomplete evacuation. Constipation is the most familiar complaint in the older patient, with at least 60% of patients relating some form of laxative usage.

Causes of constipation include medications, immobility, muscle weakness, neuromuscular dysfunction, alterations in mental status, metabolic disorders, and decreased food and fluid intake. Alterations in the digestive process affected by the aging process include changes in enzyme and acid secretion, reduction of nutrients, absorption, transport, and motility. Nervous system changes contribute to the control of organic functions by the changes in sensory and motor losses affecting peripheral nerve conduction. Parasympathetic and sympathetic function that affects intestinal motility and enzymatic release and decreased vasomotor responses also affect ingestion of adequate and appropriate nutrition.

Diarrhea may be an individualized symptom because some elderly patients equate diarrhea with fecal incontinence. Diarrhea is actually abnormal looseness of the stool that may be associated with changes in frequency or amount. Dysentery alludes to painful, bloody diarrhea. The elderly patient may be more susceptible to diarrhea of the infectious type because of a decrease in gastric acid, motility disorders, or decreases in immune function. Morbidity in the elderly with severe diarrhea is increased by their inability to compensate for volume and fluid losses, resulting in intravascular hypovolemia.

Diarrhea may be classified as being acute (less than two weeks in duration) or chronic (more than four weeks in duration). The main causes of diarrhea occurring in the elderly include: infection, drug changes, food intolerances, ischemia of the mesentery or colon, diverticulitis, inflammatory bowel disease, malabsorption of bile acids or carbohydrates, diet, endocrine or hormonal disorders, or surgery.

MEDICAL CARE

Laboratory: CBC used to identify presence of infections or anemias or identify fluid dehydration status; chemistry profiles, renal profiles, liver profiles, thyroid profiles, and coagulation profiles used to evaluate for metabolic conditions and/or dysfunctions; cultures of stool for identification of bacteria, viruses, or parasites; stool testing for guaiac to determine presence of occult blood, for white blood cells, qualitative fat, or *Clostridium difficile* toxin; stool samples may also be tested for sodium and potassium to calculate the osmotic gap; stool testing for immunosorbent assay for *Giardia* antigen may be a more sensitive test than routine ova and parasitic evaluation; 72-hour stool collection for fecal fat to identify pancreatic insufficiency or biliary steatorrhea

Radiography: abdominal X-rays used to identify bowel distention or obstruction, the amount and distribution of stool in the colon, pancreatic calcifications, and/or the presence of free air in the abdominal cavity; upper gastrointestinal series and barium enema exams may be performed to identify lesions, strictures, neoplasms, ileal disease, mucosal thickening, or other abnormalities

Sigmoidoscopy: used to identify rectal or sigmoid pathology, such as pseudomembranous colitis or ischemia

Upper gastrointestinal endoscopy: may be used to acquire small bowel biopsies for potential mucosal disease, presence of ulcerations, or neoplasms

Colonoscopy: used to directly show colonic mucosa and obtain biopsies; the procedure of choice for identification of colorectal neoplasms, inflammatory bowel disease, and other proctologic pathology

Laxatives, suppositories, enemas: bisacodyl (Bisacolax, Dulcolax, Fleet Laxative, Fleet Enema), calcium polycarbophil (Equalactin, Fiberall, FiberCon, Mitrolan), cascara sagrada, castor oil (Emulsoil, Purge) docusate calcium or sodium (DC Softgels, Sulfolax, Surfak, Colace, Coloxyl, Diocto, DOS, DUOsol, Modane, Pro-Sof), glycerin (Fleet Babylax, Sani-Supp), lactulose (Cephulac, Cholac, Chronulac, Constilac, Duphalac, Enulose), magnesium citrate, hydroxide or sulfate (Citroma, Citro-Mag, Milk of Magnesia, Epsom salts), methylcellulose (Citrucel), psyllium (Fiberall, Genfiber, Hydrocil, Konsyl, Metamucil, Perdiem, Prodiem, Serutan, Unilax, V-Lax), senna (Black-Draught, Fletcher's Castoria, Senexon, Senokot), or sodium phosphate (Fleet Phospho-Soda); bulk laxatives used to provide sufficient bulk to stool to promote peristalsis and bowel elimination; osmotic laxatives used to promote bowel elimination on a daily or every other day basis; laxatives that contain magnesium should be utilized on a short-term basis only and cautiously in patients with renal impairment; stimulant laxatives used for acute constipation but can result in abdominal cramping and fluid and electrolyte imbalances, and are frequently abused by laxative-dependent patients; stool softeners help to soften stools to allow for easier elimination; suppositories may be required for acute constipation or as part of a bowel program; enemas used when impaction of stool exists; soapsuds enemas may result in mucosal damage and cramping and should be avoided; oil enemas used to soften impacted stool for easier removal

Surgery: may be required if patient has abdominal free air which is an indication of bowel perforation or peritonitis; subtotal colectomy may be required if the patient has a chronic severe slow transit constipation; other procedures may be required for the presence of neoplasms or Crohn's disease

IV fluids: used as first line treatment for acute diarrhea to replace fluids and administer replacement electrolytes to prevent complications

Electrolyte replacement: may be required if fluid loss substantial enough to affect normal electrolyte balance; common replacements include sodium, potassium, chloride, phosphorus, and magnesium

Antimicrobials: metronidazole (Flagyl, Protostat), amphotericin B (Amphocin, Amophotericin B, Fungizone), neomycin sulfate (Neo-fradin, Neo-Tabs), ciprofloxacin (Cipro), vancomycin hydrochloride (Vancocin, Vancoled), among others used in the treatment for infectious diarrhea based on culture results

Antidiarrheals: attapulgite (Diasorb, Donnagel, Kaopectate, Parepectolin, Rheaban), bismuth subsalicylate (Bismatrol, Pepto-Bismol, Pink Bismuth), diphenoxylate hydrochloride and atropine sulfate (Logen, Lomotil, Lonox), loperamide (Imodium), octreotide acetate (Sandostatin) or opium tincture (Paregoric); opioids decrease motility and relax smooth muscle to decrease diarrhea; cholestyramine may be used if bile acid diarrhea determined to be the cause; kaolin and pectin help consolidate the stool and reduce diarrhea

COMMON NURSING DIAGNOSES

RISK FOR IMPAIRED SKIN INTEGRITY (see PERIPHERAL VASCULAR DISEASE)

Related to: aging process changes to skin, pressure on skin surfaces, bed rest, immobility, excretions on skin, diarrhea, alterations in tissue perfusion

Defining Characteristics: thin, dry skin on extremities, redness to perianal skin, burning and soreness of perianal skin, swelling, warmth to area, disruption of skin surface, excoriation of skin, abrasions, lesions, redness to bony prominences, open wounds

CONSTIPATION (see HEART FAILURE)

Related to: changes related to aging, such as immobility, less than adequate physical activity, lack of dietary bulk, neuromuscular impairment, dysphagia, paralysis, less than adequate dietary intake, chronic use of medications and enemas, weak abdominal musculature, musculoskeletal impairment

Defining Characteristics: passage of hard, formed stool, decreased bowel sounds, inability to evacuate stool, abdominal pain, abdominal distention, ileus, absent bowel sounds, nausea, vomiting, frequency of stool less than normal, less than usual amount of stool, palpable mass, feelings of rectal fullness, inability to ingest bulk-containing foods, use of laxatives, frequent bouts of constipation, impaired peristalsis, lack of awareness of defecation urge, straining at stool, weakness, fatigue, confusion, cognitive deficit, appetite impairment, depression, inability to use commode/toilet, activity intolerance, pain, discomfort, medications

ADDITIONAL NURSING DIAGNOSES

 ### RISK FOR IMBALANCED FLUID VOLUME

Related to: changes in GI system related to aging, excessive losses through normal routes, loss of fluid through abnormal routes, alterations in absorption of fluids, lack of intake of sufficient fluids, medications, failures of regulatory mechanisms, increased or decreased motility in GI tract

Defining Characteristics: weight gain or loss, diarrhea, vomiting, nausea, output greater than intake, thirst, dry skin, dry mucous membranes, weakness, change in mental status, presence of indwelling tubes, catheters, or nasogastric tubes, immobility, cognitive deficits, hypermetabolic state, active loss of fluids, diuretics, urinary frequency, renal insufficiency, pituitary abnormality, abnormal electrolytes, changes in vital signs, dehydration, abnormal stool evacuation, anorexia

Outcome Criteria

✔ Patient will have intake and output within baseline determinations, with no signs or symptoms of dehydration and with no electrolyte imbalances.

NOC: *Fluid Balance*

INTERVENTIONS	RATIONALES
Monitor vital signs every 4 hours and prn.	Fever, tachycardia, dyspnea, or hypotension may be a symptom of hypovolemia and dehydration.

INTERVENTIONS	RATIONALES
Measure intake and output every 2–4 hours. Notify physician if urinary output is less than 30 cc/hr for 2 hours, or if 8-hour I&O totals do not equilibrate.	Estimates patient's fluid balance. The elderly patient needs at least 1750 cc of fluids daily to maintain a normal fluid balance and to carry out physiologic body processes. Decreased urinary output may indicate reduced fluid volume.
Measure all output sources, including significant wound drainage, nasogastric fluid, liquid stools, and so forth.	Provides for accurate measurement of insensible loss of fluids that can add to fluid imbalances.
Assess patient for presence of nausea, vomiting, diarrhea, diaphoresis, thirst, hot, dry skin, dry mucous membranes, poor skin turgor, weakness, and sunken, mushy eyeballs.	May indicate fluid imbalance. The elderly patient is more susceptible to fluid and electrolyte imbalance, acidosis, and alkalosis, and these problems are caused by fluid losses.
Monitor patient's medications being taken and evaluate their effect on patient's intake and output.	Diuretics increase fluid elimination and loss, sedatives may affect the ability to obtain and take in adequate fluids, and urinary retention may result from the use of antihistamines and phenothiazines.
Evaluate patient for complaints of weakness, paresthesias, leg cramps, muscle fatigue, and irregular pulses.	May be signs and symptoms of hypokalemia associated with potassium loss from excessive fluid losses.
Weigh patient daily, at same time, on same scale if possible.	Monitors for weight loss resulting from fluid losses. Utilizing the same scale and time provides for consistent data.
Encourage fluids of at least 2 L/day, including fruit juices, high-caloric beverages, and slushes.	Replaces fluid loss and ensures adequate fluid intake. Increases caloric intake.
Monitor patient for confusion, sensory deficits, cognitive deficits, mobility deficits, and depression.	May indicate an inability to express thirst and inability to obtain needed fluids.
Administer IV fluids as ordered.	Replaces fluid losses if swallowing is impaired or if patient is unable or unwilling to take in adequate fluid volume. May be required if patient is unable to retain fluids.
Increase fluid amounts if patient has fever or is in hot environmental temperature.	Heat increases fluid loss for every 1° C.

INTERVENTIONS	RATIONALES
Administer electrolyte replacement as ordered.	May be required to prevent complications from imbalances that may occur due to fluid shifting, inadequate intake, or other factors.
Monitor lab work for electrolytes, BUN, creatinine, osmolality, urine specific gravity.	May indicate electrolyte imbalance as a result of fluid dehydration, or identifies renal dysfunction that can affect fluid output.
Instruct patient/family regarding need to measure intake and output, kinds of fluids to include in fluid intake, such as gelatin, custards, ice cream, and so forth.	Provides knowledge that allow for rational determination of levels that may indicate changes in intake and/or medications.
Instruct family to weigh patient weekly and report abrupt changes, such as 2–5 lbs/wk, to physician.	Provides for identification of fluid deficit or excess, and allows for prompt intervention.
Instruct family regarding need for amount of daily fluid intake and assist with scheduling intake as appropriate for patient, and to decrease amount prior to bedtime.	Ensures adequate intake, but decreases problems with nocturia.
Instruct patient/family regarding avoidance of excessive salt intake in foods.	May increase dehydration if fluid intake is not adequate by increasing water resorption in the distal tubules.

NIC: *Fluid/Electrolyte Management*

Discharge or Maintenance Evaluation

- Patient will have equivalent intake and output, with no signs or symptoms of dehydration.

- Patient will maintain weight with set parameters.

- Patient will have normal electrolytes and renal profiles.

- Patient and family will be able to accurately verbalize and demonstrate understanding of need for fluid intake, monitoring intake and output, and sodium restriction.

- Patient will maintain adequate urinary output, with no overt renal dysfunction as evident by changes in BUN and creatinine, or oliguria.

DIARRHEA

Related to: dietary intake, medications, use of laxatives, antibiotics, infection, inflammation, irritation, or malabsorption of bowel from gastrointestinal disorders

Defining Characteristics: frequent passage of stools, loose, liquid, or watery stools, abdominal pain, cramping, increased bowel sounds, changes in color of stool, fever, malaise, bloody stools, mucoid stools, fatty substances in stool, fecal urgency, presence of *Clostridium difficile* or parasites in stool

Outcome Criteria

✔ Patient will have soft, formed stool elimination based upon patient's specific baseline pattern.

NOC: *Bowel Elimination*

INTERVENTIONS	RATIONALES
Monitor patient for presence and frequency of diarrhea, characteristics of stool, presence of fecal impaction, or incontinence.	Identifies problem and severity, and facilitates establishment of plan of care. Liquid stool may pass around an impaction and be expelled as diarrhea.
Monitor I&O if diarrhea is severe.	Diarrhea can deplete fluids and electrolytes, resulting in weakness over an extended episode.
Administer antidiarrheals as ordered.	Decreases gastric motility and controls number of bowel eliminations.
Observe skin every shift, noting any decrease in skin turgor, skin excoriation in perianal region, or other skin breakdown.	Identifies skin problems and may prevent breakdown or worsening of excoriation.
Apply ointment to perianal area as ordered.	Promotes comfort and protects skin from irritation.
Obtain stool samples as ordered.	Lab examination of stool may reveal the presence of toxins, infections, or parasites, to facilitate appropriate treatment.
Maintain patient in close proximity to commode or bathroom.	Prevents embarrassment for patient if he or she has an accidental incontinent episode.
Instruct patient/family regarding factors involved with diarrhea.	Promotes knowledge and understanding of the problem.
Instruct patient to comply with fluid and dietary intake as appropriate.	Provides bulk to stool and provides for fluid replacement.

(continues)

(continued)

INTERVENTIONS	RATIONALES
Instruct patient/family regarding the use of antimicrobials that may cause diarrhea.	Use of these drugs may cause overgrowths of infection resulting in diarrhea as normal intestinal bacteria have been destroyed.
Instruct patient/family regarding use of antidiarrheals and anti-microbials as ordered.	Provides knowledge of drugs, side effects, and need for antimicrobials if diarrhea is from infectious source.
Instruct in the avoidance of caffeine drinks, spicy foods, nuts, seeds, raw foods, and gas-producing foods, such as cabbage, beans, or onions.	Dietary substances may act as diuretics and increase fluid in colon, or may be irritating to bowel and actually increase motility and diarrhea.
Instruct patient/family regarding avoidance of laxative dependence and routine enema usage.	Regular use compounds the problem by creating dependency and interfering with normal elimination reflexes and mechanisms. Mineral oil tends to be lost through the sphincter and causes soiling, and interferes with the metabolism of fat-soluble vitamins.
Instruct patient/family regarding cleaning the perianal area.	Helps to provide comfort and maintain skin integrity.
Instruct patient/family in relaxation techniques.	Helps to reduce stress and temporarily alleviates emotional distress, which can worsen diarrhea.
Prepare patient for surgery as warranted.	May require surgery for bowel perforation, unresolving ileus, adhesions, and so forth.

NIC: *Diarrhea Management*

Discharge or Maintenance Evaluation

- Patient will have diarrhea controlled, with reduced frequency and soft, formed consistency of stools.
- Patient will not exhibit any signs or symptoms of fluid or electrolyte imbalances.
- Patient/family will be compliant with dietary modifications to reduce diarrhea.
- Patient will exhibit a reduced use and/or reliance upon laxatives and enemas for routine use.

- Patient will have a return to specific baseline bowel elimination pattern.

 BOWEL INCONTINENCE

Related to: aging changes related to perceptual or cognitive impairment, neurological disorders, depression, anxiety, musculoskeletal involvement

Defining Characteristics: involuntary passage of feces, decreased rectal sphincter tone, agitation, lethargy, apathy, memory deficit, disorientation, fecal stains on clothing, inability to recognize urge to defecate, inability to delay defecation

Outcome Criteria

✔ Patient will be able to control evacuation of stool.

NOC: *Bowel Continence*

INTERVENTIONS	RATIONALES
Assess patient for presence of diarrhea, fecal impaction, patency of rectal sphincter, awareness of urge to defecate, and ability to control defecation.	Provides information regarding potential for bowel incontinence from changes associated with age, such as reduced muscle tone and reflex activity and decreased sensory perception.
Assist patient to establish a regular bowel pattern. Remind patient to use bathroom or commode each day after breakfast, or after suppository insertion.	Procedure helps to promote emptying of bowel and prevents leakage of feces. Routine scheduling assists patient to adapt physiologic function.
Provide perianal care after each incontinent occurrence.	Prevents infection from excoriation of skin, and promotes comfort.
Provide pads, diapers, or leak-proof garments if patient finds difficulty in controlling fecal leakage.	Protects clothing and prevents patient's embarrassment.
Assist patient with changing clothes if soiling occurs.	Prevents embarrassment.
Instruct patient regarding establishment of bowel regimen, sitting on commode or toilet for 30 minutes after breakfast each day, use of suppositories, and so forth.	Promotes bowel regularity and helps to prevent bowel incontinence if feces are removed from rectum.

INTERVENTIONS	RATIONALES
Instruct patient/family regarding changes that are age-related that may result in bowel elimination problems.	Age-related changes include decreased mucosal surface area of the small intestine which causes impaired absorption of nutrients, atrophy of the mucosa and muscle layers, and arteriolar sclerosis; delays in peripheral nerve transmission in the colon cause constipation or fecal incontinence; weakness of the abdominal and pelvic muscles cause difficulty in defecation; and decreases in bowel motility, gastrocolic reflex, voluntary contraction of the external sphincter, and the amount of feces all contribute to constipation or fecal incontinence.
Instruct patient/family regarding avoidance of regular use of laxatives.	May create urgency and incontinence of feces if patient is unable to reach the bathroom in time, and creates dependency on laxatives.
Instruct in Kegel exercises (perineal exercises).	Strengthens perineal muscles to increase tone and to assist in control of feces.

INTERVENTIONS	RATIONALES
Instruct family in method for removal of impaction, if needed, to assess for presence by digital examination, to remove feces that is soft by inserting lubricated gloved finger into rectum and gently removing small amounts of stool at a time.	Hard mass of stool indicates impaction. Removal of soft stool promotes comfort and prepares patient for subsequent bowel movements.

NIC: *Bowel Incontinence Care*

Discharge or Maintenance Evaluation

- Patient will achieve return of bowel control with no incontinent episodes.
- Patient will be compliant with established bowel regimen and will reduce episodes of incontinence.
- Patient will be able to use commode or toilet before bowel incontinence occurs.
- Patient/family will be able to accurately recall information about age-related changes that may contribute to bowel problems.
- Patient/family will be able to safely remove impacted stool to promote evacuation of bowel.

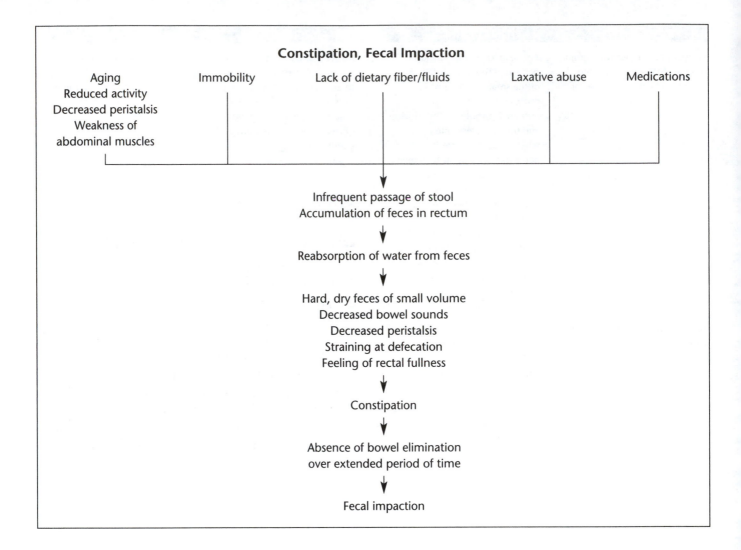

Constipation, Fecal Impaction

Aging
Reduced activity
Decreased peristalsis
Weakness of
abdominal muscles

Immobility

Lack of dietary fiber/fluids

Laxative abuse

Medications

Infrequent passage of stool
Accumulation of feces in rectum

Reabsorption of water from feces

Hard, dry feces of small volume
Decreased bowel sounds
Decreased peristalsis
Straining at defecation
Feeling of rectal fullness

Constipation

Absence of bowel elimination
over extended period of time

Fecal impaction

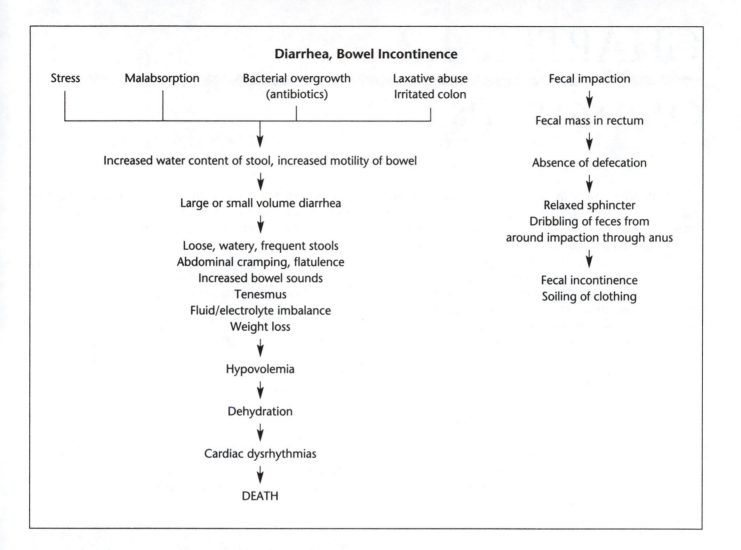

Diarrhea, Bowel Incontinence

| Stress | Malabsorption | Bacterial overgrowth (antibiotics) | Laxative abuse Irritated colon | Fecal impaction |

Fecal impaction
↓
Fecal mass in rectum
↓
Absence of defecation
↓
Relaxed sphincter
Dribbling of feces from
around impaction through anus
↓
Fecal incontinence
Soiling of clothing

Increased water content of stool, increased motility of bowel
↓
Large or small volume diarrhea
↓
Loose, watery, frequent stools
Abdominal cramping, flatulence
Increased bowel sounds
Tenesmus
Fluid/electrolyte imbalance
Weight loss
↓
Hypovolemia
↓
Dehydration
↓
Cardiac dysrhythmias
↓
DEATH

CHAPTER 4.2

CHOLECYSTITIS

Gallbladder abnormalities are common in the aged because of physiologic problems associated with the emptying of bile. Syndromes involving the gallbladder and biliary system are noted in approximately one-third of all elderly patients over the age of 70, with the most common being cholelithiasis, acute cholangitis, and cholecystitis (Beers & Berkow, 2000). The greatest risk to the elderly is obstruction of the cystic, or common bile, duct with gallstones that causes jaundice, a decrease in absorption of fat-soluble vitamins, and a decrease in fat digestion.

Acute cholecystitis is a severe inflammation of the gallbladder, frequently as a direct complication of gallstones, and is normally presented with the symptoms of increased tenderness to the right upper quadrant of the abdomen, fever, and leukocytosis. If a gallstone drifts into the common duct, severe biliary colic is noted in the right subcostal area with frequent radiation into the right scapular or right shoulder area. This can result in jaundice as a result of backed up bile migrating systemically, fever, and gallstone pancreatitis.

Gallstones are basically crystallized formations that develop in the gallbladder and are usually made up of cholesterol and calcium salts. Gallstones can also be made up of different amounts of calcium salts, and bilirubin, which is a substance formed by the deterioration of red blood cells. Studies have shown that estrogen and progesterone stimulate cholesterol synthesis and secretion, which enables the bile that is stored in the liver to become supersaturated with cholesterol and allows the bile salts to precipitate and form stones. Progesterone decreases the amount of bile that is drained out of the gallbladder.

The treatment of choice for symptomatic gallstones is surgery. Laparoscopic cholecystectomy is commonly utilized, but may involve damage to the common bile duct more often than open cholecystectomy. In asymptomatic patients, doctors usually advise the patient against surgical treatment, except in very rare cases. Lithotripsy uses high-energy shock waves directed toward the gallbladder from the outside of the body to attempt to break up the stones into smaller parts that can be dissolved or passed through the common bile duct. This procedure can be performed only if the stones are small enough and of a limited amount, and frequently is not a long-term, lasting solution as a large percentage of patients redevelop symptoms within a few years.

Acute cholangitis results when a gallstone obstructs the ampulla of Vater or secondary to pancreatic cancer. A type of cholangitis that occurs in the Far East is the product of an intestinal tract parasitic infection usually as a result of poorly cooked or undercooked meat or seafood.

Acalculous cholecystitis, in which there are no gallstones, is produced by the combination of biliary stasis, bacterial overgrowth, and ischemia, and is typically found in critically ill patients and in patients who have poor oral fluid intake.

MEDICAL CARE

Laboratory: CBC used to identify infection process, leukocytosis, and hydration status; liver function studies done to evaluate for dysfunction, especially seen with blockage of common bile duct; bilirubin usually elevated with obstruction caused by jaundice, and increase in serum amylase; electrolytes used to identify imbalances; glucose levels used to monitor patients, especially those with diabetes; cardiac isoenzymes used to rule out myocardial ischemia that may mimic pain of gallstones/cholecystitis; drug levels used to monitor efficacy and toxicity of antimicrobials used; fecal urobilinogen used to identify decreases with obstruction because bilirubin is not present to convert to urobilinogen in the intestine

Radiography: abdominal X-rays used to identify calcified stone in the gallbladder; cholangiography used to identify patency of the gallbladder and common duct, as well as presence of gallstones

CT scan: used to show changes in the bile duct, and presence of obstruction

Ultrasonography: used to show gallstones in the gallbladder

Antimicrobials: used in the treatment of acute cholangitis based on type of infection

Narcotic analgesics: buprenorphine hydrochloride (Buprenex), butophanol tartrate (Stadol), codeine phosphate, hydromorphone hydrochloride (Dilaudid), meperidine hydrochloride (Demerol), methadone hydrochloride (Dolophine), morphine hydrochloride or sulfate (Duramorph, Infumorph, Morphine, MS Contin, Roxanol, Statex), nalbuphine hydrochloride (Nubain), oxycodone hydrochloride (OxyContin), oxymorphone hydrochloride (Numorphan), pentazocine hydrochloride or lactate (Talwin), or tramadol hydrochloride (Ultram) used to relieve the pain of inflammation and infection

Anticholinergics: dicyclomine hydrochloride (Bentyl, Byclomine, Dibent, Di-Spaz), glycopyrrolate (Robinul), hyoscyamine sulfate (Cystospaz, Anaspaz, Gastrosed, Levbid, Neoquess), propantheline bromide (Pro-Banthine), or scopolamine (Scopolamine Hydrobromide) used to relieve spasms of the gallbladder by inhibiting the action of acetylcholine on the postganglionic parasympathetic muscarinic receptors, local anesthetic action, and decreasing GI motility

Antiemetics: chlorpromazine hydrochloride (Thorazine), dimenhydrinate (Dramamine, Dramanate, Dymenate), dolesetron mesylate (Anzemet), dronabinol (Marinol), granisetron hydrochloride (Kytril), meclizine hydrochloride (Antivert, Bonine, Vergon), metoclopramide hydrochloride (Clopra, Reclomide, Reglan), ondansetron hydrochloride (Zofran), prochlorperazine (Compazine, PMS), thiethylperazine maleate (Torecan), trimethobenzamide hydrochloride (Arresting, Tebamide, Ticon, Tigan, Triban), used to reduce nausea and vomiting by depressing the chemoreceptor trigger zone or by inhibiting serotonin receptors to block nausea response

Gallstone solubilizers: ursodiol (Actigall) is used for dissolving gallstones that are less than 20 mm in diameter by suppression of liver synthesis and secretion of cholesterol, and inhibition of intestinal absorption of cholesterol

Surgery: surgical cholecystectomy, either laparascopically or open, done to remove the gallbladder;

common bile duct exploration also done; lithotripsy abandoned as the re-emergence of gallstones was increased; sometimes an endoscopic papillotomy and basket removal of an obstructive stone, or ERCP may be done if the patient continues to remain ill with an obstructing stone after the gallbladder has been removed; lithotripsy can be attempted if gallstones are few in number and small enough to break into small pieces that can be dissolved or passed through the common duct

COMMON NURSING DIAGNOSES

 ### ACUTE PAIN (see CAD)

Related to: gallstones, inflammation, infection, obstruction, spasm, sepsis

Defining Characteristics: communication of pain, fever, body aches, malaise, epigastric pain in the right upper quadrant of the abdomen, heart burn, feeling of heaviness, intolerance to fatty foods, abdominal pain, abdominal distention, elevated white blood cell count, jaundice

IMBALANCED NUTRITION: LESS THAN BODY REQUIREMENTS (see COPD)

Related to: inability to take in enough food, increased metabolism caused by disease process, decreased level of consciousness, inability to absorb nutrients because of biologic or psychological factors, inability to digest or ingest nutrients because of obstruction of bile flow

Defining Characteristics: actual inadequate food intake, altered taste, weight loss, body weight 20% or more under ideal for height and frame, anorexia, absent bowel sounds, decreased peristalsis, muscle mass loss, decreased muscle tone, changes in bowel habits, nausea, vomiting, abdominal distention, lack of interest in food, abdominal pain or discomfort, steatorrhea, bleeding tendency, intolerance of fatty foods, epigastric pain after eating, jaundice

 ### RISK FOR IMPAIRED SKIN INTEGRITY (see PERIPHERAL VASCULAR DISEASE)

Related to: aging process changes to skin, pressure on skin surfaces, bed rest, immobility, excretions on skin, altered pigmentation from common bile duct obstruction, alterations in tissue perfusion

Defining Characteristics: thin, dry skin on extremities, warmth to area, disruption of skin surface, excoriation of skin, jaundice, pruritis, scratching

 IMPAIRED SKIN INTEGRITY (see PACEMAKERS)

Related to: cholecystectomy, alteration in activity, changes in mobility, aging process changes, such as loss of elasticity of skin

Defining Characteristics: disruption of skin tissue from incisional sites, insertion sites, destruction of skin layers, open wounds, drain sites

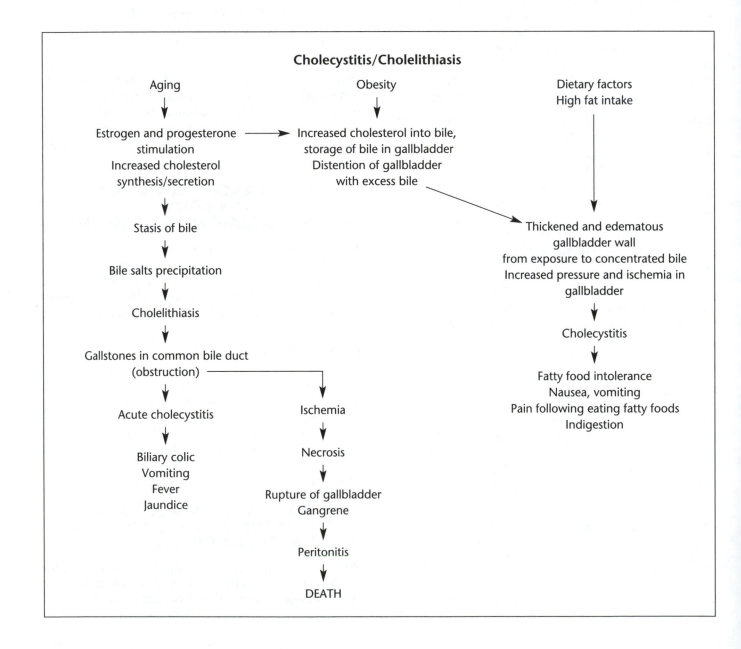

Cholecystitis/Cholelithiasis

Aging
↓
Estrogen and progesterone stimulation
Increased cholesterol synthesis/secretion ——→ Increased cholesterol into bile, storage of bile in gallbladder
↓   Distention of gallbladder
Stasis of bile   with excess bile
↓
Bile salts precipitation
↓
Cholelithiasis
↓
Gallstones in common bile duct (obstruction)
↓
Acute cholecystitis
↓
Biliary colic
Vomiting
Fever
Jaundice

Obesity
↓
(Increased cholesterol into bile, storage of bile in gallbladder; Distention of gallbladder with excess bile)

Ischemia
↓
Necrosis
↓
Rupture of gallbladder
Gangrene
↓
Peritonitis
↓
DEATH

Dietary factors
High fat intake
↓
Thickened and edematous gallbladder wall from exposure to concentrated bile
Increased pressure and ischemia in gallbladder
↓
Cholecystitis
↓
Fatty food intolerance
Nausea, vomiting
Pain following eating fatty foods
Indigestion

CHAPTER 4.3

DIVERTICULAR DISEASE

Diverticulosis is a condition in which mucosal sacs protrude through the muscular stratum of the gastrointestinal tract, and these diverticula, or protrusions, are present, but without inflammation, and the patient is asymptomatic. These out-pouchings form in the colon and are believed to be a consequence of slow-moving stools that increase the pressure within the colon.

At times, feces lodge in the diverticula and make them predisposed to ulceration, abscess, and bacterial infection. If the diverticula become irritated or burst, this is known as diverticulitis, an acute infection of diverticula. The inflamed areas may adhere to the bladder, small bowel, or pelvic organs, and produce a fistula from one organ to the other. The perforation can allow pus or fecal material to spread throughout the abdominal cavity and cause peritonitis.

The prevalence of diverticular disease increases with age, and a large percentage of persons over the age of 50 having some form of the disease.

Common symptoms of diverticulitis include fever, leukocytosis, localized left abdominal pain, and rebound tenderness. If the inflamed diverticula have burst and adhered to the bladder, the patient may experience pain above the pubic area or on the right side, as well as painful urination. In the elderly patient, the absence of a fever, leukocytosis, or rebound tenderness does not necessarily rule out diverticulitis.

The goal of treatment of diverticulitis is to eradicate the infection with antimicrobials. If medical therapy does not improve the patient's condition within 72 hours, surgery may be necessary. Even when patients recover, there are those with a complex diverticular disease history that require surgery, in which the damaged section of bowel is resected and the colon is anastomosed. Sometimes a colostomy may be required. In elderly patients who present with generalized peritonitis, immediate emergency surgery is required to avoid morbidity.

MEDICAL CARE

Laboratory: CBC used to identify infection and leukocytosis, and to evaluate for bleeding and peritonitis; general chemistry profiles used to identify dysfunction in other body systems; guaiac stools for identification of occult bleeding caused by inflammation; albumin, prealbumin and protein levels to identify nutritional needs and status; electrolyte panels to identify imbalances

Radiography: barium enema may be done after the acute inflammation has subsided, to identify diverticula, fistulas, or other lesions

CT scan: abdominal CT scan used to show colonic wall thickness, structures, and to identify diverticulitis and/or the presence of abscesses; occasionally CT scans may be done in conjunction with percutaneous drainage of abscesses

Ultrasonography: used to identify colon wall thickness and extraluminal structures in diverticulitis

Colonoscopy: used after an acute episode to rule out tumors or other medical conditions, or if the patient has rectal bleeding, to identify the source

Angiography: used if the patient has gastrointestinal bleeding that cannot be located, or if the bleeding is vigorous, or if the patient is hemodynamically unstable; a mesenteric angiogram may be used to detect the site of bleeding and potentially allow vasoactive substances to be infused at the site

Antimicrobials: used to treat the specific organism when infection develops

Anticholinergics: dicyclomine hydrochloride (Bentyl, Byclomine, Dibent, Di-Spaz), glycopyrrolate (Robinul), hyoscyamine sulfate (Cystospaz, Anaspaz, Gastrosed, Levbid, Neoquess), propantheline bromide (Pro-Banthine), or scopolamine (Scopolamine Hydrobromide) used to relieve spasms of the gallbladder by inhibiting the action of acetylcholine on the post-ganglionic parasympathetic muscarinic receptors, its local anesthetic action, and decreasing GI motility

Laxatives, stool softeners: bisacodyl (Bisacolax, Dulcolax, Fleet Laxative, Fleet Enema), calcium polycarbophil (Equalactin, Fiberall, FiberCon, Mitrolan), cascara sagrada, castor oil (Emulsoil, Purge) docusate calcium or sodium (DC Softgels, Sulfolax, Surfak, Colace, Coloxyl, Diocto, DOS, DUOsol, Modane, Pro-Sof), glycerin (Fleet Babylax, Sani-Supp), lactulose (Cephulac, Cholac, Chronulac, Constilac, Duphalac, Enulose), magnesium citrate, hydroxide or sulfate (Citroma, Citro-Mag, Milk of Magnesia, Epsom salts), methylcellulose (Citrucel), psyllium (Fiberall, Genfiber, Hydrocil, Konsyl, Metamucil, Perdiem, Prodiem, Serutan, Unilax, V-Lax), senna (Black-Draught, Fletcher's Castoria, Senexon, Senokot), or sodium phosphate (Fleet Phospho-Soda); bulk laxatives are used to provide sufficient bulk to stool to promote peristalsis and bowel elimination; osmotic laxatives are used to promote bowel elimination on a daily or every other day basis; laxatives that contain magnesium should be utilized on a short-term basis only and cautiously in patients with renal impairment; stimulant laxatives used for acute constipation but can result in abdominal cramping and fluid and electrolyte imbalances, and are frequently abused by laxative-dependent patients; stool softeners help soften stools to allow for easier elimination; suppositories may be required for acute constipation or as part of a bowel program; enemas used when impaction of stool exists; soapsuds enemas may result in mucosal damage and cramping and should be avoided; oil enemas used to soften impacted stool for easier removal

Surgery: may be required for bowel obstruction, generalized peritonitis, unrelenting gastrointestinal bleeding, or bowel resection for the diseased segment of the colon involved or for removal of abscesses; colostomy may be required depending on the severity of the condition

COMMON NURSING DIAGNOSES

ACUTE PAIN (see CAD)

Related to: diverticulitis, inflammation, infection, obstruction, spasm, sepsis, peritonitis, surgery

Defining Characteristics: communication of pain, fever, body aches, malaise, abdominal pain, abdom-

inal distention, elevated white blood cell count, pelvic pain, dysuria, left lower quadrant abdominal pain, surgical wound, drains, abdominal guarding, tachycardia, hypotension, bradypnea

IMBALANCED NUTRITION: LESS THAN BODY REQUIREMENTS (see COPD)

Related to: changes related to aging, such as decreased GI motility, inability to take in enough food, increased metabolism caused by disease process, decreased level of consciousness, inability to absorb nutrients because of biologic factors, inability to digest food because of biologic factors from diverticular formation

Defining Characteristics: actual inadequate food intake, nutrients caught in diverticula, inflammation of diverticula, weight loss, body weight 20% or more under ideal for height and frame, anorexia, absent bowel sounds, decreased peristalsis, muscle mass loss, decreased muscle tone, changes in bowel habits, nausea, vomiting, abdominal distention, lack of interest in food, abdominal pain or discomfort, cramping, low residue dietary intake, decreased GI motility, gastric paresis, ileus, obstruction, increased WBC count, decreased albumin and prealbumin levels, decreased protein levels

IMPAIRED SKIN INTEGRITY (see HEMORRHOIDS)

Related to: surgical wounds, alteration in activity, changes in mobility, changes in skin elasticity and healing ability associated with aging process

Defining Characteristics: disruption of skin tissue from incisional sites, insertion sites, destruction of skin layers, open wounds, drain sites

CONSTIPATION (see HEART FAILURE)

Related to: low residue dietary intake, lack of dietary bulk, dysphagia, diverticulitis, medications

Defining Characteristics: passage of hard, formed stool, decreased bowel sounds, inability to evacuate stool, abdominal pain, abdominal distention, ileus, absent bowel sounds, nausea, vomiting, frequency of stool less than normal, less than usual amount of stool, palpable mass, feelings of rectal fullness, inability to ingest bulk-containing foods, flatulence, episodes alternating with diarrhea

DIARRHEA
(see BOWEL DISORDERS)

Related to: diverticulosis, diverticulitis, dietary intake, medications, infection, inflammation, irritation, or malabsorption of bowel from gastrointestinal disorders, irritation of bowel from rough or spicy foods

Defining Characteristics: frequent passage of stools, loose, liquid, or watery stools, abdominal pain, cramping, increased bowel sounds, changes in color of stool, fever, malaise, episodes alternating with constipation episodes

ADDITIONAL NURSING DIAGNOSES

DEFICIENT KNOWLEDGE

Related to: lack of exposure to information, potential for infection, or diverticulitis

Defining Characteristics: request for information, cognitive limitation, noncompliance of previous instruction, presence of preventable complications

Outcome Criteria

✔ Patient will be compliant with preventive measures for diverticulosis/diverticulitis.

NOC: *Knowledge: Disease Process*

INTERVENTIONS	RATIONALES
Assess patient for knowledge of signs and symptoms of disease, preventive measures, and treatment of disease.	Provides basis for teaching plan and promotes compliance.
Assess past episodes of bowel infection and lifestyle changes.	Prevents recurrence of diverticulitis by teaching prevention of disease exacerbations.
Instruct patient/family regarding risk factors associated with diverticulosis/diverticulitis.	Provides information to help eliminate risk factors and reduce the possibility of complications or exacerbations.

INTERVENTIONS	RATIONALES
Instruct patient regarding dietary modifications, such as eating high-fiber foods and to avoid nuts, seeds, raw fruits, and vegetables.	Prevents constipation and slow-moving stools, helps to prevent irritation to bowel mucosa, and prevents retention of small particles in diverticula that could lead to infection.
Instruct patient in maintaining daily exercise program.	Helps to promote bowel motility.
Instruct patient to avoid stressful situations. Teach relaxation techniques, guided imagery, meditation, biofeedback, and so forth.	Helps to reduce stress and anxiety, that may predispose patient to diverticular disease.
Instruct patient to maintain adequate fluid intake of at least 2 L/day, unless contraindicated.	Promotes hydration and soft stools that are easier to expel.
Instruct patient/family regarding bowel elimination programs.	Helps to establish routine to eliminate feces and prevent episodes of diverticulitis.
Instruct patient to report any bleeding from rectum, abdominal pain, especially left lower quadrant pain, alternating diarrhea and constipation, or elevation of temperature.	May be indication of recurring diverticulitis and infection. Prompt recognition may prevent peritonitis spread and severity of recurrence.

NIC: *Teaching: Disease Process*

Discharge or Maintenance Evaluation

■ Patient will be compliant with dietary, fluid, and exercise programs.

■ Patient will be able to avoid exacerbations of diverticulitis.

■ Patient will exhibit no signs or symptoms of diverticular disease.

■ Patient/family will be able to accurately verbalize understanding of information given to them, and will be able to prevent or reduce recurrences.

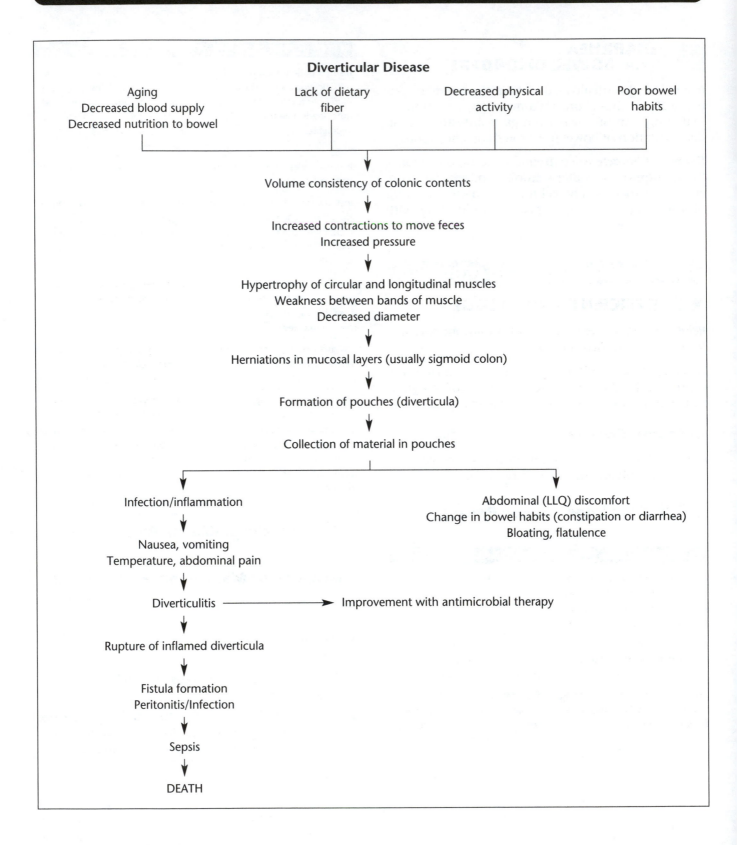

Diverticular Disease

| Aging
Decreased blood supply
Decreased nutrition to bowel | Lack of dietary
fiber | Decreased physical
activity | Poor bowel
habits |

Volume consistency of colonic contents

Increased contractions to move feces
Increased pressure

Hypertrophy of circular and longitudinal muscles
Weakness between bands of muscle
Decreased diameter

Herniations in mucosal layers (usually sigmoid colon)

Formation of pouches (diverticula)

Collection of material in pouches

Infection/inflammation

Nausea, vomiting
Temperature, abdominal pain

Diverticulitis   ⟶   Improvement with antimicrobial therapy

Rupture of inflamed diverticula

Fistula formation
Peritonitis/Infection

Sepsis

DEATH

Abdominal (LLQ) discomfort
Change in bowel habits (constipation or diarrhea)
Bloating, flatulence

CHAPTER 4.4

GASTROESOPHAGEAL REFLUX

Gastroesophageal reflux disease, or GERD, occurs when gastric contents make contact with the esophageal mucosa for a sustained length of time and suppress the normal esophageal defense system and tissue resistance. This occurs as gastric contents reflux into the esophagus because of relaxation of the esophageal or stomach sphincters. The syndrome is common, occurring in approximately 45% of the population at some point (Beers & Berkow, 2000). Most patients have mild disease, but some develop damage with reflux esophagitis, or potential severe complications.

The most universal symptom is substernal burning that occurs after meals or when the patient is in a reclining position. The severity of heartburn does not correlate with the severity of the esophagitis or tissue injury. Atypical chest pain that occurs with GERD must be distinguished from cardiac conditions. Regurgitation of gastric acids causes a bitter or sour taste, and salivary production that is stimulated by acid reflux can also occur. Oropharyngeal inflammation can result in sore throat, earaches, and gingivitis, and laryngeal or respiratory irritation can result in hoarseness, wheezing, bronchitis, asthma, and aspiration pneumonia.

Strictures can result at the sites of recurrent inflammatory injury, and Barrett's esophagus occurs when normal squamous cells in the esophagus are replaced by metaplastic columnar epithelium containing goblet and columnar cells. It is a premalignant state that can develop into adenocarcinoma and is found in patients who suffer with erosive esophagitis and peptic strictures. Hemorrhage can occur as a result of erosion, ulceration, or severe mucosal injury, and infrequently, deep esophageal ulcerations can perforate the esophagus.

Some of the factors that play a role in the development of GERD include an incompetent lower esophageal sphincter that results in free reflux or stress reflux during increased intra-abdominal pressure, the type of the reflux mixture, whether it is acid gastric fluid, bile, and/or pancreatic secretions, and the amount of time it is in direct contact with the mucosa. Reduced peristaltic clearance and an impairment of gastric emptying result from gastroparesis or partial gastric outlet obstruction.

Zollinger-Ellison syndrome is one of the more severe manifestations of GERD, in which a gastrin-producing tumor in the pancreas or the duodenum causes increased secretion of gastric acids and peptic ulceration results. Treatment of this syndrome is usually either surgical removal of the gastrinoma or pharmacologic treatment utilizing omeprazole.

A significant percentage of all patients with severe erosive esophagitis have concurrent hiatal hernias. The hernia, which is really a protrusion of the stomach above the diaphragm, tends to slow down clearance of esophageal acids.

The aging esophagus decreases in motility and the synchronization and relaxation of its sphincters which delays the emptying of the esophagus of its contents into the stomach. This delay in emptying causes putrifaction of the food in the esophagus and results in spasms and reflux. Hiatal hernia may cause or accompany gastric reflux. Both have a high incidence in the elderly population.

MEDICAL CARE

Laboratory: CBC used to identify the presence of anemia that must be ruled out; cardiac enzymes used to rule out myocardial pain related to the atypical pain felt with GERD; serum iron to identify presence of iron-deficiency anemia; gastrin levels to identify toxicity of proton pump inhibitors or to diagnose Zollinger-Ellison syndrome; with Zollinger-Ellison, serum gastrin levels are normally over 150 pg/ml and can range up to 1,000 pg/ml; gastric acid secretory analysis used to determine if failure with pharmacologic agents is caused by inadequate suppression of gastric acid secretion, which may signify bile reflux or pill-induced disease; calcium testing which uses a calcium gluconate infusion given for 3 hours, and then serum gastrin levels are measured at specific intervals

Upper gastrointestinal endoscopy: used to identify the type and extent of tissue damage; normally patients with GERD will have mucosal abnormalities, and Barrett's esophagus or peptic stricture can be viewed

Barium swallow (UGI series): may have a restricted part in the evaluation for GERD; can be used to identify strictures and hiatal hernias

Esophageal pH monitoring: used to document pathologic acid reflux, especially for patients who have atypical symptoms; data are collected regarding the frequency and duration of acid reflux, and can be used to assess if the patient has an abnormal amount of reflux

Esophageal manometry: used in patients that plan on having surgical intervention; determines the esophageal sphincter pressure and presence of adequate esophageal peristalsis

Radionuclide scans: may be used to identify radiolabeled colloid in the area of the esophagus

Surgery: esophagectomy may be required for severe dysplasia; photodynamic ablation, laser therapy, or electrocauterization has been utilized for patients with Barrett's esophagus; fundoplication or posterior gastropexy extensively used for patients who have symptoms that are nonresponsive to other therapy, or have severe complications

Dietary modification: foods that affect esophageal sphincter pressure or irritate the esophagus should be avoided (fried foods, fatty foods, coffee, alcohol, tomato products, citrus juices, peppermint, cola drinks, and chocolate); overeating should be avoided, and those patients who are overweight should be encouraged to reduce

Antacids: aluminum carbonate (Basaljel), aluminum hydroxide (AlternaGEL, Amphojel, Dialume), calcium carbonate (Alka-Mints, Amitone, Chooz, Dicarbosil, Maalox, Rolaids, Tums), magaldrate (Lowsium, Riopan), and magnesium oxide (Mag-Ox, Maox, Uro-Mag) used to help neutralize gastric acid; Gaviscon may be superior to antacids alone because it also contains alginic acid which floats on the gastric acid collection in the stomach and helps decrease reflux if the patient is upright

H₂-receptor antagonists: cimetidine (Tagamet), famotidine (Pepcid), nizatidine (Axid), ranitidine bismuth citrate (Tritec), and ranitidine hydrochloride (Zantac) used to inhibit histamine at the receptor sites in the parietal cells, which results in gastric acid secretion being inhibited; should not be utilized at the same time with antacids because of absorption interference

Proton pump inhibitors: esomeprazole magnesium (Nexium), lansoprazole (Prevacid), omeprazole (Prilosec), pantoprazole sodium (Prontonix), and rabeprazole sodium (Aciphex) used to suppress gastric secretion by inhibiting hydrogen/potassium ATPase enzyme system in the gastric parietal cell; blocks the final step of acid production

Prostaglandin E₁ analogues: misoprostol (Cytotec) used to replace gastric prostaglandins that have been depleted by the use of NSAIDs; decreases basal gastric acid secretion and increases gastric mucus and bicarbonate production

Sucralfate: Carafate used to help ulcer healing by forming a protective barrier on the surface of the ulcer

Promotility agents: metoclopramide hydrochloride (Clopra, Reclomide, Reglan) used to increase the lower esophageal pressure and improve gastric emptying

COMMON NURSING DIAGNOSES

IMBALANCED NUTRITION: LESS THAN BODY REQUIREMENTS (see COPD)

Related to: inability to take in enough food because of reflux, increased metabolism caused by disease process, early satiety, heartburn

Defining Characteristics: actual inadequate food intake, altered taste, weight loss, body weight 20% or more under ideal for height and frame, anorexia, absent bowel sounds, decreased peristalsis, muscle mass loss, decreased muscle tone, changes in bowel habits, nausea, vomiting, abdominal distention, lack of interest in food, abdominal pain or discomfort, intolerance of fatty foods, epigastric pain after eating, heartburn, regurgitation, dysphagia, early satiety after eating

ACUTE PAIN (see CAD)

Related to: GERD, coughing, aspiration, irritated esophageal mucosa, irritated oral cavity from reflux

Defining Characteristics: communication of pain, fever, cough with or without production, heartburn, dysphagia, regurgitation of acidic, putrified material, referred pain, atypical chest pain, abdominal pain, pelvic pain

 ## ANXIETY (see CAD)

Related to: changes in health, hiatal hernia, persistent reflux, potential for Barrett's esophagus, threat of change in health status, life-threatening crises, chronic nature of disease and effect on lifestyle, change in role functioning, decreased energy

Defining Characteristics: fear, restlessness, muscle tension, helplessness, communication of uncertainty and apprehension, feeling of suffocation, feelings of inadequacy, feelings of exhaustion, insomnia, sleep apnea, verbalizations of fear of complications

ADDITIONAL NURSING DIAGNOSES

IMBALANCED NUTRITION: MORE THAN BODY REQUIREMENTS

Related to: decreased physical activity, GERD, eating to try to assuage pain, decreased metabolic rate

Defining Characteristics: body weight 10% or more over ideal weight, triceps skin-fold measurement more than 15 mm in men and 25 mm in women, eating in response to social situations, eating in response to abdominal pain, eating in response to cues other than hunger, pairing food with other activities, sedentary lifestyle

Outcome Criteria

✔ Patient will achieve and maintain an adequate body weight.

✔ Patient will carry out exercise program and weight reduction plan as devised.

NOC: *Weight Control*

INTERVENTIONS	RATIONALES
Assess patient for dietary history intake, eating patterns, importance of eating, and potentials for where dietary excesses can be limited.	Provides information regarding factors associated with being overweight or obesity problems and assists in establishing a plan of care for weight reduction. The elderly tend to gain weight easily because of decreased activity and a lower metabolic rate.
Identify amount of weight loss needed for optimal body size and frame.	Provides basis for dietary planning.
Weigh patient every day, on same scale, at same time if possible.	Provides goal achievement weight loss information, or lack of progress that may require changes in the plan of care. Weighing on same scale each day helps to obtain consistent data.
Establish a dietary plan for weekly goals of weight loss of one pound. Encourage patient to make gradual changes in dietary habits.	Prevents frustration from lack of achieving goals. One pound equals approximately 3,500 calories, so a reduction of approximately 500 calories/day will achieve the prescribed goal. The elderly patient has developed current eating habits over several years and gradual changes increase the potential for success.
Provide activities for the patient that do not center around or are associated with meals or snacks.	Utilizes calories and provides diversion from eating.
Commend patient for his success and efforts in losing weight.	Weight reduction may alleviate some of patient's physical symptoms, and praise encourages continued progress.
Assist patient and develop a modified exercise program, such as walking, or low-impact exercises.	Increases utilization of calories, increases endurance, and maintains musculoskeletal strength. Regularly scheduled exercise facilitates improvement of self-worth and self-esteem.
Instruct patient/family regarding dietary restrictions, modifying favorite foods to use lower calorie substitute ingredients, and to make choices that provide for adequate nutritional intake.	Promotes weight reduction plan by allowing the patient to use familiar foods that have had calories cut down.

(continues)

(continued)

INTERVENTIONS	RATIONALES
Instruct patient to keep a dietary log of intake for calorie counting.	Facilitates adequate nutritional intake and calorie reduction. Many patients are unaware of many "hidden" calories in foods they actually ingest.
Instruct patient regarding community resources, weight reduction programs, or support groups.	Provides support for weight loss and behavior modification for reduced food intake postdischarge.
Instruct patient/family regarding changes in nutrition that occur with aging, such as a decrease in the feeding drive, early satiety, lack of physical activity, lowered resting metabolic rate, and so forth.	Dietary requirements usually decrease with age by approximately 10–25%. Overeating, together with a reduction in metabolic rate, contributes to obesity.
Consult with dietician for meal planning and food preparation.	Provides meal planning and appropriate nutritional guidance based on physical, psychological, socioeconomic, and cultural factors.

NIC: *Nutritional Counseling*

Discharge or Maintenance Evaluation

- Patient will achieve a weight loss of at least 1 lb/week until weight is at desired level.
- Patient will maintain adequate nutritional intake with reduced calories to meet metabolic needs.
- Patient will eliminate higher calorie foods and substitute lower calorie alternatives for familiar foods.
- Patient will be able to participate in activity programs and exercise programs to facilitate weight loss.
- Patient/family will be able to accurately verbalize and understand need for weight loss, goals, and methods of obtaining goals.

DEFICIENT KNOWLEDGE

Related to: lack of information regarding reduction in reflux activity, lack of information about disease process

Defining Characteristics: request for information, verbalization of the problem, presence of preventable complications

Outcome Criteria

✔ Patient will have increased knowledge of actions that reduce reflux.

NOC: *Knowledge: Health Behaviors*

INTERVENTIONS	RATIONALES
Assess patient for information needed and ability to perform actions independently.	Provides basis for teaching.
Assist with reduction in caloric intake.	Overweight increases intra-abdominal pressure.
Provide patient with information regarding disease process, changes that can be made, and medications to be utilized.	Provides knowledge and facilitates compliance.
Instruct patient regarding eating small amounts of bland food, followed by small amount of water. Instruct to remain in upright position at least 1–2 hours after meals, and to avoid eating within 2–4 hours of bedtime.	Gravity helps to control reflux and causes less irritation from reflux action into esophagus.
Instruct patient to avoid bending over, coughing, straining at defecation, and other activities that increase reflux.	Promotes comfort by decrease in intra-abdominal pressure, which reduces the reflux of gastric contents.
Instruct patient to eat slowly, chew foods well, and maintain a high-protein, low-fat diet.	Prevents reflux.
Instruct patient to avoid temperature extremes of food, spicy foods, citrus, and gas-forming foods.	These food items increase acid production that precipitates heartburn and increased reflux.
Instruct patient regarding avoiding alcohol, smoking, and caffeinated beverages.	Increases acid production and may cause esophageal spasms.
Instruct patient to raise both arms fully extended toward the ceiling prior to eating.	Relieves spasms and allows for more comfort when eating.
Instruct patient in medications, effects, side effects, and to report to physician if symptoms persist despite medication treatment.	Promotes knowledge, facilitates compliance with treatment, and allows for prompt identification of potential need for changes in medication regimen to prevent complications.

NIC: *Teaching: Disease Process*

Discharge or Maintenance Evaluation

■ Patient will be able to verbalize understanding of disease process and actions to take to prevent and reduce reflux.

■ Patient will be compliant with dietary limitations and inclusions of positioning and stretching prior to and after meals.

■ Patient will be compliant with medication regimen, and will notify physician if symptoms persist despite correct use of medicines.

■ Patient will be able to accurately recall all information and have increased understanding of positioning after meals.

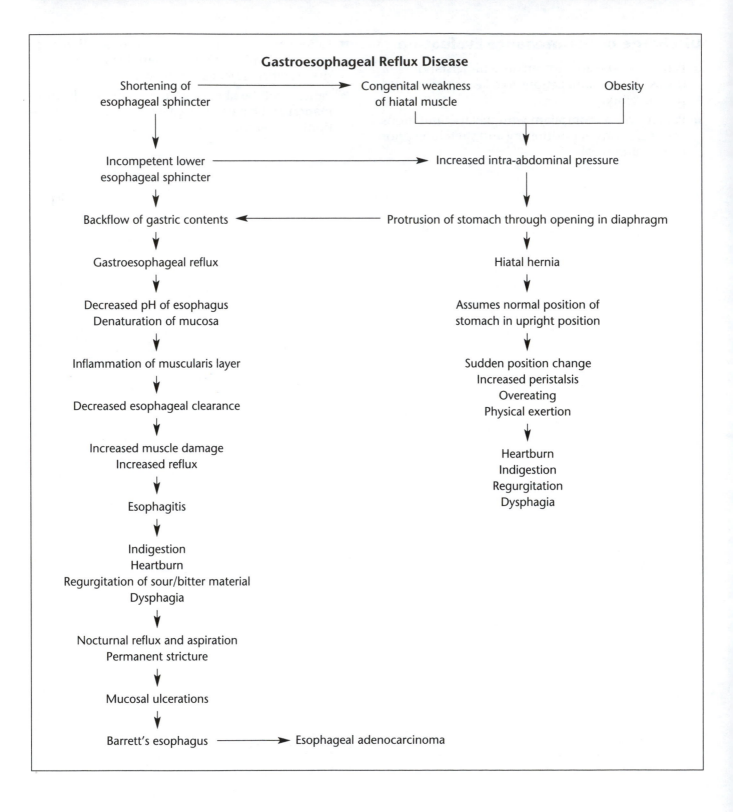

Gastroesophageal Reflux Disease

Shortening of esophageal sphincter → Congenital weakness of hiatal muscle   Obesity

Shortening of esophageal sphincter ↓
Incompetent lower esophageal sphincter

Congenital weakness of hiatal muscle / Obesity ↓
Increased intra-abdominal pressure

Incompetent lower esophageal sphincter → Increased intra-abdominal pressure

Incompetent lower esophageal sphincter ↓
Backflow of gastric contents

Protrusion of stomach through opening in diaphragm → Backflow of gastric contents

Increased intra-abdominal pressure ↓
Protrusion of stomach through opening in diaphragm

Backflow of gastric contents ↓
Gastroesophageal reflux

Protrusion of stomach through opening in diaphragm ↓
Hiatal hernia

Gastroesophageal reflux ↓
Decreased pH of esophagus
Denaturation of mucosa

Hiatal hernia ↓
Assumes normal position of stomach in upright position

Decreased pH of esophagus / Denaturation of mucosa ↓
Inflammation of muscularis layer

Assumes normal position of stomach in upright position ↓
Sudden position change
Increased peristalsis
Overeating
Physical exertion

Inflammation of muscularis layer ↓
Decreased esophageal clearance

Sudden position change / Increased peristalsis / Overeating / Physical exertion ↓
Heartburn
Indigestion
Regurgitation
Dysphagia

Decreased esophageal clearance ↓
Increased muscle damage
Increased reflux

Increased muscle damage / Increased reflux ↓
Esophagitis

Esophagitis ↓
Indigestion
Heartburn
Regurgitation of sour/bitter material
Dysphagia

Indigestion / Heartburn / Regurgitation of sour/bitter material / Dysphagia ↓
Nocturnal reflux and aspiration
Permanent stricture

Nocturnal reflux and aspiration / Permanent stricture ↓
Mucosal ulcerations

Mucosal ulcerations ↓
Barrett's esophagus → Esophageal adenocarcinoma

CHAPTER 4.5

GASTROINTESTINAL BLEEDING

Gastrointestinal bleeding may be massive and acute, or occult and chronic in nature. GI bleeding results when irritation of the mucosal lining results in erosion through to the submucosal layer. Upper GI hemorrhage is considered to be a bleed from any site proximal to the cecum, and all ulcerative bleeding is arterial with the exception of a tear that cuts across all vessels, malignant tumors, and in patients with esophagitis.

When erosion into an artery occurs, it usually produces two bleeding sites because of arterio-arterial anastomoses. When the bleeding occurs at the ulcer base artery, it may be a life-threatening emergency.

Bleeding may occur from the lower gastrointestinal tract as well. Causes of lower GI bleeding include hemorrhoids, diverticulosis, inflammatory bowel disease, rectal perforation, or intussusception.

Acute upper GI bleeding may result from many causes, such as gastritis, peptic ulcer, stress, drugs, hormones, trauma, head injuries, burns, and esophageal varices.

Differential diagnosis between gastric and duodenal ulcers must be obtained. Duodenal ulcers usually account for approximately 80% of all ulcers noted and rarely become cancerous. Gastric ulcers, on the other hand, may become cancerous and are more likely to bleed.

Initial presenting symptoms of a GI bleed include at least one of the following: hematemesis, melena, or hematochezia. An acute bleed will comprise more than 60 cc/day of black tarry stool, and usually greater than 500 cc, whereas occult bleeding amounts are normally 15–30 cc/day. Stools can be positive for occult blood up to 12 days after an acute bleed. Of all GI hemorrhages, 80% usually stop spontaneously.

In the elderly, the most common causes of minor GI bleeding are hemorrhoids and colorectal cancers. The most common causes of major GI bleeding are peptic ulcer disease, diverticular disease, and angiodysplasia. Substantial GI bleeding is not tolerated well by the elderly because of their inability to compensate for massive losses of blood and circulating volume, and these bleeding episodes have a high morbidity. Aged patients may continue to have urinary output even with decreasing intravascular volume up to such a point that they have no urinary output and cannot be fluid resuscitated, which results in circulatory collapse.

The goal of treatment is initially prevention and treatment of shock, with fluid volume replacement. Maintenance of circulating blood volume is imperative to prevent myocardial infarction, sepsis, and death. Endoscopic examination is the primary diagnostic procedure utilized. Once the lesion has been identified, treatment may be used to control bleeding.

MEDICAL CARE

Laboratory: CBC used to identify changes in blood volume and concentration, but may be normal during rapid loss because of the lapsed time required for equilibration of intravascular with extravascular spaces; MCV is useful to identify prolonged chronic loss with iron deficiency; B_{12} and folic acid levels used to identify anemia type; reticulocyte count may identify new RBC formation that occurs with an old bleed; platelet count, PT, PTT, and bleeding times to evaluate clotting status and platelet dysfunction; BUN and creatinine to evaluate effect on renal status; electrolyte profiles to evaluate imbalances and treatment; ammonia levels may be used to identify liver dysfunction; gastric analysis to determine presence of blood and assess secretory activity of gastric mucosa; amylases is elevated if duodenal ulcer has posterior penetration; pepsinogen level used to help identify type of bleeding, with elevations seen in duodenal ulcer, and decreased levels seen in gastritis; stool specimens for guaiac

Arterial blood gases: may be used to identify acid–base imbalances, compensation for decreased blood flow; initially respiratory alkalosis occurs and changes to metabolic acidosis as metabolic wastes accumulate

Esophagogastroduodenoscopy (EGD): used as the primary diagnostic tool for upper GI bleeding to visually identify the lesion; can be performed as soon as lavage controls bleeding

Angiography: used when bleeding cannot be cleared for endoscopy; can identify bleeding site and allows for injection of vasopressin for active mucosal bleeding

Radiography: chest X-rays may be done to evaluate for free air/perforation; upper GI series may be done after endoscopy, but is never done prior because of the fact that the contrast media will adhere to the mucosa and prevent further examination; may be done to identify other diagnoses; barium enema may be done once lower GI bleeding is stopped; radionuclide scanning, such as Red Cell Tags, identify sources of bleeding, but may take an extended time for results to show

Electrocardiogram: used to identify changes in heart rate and rhythm, and identify conduction problems or dysrhythmias that may occur with fluid shifting or electrolyte imbalances

IV fluids: used for fluid resuscitation, to provide hydration, and for the administration of medications and blood products

Blood products: blood, plasma, and platelets may be required for replacement based on the severity of the bleed

Nasogastric tubes: large bore NG tubes or Ewald tube may be inserted to allow for iced/saline lavage, confirmation of bleeding, and for decompression of the stomach

Levophed: may be used in solution with saline for lavage when plain saline not effective in stopping bleeding because of its vasoconstrictor effects; must be used cautiously in the elderly

Vasopressin: may be used for direct infusion into the gastric artery to control bleeding, or via intravenous route for specified length of time; cardiac side effects must be considered; this usually controls bleeding in approximately 80% of cases

Antacids: aluminum carbonate (Basaljel), aluminum hydroxide (AlternaGEL, Amphojel, Dialume), cal-

cium carbonate (Alka-Mints, Amitone, Chooz, Dicarbosil, Maalox, Rolaids, Tums), magaldrate (Lowsium, Riopan), and magnesium oxide (Mag-Ox, Maox, Uro-Mag) used to help neutralize gastric acid; Gaviscon may be superior to antacids alone because it also contains alginic acid which floats on the gastric acid collection in the stomach and helps decrease reflux if the patient is upright; antacids are used to alter pH so that platelets can aggregate and stop bleeding, and to prevent digestion of raw mucosal surfaces

H_2-receptor antagonists: cimetidine (Tagamet), famotidine (Pepcid), nizatidine (Axid), ranitidine bismuth citrate (Tritec), and ranitidine hydrochloride (Zantac) used to inhibit histamine at the receptor sites in the parietal cells, which results in gastric acid secretion being inhibited; should not be utilized at the same time with antacids because of absorption interference

Proton pump inhibitors: esomeprazole magnesium (Nexium), lansoprazole (Prevacid), omeprazole (Prilosec), pantoprazole sodium (Prontonix), and rabeprazole sodium (Aciphex) used to suppress gastric secretion by inhibiting hydrogen/potassium ATPase enzyme system in the gastric parietal cell; blocks final step of acid production

Prostaglandin E_1 analogues: misoprostol (Cytotec) used to replace gastric prostaglandins depleted by the use of NSAIDs; decreases basal gastric acid secretion and increases gastric mucus and bicarbonate production

Sucralfate: used to help heal ulcer by forming protective barrier at site; must not be used with any other medication as it will also form barrier around that medicine and prevent absorption

Surgery: may be required for control of hemorrhage, or laparotomy may be required to identify the source of the lesion

COMMON NURSING DIAGNOSES

IMBALANCED NUTRITION: LESS THAN BODY REQUIREMENTS (see COPD)

Related to: nausea, vomiting, nasogastric tube, gastrointestinal bleeding, increased metabolism caused by disease process, decreased level of consciousness, inability to absorb nutrients because of biologic or psychological factors

Defining Characteristics: actual inadequate food intake, altered taste, altered smell sensation, weight loss, body weight 20% or more under ideal for height and frame, anorexia, absent bowel sounds, decreased peristalsis, muscle mass loss, decreased muscle tone, changes in bowel habits, nausea, vomiting, abdominal distention, lack of interest in food, abdominal pain or discomfort, sore, inflamed buccal cavity, depression, anxiety, social isolation, changes in mental status, fatigue from work of breathing, weakness

ACUTE PAIN (see CAD)

Related to: gastrointestinal bleeding, gastric mucosal irritation, inflammation, infection, obstruction, spasm, sepsis, peritonitis, surgery

Defining Characteristics: communication of pain, fever, malaise, abdominal pain, abdominal distention, elevated white blood cell count, surgical wound, drains, abdominal guarding, tachycardia, hypotension, hypertension, bradypnea, tachypnea, facial grimacing, crying, moaning

INEFFECTIVE TISSUE PERFUSION: CARDIOPULMONARY, CEREBRAL, PERIPHERAL, GASTRO-INTESTINAL, RENAL (see CAD)

Related to: reduced oxygen supply, hypovolemia, hypoxia, vasoconstrictive therapy, hypoperfusion, myocardial infarction, angina, dysrhythmias, coexisting disease processes, age-related vascular structure changes, inactivity, surgery

Defining Characteristics: chest pain, conduction disturbances, dysrhythmias, vital sign changes, ECG changes, delayed capillary refill time, chest retractions, dyspnea, nasal flaring, use of accessory muscles, increased work of breathing, tachypnea, bradypnea, changes in mental status, weakness, paralysis, behavioral changes, abdominal distention, ileus, hypoactive or absent bowel sounds, nausea, vomiting, edema, weak or absent peripheral pulses, skin temperature changes, skin color changes, decreased peripheral tactile sensation, hematuria, oliguria, anuria, increased BUN and creatinine, confusion, headache

DEFICIENT KNOWLEDGE (see CAD)

Related to: lack of information about gastrointestinal bleeding, hypovolemia, hypoxia, cognitive limita-

tions, medications, neurologic impairment, lack of recall

Defining Characteristics: request for information, anxiety regarding potential errors, presence of preventable complications, noncompliance with instructions, misperceptions about illness

ADDITIONAL NURSING DIAGNOSES

DEFICIENT FLUID VOLUME

Related to: gastrointestinal bleeding

Defining Characteristics: hypotension, tachycardia, decreased skin turgor, weakness, decreased urinary output, pallor, diaphoresis, decreased capillary refill, mental changes, restlessness, decreased filling pressures, decreased hemoglobin and hematocrit, dry mucous membranes, increased hematocrit initially, concentrated urine, thirst, weakness

Outcome Criteria

✔ Patient will have no further bleeding and vital signs will be stable.

NOC: *Fluid Balance*

INTERVENTIONS	RATIONALES
Monitor vital signs, including orthostatic changes when feasible.	Patients with major GI blood losses will present with supine hypotension and resting tachycardia greater than 110/minute, orthostatic diastolic BP decreases of at least 10 mm Hg, and orthostatic pulse increases of at least 15/min. Changes in vital signs may help approximate amount of blood loss and reflect decreasing circulating blood volume.
Measure I&O every 1–4 hours and notify physician of significant changes. Measure specific gravity as ordered.	Oliguria and increased specific gravity indicate hypovolemia.
Insert nasogastric tube for acute bleeding episodes, and monitor drainage for changes in bleeding character.	Facilitates removal of gastric contents, blood, and clots, relieves gastric distention, decreases nausea and vomiting, and provides for lavaging of

(continues)

(continued)

INTERVENTIONS	RATIONALES
	stomach. Blood left in the stomach can be metabolized into ammonia and result in neurologic encephalopathy.
Actively lavage stomach via NG or Ewald tube per protocol with cold or room temperature saline until return is light pink or clear.	Saline solution is utilized to reduce washout of electrolytes that may occur with use of water. Flushing facilitates removal of clots to assist with visualization of bleeding site, and may assist with control of bleeding through a vasoconstrictive effect. The current consensus of opinion is that differences between using cold versus room temperature solution is negligible, and, in fact, iced solution may actually inhibit platelet function by lowering core body temperature.
Notify physician if bleeding clears and then becomes bright red again.	May indicate further bleeding or renewed bleeding.
Monitor amounts of lavage fluid, bloody aspirate, blood products, and vomitus, and include in I&O totals.	Helps facilitate estimation of fluid replacement required. Lavage amounts facilitate estimation of the magnitude of bleeding based on the volume of solution needed to clear the gastric return, and how long lavage is required before the aspirate clears.
Administer IV fluids as ordered, through large bore catheters. Many facilities recommend at least 2 IV sites for patients with active bleeding.	Facilitates rapid replacement of circulating volume prior to availability of blood products. Solutions of choice are normal saline or lactated Ringer's, and should be run wide open until blood pressure is stabilized, and titrated to match volume requirements after that.
Administer blood transfusions, fresh frozen plasma, platelets, or whole blood as ordered.	Fresh whole blood may be ordered when bleeding is acute and the patient is in shock so as to ensure that clotting factors are not deficient. Packed red blood cells are utilized most often for replacement, especially when fluid shifting may create overload. Frequently, fresh frozen plasma (FFP) will be concurrently administered to replace clotting factors, and

INTERVENTIONS	RATIONALES
	facilitate cessation of an acute bleed. For each unit of blood transfused, a 3 point increase in the hematocrit should be noted. If this elevation is not noted, continued bleeding should be suspected.
Administer albumin as ordered.	May be used for volume expansion until blood products are available.
Administer vasopressin as ordered.	Intra-arterial infusion may be required for severe active bleeding and the patient must be monitored closely for development of complications from the infusion. ICU placement is preferred.
Administer histamine blockers and/or proton pump inhibitors as ordered.	Histamine blockers decrease acid production, increase pH, and decrease gastric mucosal irritation. Proton pump inhibitors act at the parietal cell level to block the final step in acid production.
Administer sucralfate as ordered.	Decreases gastric acid secretion and provides a protective layer over the ulcer site. May decrease or inhibit absorption of other medications.
Administer antacids as ordered.	Facilitates maintenance of pH level to decrease the potential for rebleeding. Antacids should not be concurrently given with histamine blockers.
Monitor lab work for changes and/or trends.	Hemoglobin and hematocrit help to identify blood replacement needs, but may not initially change as a result of loss of plasma and RBCs. BUN levels greater than 40 in the presence of a normal creatinine may signify major bleeding, and BUN should normalize within 12 hours after bleeding has ceased.
Administer antimicrobials as ordered.	May be indicated when infection is thought to be the cause of the gastritis or ulcer.
Instruct patient/family regarding procedures, surgery, and care needed to treat GI bleeding.	Provides knowledge and enhances compliance. Patient may be too ill for education because of hypovolemia.

INTERVENTIONS	RATIONALES
Instruct patient/family regarding EGD and sclerotherapy.	EGD provides direct visualization of an upper GI bleeding site, and a sclerosing substance may be injected at the site to stop bleeding or prevent a recurrence.
Instruct patient/family regarding colonoscopy.	Colonoscopy may be required to identify a lower GI bleeding site and for removal of biopsy tissue or polyps.
Prepare patient for surgery.	May be required to control gastric hemorrhage. Vagotomy, pyloroplasty, oversewing of the ulcer, and total or subtotal gastrectomy may be the procedure of choice based on the severity of the bleed and site of the bleed.

NIC: *Hypovolemia Management*

Discharge or Maintenance Evaluation

■ Patient will achieve and have stable fluid balance with normal vital signs based on specific patient parameters.

■ Patient will have adequate urinary output and an equivalent intake and output.

■ Patient will have no complications from fluid or blood replacement therapy, such as pulmonary edema or congestive heart failure.

■ Patient will have lab work within normal limits.

■ Patient will have no active bleeding or occult blood in stools.

■ Patient/family will be able to accurately verbalize understanding of procedures required.

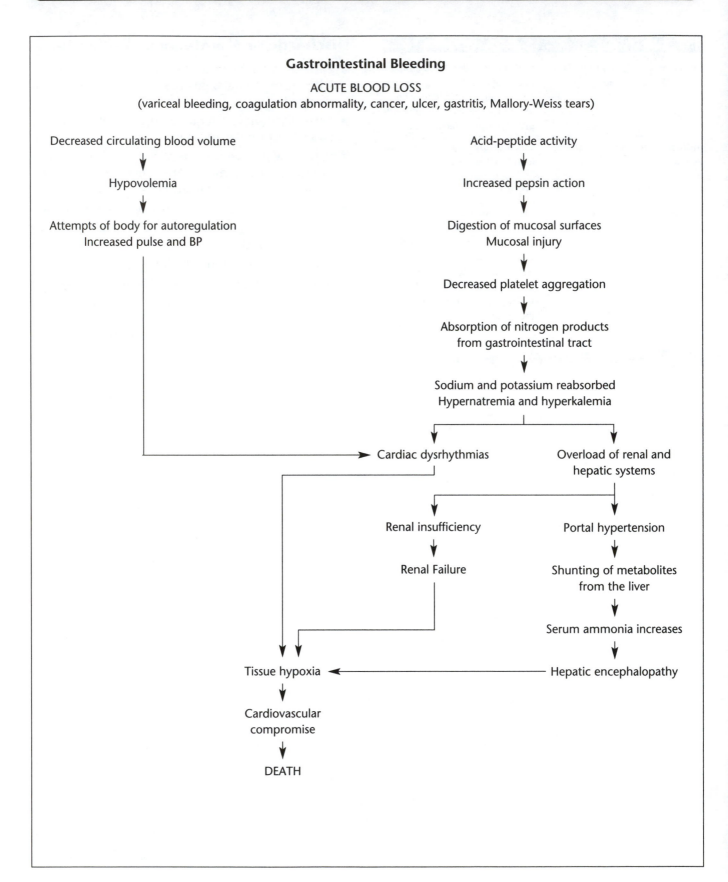

Gastrointestinal Bleeding

ACUTE BLOOD LOSS
(variceal bleeding, coagulation abnormality, cancer, ulcer, gastritis, Mallory-Weiss tears)

Decreased circulating blood volume

↓

Hypovolemia

↓

Attempts of body for autoregulation
Increased pulse and BP

Acid-peptide activity

↓

Increased pepsin action

↓

Digestion of mucosal surfaces
Mucosal injury

↓

Decreased platelet aggregation

↓

Absorption of nitrogen products
from gastrointestinal tract

↓

Sodium and potassium reabsorbed
Hypernatremia and hyperkalemia

Cardiac dysrhythmias

Overload of renal and
hepatic systems

Renal insufficiency

↓

Renal Failure

Portal hypertension

↓

Shunting of metabolites
from the liver

↓

Serum ammonia increases

↓

Tissue hypoxia ← Hepatic encephalopathy

↓

Cardiovascular
compromise

↓

DEATH

CHAPTER 4.6

HEMORRHOIDS

Hemorrhoids, also known as piles, are abnormally swollen or dilated collections of blood veins that are located at the anal opening or just inside the opening. Internal hemorrhoids are varicose veins above the notched line above the anus that involves the rectal mucosa. External hemorrhoids are ones that involve the distal portion that is covered with anorectal skin. A thrombosed external hemorrhoid occurs when a clot localizes in the vein of an external hemorrhoid or appears as a result of a ruptured hemorrhoidal blood vessel.

Hemorrhoids are created when increased pressure in the veins destroy the valves and allows blood to pool in the veins, distending the walls and predisposing them to rupture and bleeding during a bowel movement. Constipation is a significant contributing factor to the development of hemorrhoids, and pregnancy, obesity, and other conditions that increase abdominal pressure are also factors.

Symptoms of hemorrhoids include an initial observation of bright red blood noted after a bowel movement, either on the stool or on the toilet paper. Burning and itching around the anus also occurs. Significant bleeding rarely occurs, but continued blood loss may lead to anemia. Severe, exquisite type pain may be felt if internal hemorrhoids prolapse or external hemorrhoids become thrombosed.

The goals of treatment include reducing pain, swelling, and bleeding, and prevention of recurrences. Establishment of regular bowel routines, prevention of constipation, and Kegel exercises have been found to be helpful in the prevention and improvement of hemorrhoids. If conservative methods of treatment are not effective, surgical intervention may be necessary.

Sclerotherapy, in which a chemical solution is injected into the distended veins, can be performed and causes the vessel to become inflamed, swelling of the lining, and ultimately closing off the vessel. The blood-deprived vein collapses and is absorbed into the body. Banding the hemorrhoids is another procedure that involves tying off the blood vessels with a rubber band until it falls off after several days.

MEDICAL CARE

Laboratory: CBC may be used to identify significant blood loss or anemia as a result of continued hemorrhoidal bleeding

Proctoscopy/anoscopy: used to identify and visualize the presence and condition of hemorrhoids

Dietary modifications: increasing bulk in the diet, and increasing fluid intake to decrease constipation helps prevent hemorrhoids

Stool softeners: calcium polycarbophil (Equalactin, Fiberall, FiberCon, Mitrolan), docusate calcium or sodium (DC Softgels, Sulfolax, Surfak, Colace, Coloxyl, Diocto, DOS, DUOsol, Modane, Pro-Sof), glycerin (Fleet Babylax, Sani-Supp), lactulose (Cephulac, Cholac, Chronulac, Constilac, Duphalac, Enulose), methylcellulose (Citrucel), psyllium (Fiberall, Genfiber, Hydrocil, Konsyl, Metamucil, Perdiem, Prodiem, Serutan, Unilax, V-Lax); bulk laxatives used to provide sufficient bulk to stool to promote peristalsis and bowel elimination; osmotic stool softeners help soften stools to allow for easier elimination; suppositories may be required for acute constipation or as part of a bowel program; enemas used when impaction of stool exists; soapsuds enemas may result in mucosal damage and cramping and should be avoided; oil enemas used to soften impacted stool for easier removal; may be used to reduce hemorrhoid discomfort and preventing recurrence by assisting with bowel elimination that avoids straining and increasing intra-abdominal pressures

Topical medications: hydrocortisone (Anusol HC, Hemril-HC, ProctoCream-HC) is a cortisone-based drug used to reduce inflammation, pruritis, and vasoconstriction to rectal tissues and vasculature;

ointments, such as Hemorid or Preparation H, that contain benzocaine or other local anesthetics help to alleviate the exquisite pain, and some ointments can help reduce the swelling and itching also associated with hemorrhoids

Surgery: rubber banding of mildly prolapsed or bleeding internal hemorrhoids sometimes performed which effectively ligates the hemorrhoid and then falls off a few days later; sclerotherapy, utilizing a chemical that is injected into the vein, seals off the internal hemorrhoid to prevent further bleeding, but frequently secondary hemorrhoids develop; laser surgery or cryotherapy can be used for external hemorrhoids; hemorrhoidectomy is treatment of choice when both internal and external hemorrhoids are involved

COMMON NURSING DIAGNOSES

 ### ACUTE PAIN (see INFLUENZA)

Related to: hemorrhoidal pain, gastrointestinal bleeding, gastric mucosal irritation, inflammation, infection, constipation, spasm, surgery

Defining Characteristics: communication of pain, fever, malaise, rectal pain, elevated white blood cell count, surgical wound, drains, tachycardia, hypertension, tachypnea, facial grimacing, crying, moaning, exquisite rectal pain, rectal bleeding, rectal pruritis, rectal burning

 ### CONSTIPATION (see HEART FAILURE)

Related to: low residue dietary intake, lack of dietary bulk, hemorrhoidal pain, medications

Defining Characteristics: passage of hard, formed stool, decreased bowel sounds, inability to evacuate stool, severe, exquisite rectal pain, abdominal pain, abdominal distention, ileus, absent bowel sounds, nausea, vomiting, frequency of stool less than normal, less than usual amount of stool, palpable mass, feelings of rectal fullness, inability to ingest bulk-containing foods, flatulence

 ### RISK FOR INFECTION (see TB)

Related to: inadequate primary defenses, perianal sepsis following hemorrhoidal banding procedure, chronic disease process, immunosuppression, poor nutrition

Defining Characteristics: increased temperature, chills, elevated white blood cell count, purulent drainage, prolonged rectal pain, urinary retention, sepsis, positive blood cultures

ADDITIONAL NURSING DIAGNOSES

 ### IMPAIRED SKIN INTEGRITY

Related to: hemorrhoidal surgery, hemorrhoidal procedures, alteration in activity, changes in mobility, aging process, loss of elasticity of skin

Defining Characteristics: disruption of skin tissue from incisional sites, destruction of skin layers, thrombosed hemorrhoids, internal prolapsed hemorrhoids, pain, swelling, drainage

Outcome Criteria

✔ Patient will have intact skin, with no signs or symptoms of rectal prolapse or bleeding.

✔ Hemorrhoids will be reduced or removed.

NOC: *Tissue Integrity: Skin and Mucus Membranes*

INTERVENTIONS	RATIONALES
Assess patient for presence of hemorrhoids, discomfort associated with hemorrhoids, diet, fluid intake, and presence of constipation.	Provides information as to type of hemorrhoids (external versus internal), degree of venous thrombosis, presence of complications, including bleeding, and risk factors that preclude patient to hemorrhoids to enable initiation of care plan appropriate for patient.
Administer topical medications as ordered.	Reduces swelling, pain, and itching in order to make patient more comfortable.
Provide "donut" for patient to sit on if needed.	Hemorrhoids are exquisitely painful and patient may not be able to sit in chair and apply pressure to delicate tissues. Rubber donuts can help to remove pressure from hemorrhoid, but caution should be employed to ensure that other pressure areas do not develop.
Administer stool softeners as ordered.	Helps to prevent further straining and increased pressure that may

INTERVENTIONS	RATIONALES
	cause clotted vessel to rupture or cause further hemorrhoids to develop. Helps to relieve pain by avoiding passage of hard fecal material.
Assist with procedures for treatment of hemorrhoids.	Sclerotherapy may be used if hemorrhoidal problem is noted early, with injection of quinine urea hydrochloride or other agent into sclerosed vessels, with resultant swelling and dying of the vessel, with reabsorption within the body. Banding the hemorrhoids may be performed by application of a rubber band around the base of each hemorrhoid, which ultimately results in the death and necrosis of the hemorrhoid. Laser surgery may be performed but symptomatic relief is not obtained quickly. Hemorrhoidectomy is performed if the patient has internal hemorrhoids with prolapse, or if the patient has both internal and external hemorrhoids. It relieves symptoms immediately, but current thoughts are that this surgery creates scar tissue that can lead to fissures, tears, and other complications, and should be done only as a last resort.
Instruct patient/family regarding causes of hemorrhoids, methods of avoiding hemorrhoids, and treatments that can be performed.	Hemorrhoids are caused by heavy lifting, straining, obesity, pregnancy, and any activity that distends rectal veins and causes them to prolapse. Rubber banding, sclerotherapy, and hemorrhoidectomy are potential treatments if medication and dietary changes are not successful at treating the problem.
Instruct patient/family regarding all procedures required.	Internal hemorrhoids are normally diagnosed by anoscopy or flexible sigmoidoscopy because digital

INTERVENTIONS	RATIONALES
	rectal exam cannot adequately detect hemorrhoids. Barium enemas or colonoscopy may be required to ensure that intestinal masses are not present as well.
Instruct patient/family in dietary management.	Increasing bulk, fiber, fluids, and eating fruits and vegetables can help by maintaining soft stools to avoid straining at bowel movements.
Instruct patient/family regarding the use of bulk producing agents, such as psyllium.	Bulk-forming laxatives, such as Fiberall, Metamucil, and Serutan, help to absorb water to increase moisture content of the stool, increase peristalsis, and help to promote soft bowel movements.
Instruct patient/family in comfort measures to use with the presence of hemorrhoids.	Use of rubber donuts remove pressure directly placed on the hemorrhoid. Warm sitz baths or suppositories/creams containing anesthetic agents can help to alleviate pain temporarily.

NIC: *Skin Care: Topical Treatments*

NIC: *Skin Surveillance*

Discharge or Maintenance Evaluation

- Patient will exhibit no evidence of thrombosed hemorrhoids or rectal bleeding.
- Patient will have normal CBC with no noted anemias.
- Patient will be able to accurately verbalize understanding of causes of hemorrhoids, methods of controlling worsening hemorrhoids, and comfort measures to employ if hemorrhoids are present.
- Swollen hemorrhoids will be reduced in size, with no pain evoked.
- Patient will be able to tolerate procedures to diagnose problem and to treat hemorrhoids without the presence of any complication.

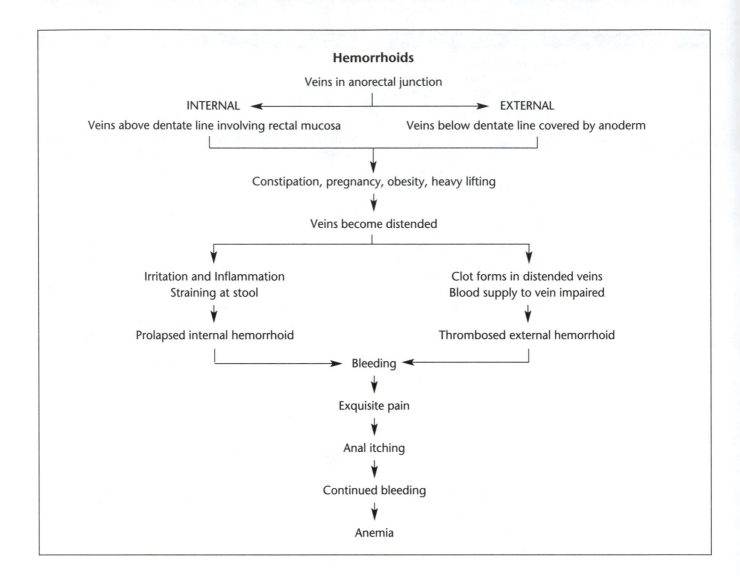

Hemorrhoids

Veins in anorectal junction

INTERNAL ←———————————————→ EXTERNAL

Veins above dentate line involving rectal mucosa   Veins below dentate line covered by anoderm

Constipation, pregnancy, obesity, heavy lifting

Veins become distended

Irritation and Inflammation   Clot forms in distended veins
Straining at stool   Blood supply to vein impaired

Prolapsed internal hemorrhoid   Thrombosed external hemorrhoid

Bleeding

Exquisite pain

Anal itching

Continued bleeding

Anemia

CHAPTER 4.7

HEPATITIS

Acute hepatitis is an infection of the liver that usually is viral in origin but may be induced by drugs or toxins. There are currently five types of hepatitis, denoted HAV, HBV, NANB or hepatitis C, HDV, and HEV, with HAV being the most common type. Hepatitis B, or HBV, is more severe and because it can be acquired from exposure to individuals who are asymptomatic, the potential for transmission is increased many-fold. Acute hepatitis A, B, and C are much less commonly seen in the elderly than in younger patients.

Hepatitis A, or HAV, is transmitted via the fecal-oral route, with poor sanitation practices, with contamination of food, water, milk, and shellfish, or oral-anal sexual practices. HAV patients may exhibit no acute symptoms or have symptoms that are related to other causes. It is the most common and least dangerous form of the disease. Once a person has had hepatitis A, he or she becomes immune to future infection. The elderly patient may not recover as easily as a younger, more healthy person, with this illness, especially if he or she has other concurrent medical diseases.

Hepatitis B, or HBV, is transmitted via blood and blood products, breaks in the skin or mucous membranes, via any bodily fluid, from contaminated needles, or from an asymptomatic carrier with Hepatitis B surface antigen (HbsAg) (Bockhold, 2000). This type of hepatitis accounts for approximately 10% of all deaths worldwide, and is approximately 100 times more contagious than the HIV (AIDS) virus. Treatment with lamivudine therapy in the elderly results in less response than with younger patients. The majority of patients who are infected with Hepatitis B recover and have a lifelong immunity, with the exception of approximately 10% who become carriers of the virus.

Hepatitis C, or Non-A, Non-B hepatitis, is transmitted via intravenous drug use, sexual contact,

blood or blood products, and from asymptomatic carriers. Treatment with interferon, either alone or in combination with ribavirin, usually results in less clearance of the virus in the elderly as compared with treatment in a younger population, and is caused by a decrease in immune system function and progressive destruction of T-lymphocyte activity. Hepatitis C can become chronic in nature and produce carriers of the disease.

Hepatitis D, or HDV, is transmitted through the same routes as HBV but must have hepatitis B surface antigen to replicate.

Hepatitis E, or HEV, is seen in developing countries and not usually encountered in the United States. It is transmitted through food or water contamination.

Once the disease has been contracted, treatment is symptomatic. Prophylactic therapy may assist in prevention of hepatitis from developing after being exposed to the virus. Immune globulin (IG) is generally given to provide temporary passive immunity. Hepatitis B vaccine provides active immunity and offers protection to people who are at high risk.

MEDICAL CARE

Laboratory: CBC shows decreased RBCs as a result of decreased life span from enzyme alterations or from hemorrhage; white blood cell count usually shows leukocytosis, atypical lymphocytes, and plasma cells; liver function studies abnormal, up to 10 times the normal values in some cases, albumin is decreased; blood glucose may be decreased or elevated transiently because of liver dysfunction; Anti-HAV IgM presence shows either current infection or after 6 weeks may indicate immunity; hepatitis B surface antigen and hepatitis Be antigen show presence of HBV; Anti-HBc in serum indicates carrier status;

Anti-HbsAg indicates HBV immunity; anti-delta anti-bodies present without HbsAg indicates HDV; urine bilirubin is elevated; prothrombin time may be elevated with liver dysfunction

Liver biopsy: used to delineate type of hepatitis and degree of liver necrosis

Liver scans: may be used to identify level of parenchymal damage

Hepatitis vaccine: used against Hepatitis B for people who are at high risk; provides immunity for 5 years or more

Immunoglobulin (IG): may be given prophylactically to prevent the spread of the virus; has been shown to help prevent Hepatitis A but lasts for only a few weeks

Ribavirin: Virazole helps to inhibit RNA and DNA synthesis by decreasing the intracellular nucleotide collection, and may be helpful in some cases of hepatitis

COMMON NURSING DIAGNOSES

 ### ACTIVITY INTOLERANCE (see CAD)

Related to: infective process, fatigue, weakness, decreased endurance, inadequate rest

Defining Characteristics: dyspnea, decreased oxygen saturation levels with movement or activity, increased heart rate and blood pressure with movement or activity, feelings of tiredness, weakness, easy fatigability, lethargy, malaise, decreased muscle strength, reluctance to perform activities

 ### SOCIAL ISOLATION (see ALZHEIMER'S DISEASE)

Related to: changes in health status, changes in physical status, imposed physical isolation, inadequate support systems, depression, withdrawal, loneliness

Defining Characteristics: sad, dull affect, uncommunicative, withdrawn, expresses feeling of loneliness and aloneness, rejection, absence of supportive significant other(s), inability to meet expectations of others, indifference by others, lack of support systems

 ### IMBALANCED NUTRITION: LESS THAN BODY REQUIREMENTS (see LIVER FAILURE)

Related to: anorexia, inability to take in enough food, increased metabolism caused by disease process, decreased level of consciousness, inability to absorb nutrients because of biologic or psychological factors

Defining Characteristics: actual inadequate food intake, altered taste, altered smell sensation, weight loss, body weight 20% or more under ideal for height and frame, anorexia, absent bowel sounds, decreased peristalsis, muscle mass loss, decreased muscle tone, changes in bowel habits, nausea, vomiting, abdominal distention, lack of interest in food, social isolation, anorexia, malabsorption of fats, altered metabolism of protein, carbohydrates, and fat, fatigue, edema

 ### RISK FOR INFECTION (see TB)

Related to: leukopenia, immunosuppression, malnutrition, exposure to virus, risk factors that threaten physical well-being, crowded living conditions, unsanitary living conditions, presence of HIV infection, presence of chronic illnesses, history of substance abuse, immigration from Africa, Asia, or South America

Defining Characteristics: positive cultures, fever, cough, anorexia, weight loss, fatigue, jaundice, hepatomegaly, increased white blood cell count, differential with a shift to the left, chills, hypotension, tachycardia

 ### IMPAIRED SKIN INTEGRITY (see LIVER FAILURE)

Related to: bile salt accumulations on skin

Defining Characteristics: jaundice, pruritus, itching, scratching

ADDITIONAL NURSING DIAGNOSES

DEFICIENT KNOWLEDGE

Related to: lack of information about hepatitis, lack of recall, unfamiliarity of resources, misinterpretation of information received

Defining Characteristics: verbalization of questions, requests for information, statements of misperceptions, development of preventable complications

Outcome Criteria

✔ Patient will be able to verbalize understanding of hepatitis, treatment, and causative behaviors.

NOC: *Knowledge: Disease Process*

INTERVENTIONS	RATIONALES
Discuss patient's perception of his illness. Assess if patient is aware of type of hepatitis and method of transmission with regard to his illness.	Identifies knowledge base and misconceptions to facilitate establishment of appropriate teaching plan.
Consult with counselors, ministers, drug or alcohol treatment facilities, or other community resources as warranted.	May be required for assistance with substance withdrawal and for long-term support once patient is discharged.
Instruct patient on disease process, prevention and transmission of disease, and isolation requirements.	Types of isolation will vary according to the type of hepatitis and personal situation. Family members may require treatment depending on the type of hepatitis.
Instruct patient/family in appropriate home sanitation.	Dirty environment and poor sanitation methods may be responsible for transmission of the disease.
Instruct patient on activity limitations.	Complete resumption of normal activity may not take place until the liver returns to its normal size and patient begins to feel better, and this make take up to several months.

INTERVENTIONS	RATIONALES
Instruct patient/family on all medications, side effects, effects, contraindications, and dangers of administration of over-the-counter drugs without physician approval.	Promotes knowledge and facilitates compliance. Some medications are hepatotoxic or are metabolized by the liver, increasing its workload. Some over-the-counter drugs interact with prescribed medications and may inhibit or decrease their efficacy.
Instruct patient to refrain from blood and plasma donation.	Most states do not allow anyone who has a history of any type of hepatitis to donate blood or blood products to prevent possible spread of the infection.
Instruct patient/family regarding avoidance of recreational drugs and/or alcohol.	May jeopardize recovery from infection and increases liver dysfunction.

NIC: *Teaching: Disease Process*

Discharge or Maintenance Evaluation

- Patient will be able to accurately verbalize understanding of all instructions given.
- Patient/family will be able to modify environment to control the spread of disease.
- Patient will be able to effectively access community resources for treatment programs and discharge follow-up care.
- Patient will be able to effectively manage medical regimen with follow-up from physician.
- Patient will refrain from using recreational drugs and/or alcohol.

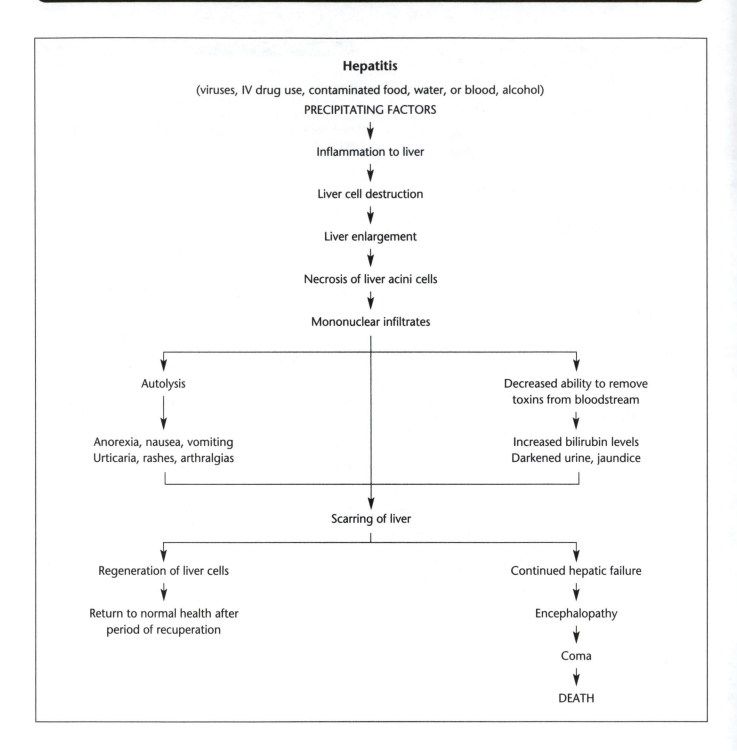

Hepatitis

(viruses, IV drug use, contaminated food, water, or blood, alcohol)

PRECIPITATING FACTORS

↓

Inflammation to liver

↓

Liver cell destruction

↓

Liver enlargement

↓

Necrosis of liver acini cells

↓

Mononuclear infiltrates

Autolysis	Decreased ability to remove toxins from bloodstream
Anorexia, nausea, vomiting Urticaria, rashes, arthralgias	Increased bilirubin levels Darkened urine, jaundice

↓

Scarring of liver

Regeneration of liver cells	Continued hepatic failure
Return to normal health after period of recuperation	Encephalopathy
	↓
	Coma
	↓
	DEATH

CHAPTER 4.8

LIVER FAILURE

The liver plays a vital role by providing multiple functions, such as, metabolism of carbohydrates, proteins, and fats, storing fat-soluble vitamins, vitamin B_{12}, copper, and iron, synthesis of blood clotting factors, amino acids, albumin, and globulins, detoxification of toxic substances, and phagocytosis of microorganisms. It also plays a role in glycolysis and gluconeogenesis. Liver functioning can be preserved until up to 75% of the hepatocytes become damaged or necrotic, at which time the liver can no longer perform its normal operation.

Liver disease is becoming more common in the elderly because of increased susceptibility to drugs and other toxic substances. The elderly person is unable to compensate for various metabolic, infectious, and immunologic abuse.

Early hepatic failure presents as a type of cirrhosis of the liver. Liver cells become inflamed and obstructed, which results in damage to the cells around the central portal vein. When the inflammation decreases, the lobule regenerates, and this cycle is repeated until the lobule is irreversibly damaged and fibrotic tissue replaces healthy normal liver tissue.

Advanced hepatic failure develops when all compensatory mechanisms fail, causing the serum ammonia level to rise. The already-damaged liver is unable to synthesize normal products, so acidosis, hypoglycemia, or blood dyscrasias develop, and the patient becomes comatose.

Acute liver failure, also known as fulminant hepatic failure, may be precipitated by a stress factor that aggravates a pre-existing chronic liver disease. Some stress factors include alcohol intake, ingestion of Amanita mushrooms, large amounts of dietary protein, gastrointestinal bleeding, and portacaval shunt surgery. An acute type of liver failure may occur as a result of viral or toxic hepatitis, biliary obstruction, cancer, acute infective processes, drugs, such as acetaminophen, isoniazid, and rifampin, severe dehydration, Reye's syndrome, or shock states.

Fulminant hepatic failure may begin as stage I hepatic encephalopathy, progressing to drowsiness and asterixis (liver flap), stupor, and incoherent communication, until progressing finally to stage IV with deep coma. The stages may progress over as little as two months. Distinguishing attributes between acute and chronic failure are the presence of cerebral edema and increases in intracranial pressure.

The goal of treatment is to halt progression of the encephalopathy that occurs with increasing ammonia levels, and is accomplished with the use of cathartics, decreasing dietary protein, and electrolyte replacement. Even with treatment, mortality rates are as high as 90%, depending on the age of the patient and the severity of the disease. The elderly have a very poor rate of survival for end-stage liver disease because of their decreased ability to recover from problems and their inability to tolerate the amount of toxic deposits and other symptoms of the disease.

MEDICAL CARE

Laboratory: CBC used to identify anemias and white blood cell count helps to identify hypersplenism or infection; thrombocytopenia may occur secondary to alcoholic bone marrow suppression, sepsis, or folate deficiency; elevated BUN; electrolytes used to identify imbalances; liver function studies are elevated; serum bilirubin is elevated; urine bilirubin may be present if direct serum bilirubin is elevated; AST and ALT elevations may result from hepatocellular necrosis or inflammation; AST levels that are double the amount of AST are typical of alcoholic liver injury; alkaline phosphatase levels used to identify cholestasis or infiltrative liver disease; albumin decreases and globulin increases with liver failure; cholesterol is elevated; PT is prolonged; toxicology screens are used to identify ingestion of alcohol or other drugs that may have precipitated failure; magnesium level may be low with alcoholic cirrhosis and toxic if magnesium replacement is utilized; ammonia levels used to identify severity of liver involvement and toxic levels

CT scans: used to identify biliary obstruction or dilation of bile ducts, hepatomegaly, intrahepatic tumors, and changes of portal hypertension

Liver scans: may be used to detect degenerative cirrhosis changes or to identify focal liver disease

Liver biopsy: may be done to establish the diagnosis by study of biopsied tissue

Hyperalimentation: may be used as nutrition method of choice because of ability to control concentration of nutrients, electrolytes, and vitamins

Medications: aminoglycosides, such as neomycin (Mycifradin Sulfate) or kanamycin (Kantrex) frequently used to prevent intestinal bacteria from converting protein and amino acids to ammonia; lactulose (Cephulac, Emulose) or sorbitol used to induce catharsis to empty the intestines of fecal matter to decrease conversion to ammonia; thiazide diuretics, such as chlorothiazide (Diuril) and hydrochlorothiazide (Esidrix, Ezide, HydroDiuril, Microzide, Oretic), as well as chlorthalidone (Hygroton, Thalitone), Indapamide (Lozol), and metolazone (Mykrox, Zaroxolyn) which are thiazide-acting diuretics that increase sodium and water excretion by inhibiting reabsorption of sodium in the cortical diluting site of the ascending loop of Henle, or inhibit sodium and chloride reabsorption in the distal segment of the nephron to decrease fluid retention

Paracentesis: may be used to remove fluid in patients with massive ascites and respiratory compromise that have been refractory to diuretic therapy; usually 4–6 L of fluid is removed

Surgery: may be required for placement of peritoneovenous shunt to provide method of returning accumulations of ascitic fluid in abdomen to the systemic circulation to provide long-term relief for ascites

COMMON NURSING DIAGNOSES

DEFICIENT FLUID VOLUME (see GI BLEEDING)

Related to: gastrointestinal bleeding, osmotic changes, hydrostatic pressure changes, ascites

Defining Characteristics: hypotension, tachycardia, decreased skin turgor, weakness, pallor, diaphoresis, decreased capillary refill, mental changes, restlessness, decreased filling pressures, decreased hemoglobin and hematocrit, dry mucous membranes, ascites, concentrated urine, oliguria, anuria, thirst, weakness, edema

INEFFECTIVE BREATHING PATTERN (see TB)

Related to: increased pressure from ascites, increased ammonia levels, decreased lung expansion, fatigue, fear of suffocation, pain, inflammatory process, inadequate oxygenation, respiratory muscle weakness

Defining Characteristics: dyspnea, tachypnea, nasal flaring, cyanosis, shallow respirations, pursed-lip breathing, changes in inspiratory/expiratory ratio, use of accessory muscles, diminished chest expansion, fremitus, anxiety, decreased oxygen saturation, adventitious breath sounds, decreased energy, fatigue, presence of ascites, abnormal arterial blood gases

DISTURBED BODY IMAGE (see PACEMAKERS)

Related to: changes in physical appearance, ascites, disease process

Defining Characteristics: fear of rejection, fear of reaction from others, negative feelings about body, refusal to participate in care, refusal to look at self, withdrawal from social contacts, withdrawal from family, presence of ascites, biophysical changes, fear of death, fear of the unknown

ADDITIONAL NURSING DIAGNOSES

DISTURBED THOUGHT PROCESSES

Related to: serum ammonia levels, hepatic encephalopathy

Defining Characteristics: increased ammonia levels, increased BUN, mental status changes, decreasing level of consciousness, changes in personality, handwriting changes, tremors, coma, asterixis (liver flap)

Outcome Criteria

✔ Patient will be conscious and stable, with ammonia levels within normal ranges.

NOC: *Neurologic Status: Consciousness*

INTERVENTIONS	RATIONALES
Monitor patient's neurologic status every 1–2 hours, and prn. Notify physician for abnormalities and/changes.	Identifies onset of problem and potential trend. May indicate acute change in condition if abrupt change in sensorium is noted.
If possible, have patient write name each day and do simple mathematic calculation.	As hepatic failure progresses, the ability to write becomes more difficult, and writing becomes illegible at precoma stage. Inability to perform mental calculations may indicate worsening liver failure.
Administer cathartics as ordered.	Lactulose minimizes the formation of ammonia and other nitrogenous byproducts by altering intestinal pH. Neomycin or kanamycin help to prevent conversion of amino acids into ammonia. Sorbitol-type cathartics cause an osmotic diarrhea to empty the intestines to decrease ammonia production.
Observe for asterixis or other tremors.	Rapid wrist flapping, called "liver flap," when the arms are raised in front of the body with hands dorsiflexed may indicate presence of hepatic encephalopathy.
Provide safe environment for patient, with furniture moved to edges of room, using sufficient lighting, keeping room uncluttered, and so forth.	Decreases risk of injury caused by altered consciousness levels.
Provide low-protein diet.	Decreased dietary protein may lessen serum ammonia levels, which ultimately leads to comatose state from the buildup of toxins.

INTERVENTIONS	RATIONALES
Avoid sedatives and narcotics, if at all possible.	May worsen decreasing levels of consciousness and make identification of cause of decreased sensorium more difficult.
Instruct patient/family in potential for altered sensorium and encephalopathy signs. Reorient patient as needed.	Provides knowledge and facilitates family involvement with maintaining optimal orientation level. Provides support with realistic expectations of disease process as outcome is poor.
Instruct patient/family in side effects of drugs used to facilitate decrease in ammonia levels.	Diarrhea will occur, and lactulose should be titrated to where patient has 3 stools per day.

NIC: *Delirium Management*

Discharge or Maintenance Evaluation

■ Patient will be awake, alert, and oriented.

■ Patient will have serum ammonia levels within acceptable ranges.

■ Patient/family will be able to accurately verbalize understanding of instructions and be able to communicate concerns.

■ Patient will be compliant with medication and dietary regimen.

IMBALANCED NUTRITION: LESS THAN BODY REQUIREMENTS

Related to: metabolism changes, increased ammonia levels, encephalopathy, ascites

Defining Characteristics: anorexia, nausea, vomiting, malabsorption of fats, malabsorption of vitamins, altered carbohydrate, fat, and protein metabolism, malnutrition, weight loss, fatigue, edema, ascites, changes in mental status, elevated ammonia levels

Outcome Criteria

✔ Patient will be able to achieve a positive nitrogen balance and have stable weight.

NOC: *Nutritional Status*

INTERVENTIONS	RATIONALES
Provide diet that has protein in ordered amounts, with supple-mentation of vitamins and other nutrients.	Protein metabolism is altered with liver disease and results in increased ammonia levels. Vitamin and nutrient supplementation may be required because of malabsorption of elements.
Ensure that patient is positioned in upright, sitting position for meals.	Decreases abdominal tenderness and fullness, and prevents potential for aspiration.
Avoid sodium intake of amounts greater than ordered.	Sodium should be restricted to less than 500 mg per day to decrease edema and ascites.
If patient is unable to ingest adequate dietary intake, admini-ster tube feedings or parenteral nutrition as ordered.	Provides needed nutrients when patient is unable to eat or when absorption is not adequate.
Weigh patient daily, on same scale, at same time if at all possible.	Provides indication of nutritional efficacy, fluid balance, and helps with accurate consistent data.
Instruct patient/family regarding need for limitations of protein and sodium.	Provides knowledge and facilitates compliance to ensure improve-ment with liver failure symptoms.
Instruct patient/family regarding need for enteral or parenteral nutrition as warranted.	Facilitates understanding of need for dietary control of nutrients to reduce encephalopathy and increasing ammonia levels.

NIC: *Nutritional Counseling*

Discharge or Maintenance Evaluation

- Patient will be able to ingest an adequate amount of prescribed diet to maintain weight and ammo-nia levels at acceptable levels.

- Patient will be compliant with dietary regimen and limitations.

- Patient will have no complications from enteral or parenteral therapies.

- Patient/family will be able to accurately verbalize understanding of need for dietary limitations to improve health status.

IMPAIRED SKIN INTEGRITY

Related to: poor nutrition, renal involvement, ascites, bile deposits on skin, liver failure, immobility

Defining Characteristics: edema, ascites, jaundice, pruritis, deposits of bile salts on skin, increased ammonia levels, decreased mental sensorium, dry, scaly skin

Outcome Criteria

✔ Patient will maintain skin integrity, with no signs of complications, such as lesions or wounds.

NOC: *Tissue Integrity: Skin and Mucous Membranes*

INTERVENTIONS	RATIONALES
Observe skin for changes, abra-sions, rashes, scaling, wounds, bleeding, redness, and so forth.	Facilitates identification of potential complications.
Turn patient at least every 2 hours and prn.	Prevents pressure and compro-mise of skin and tissues, which may result in injury.
Apply lotions frequently when providing skin care; do not use soap when bathing patient; apply cornstarch or baking soda prn.	Soaps may dry skin further and result in breach of integrity. Lotions and other agents may decrease itching.
Administer medications for pruritus as ordered.	Decreases itching, which may provoke patient to scratch and cause wounds. Bile salts that are deposited on the skin of patients with hepatic or renal involve-ment cause chronic and severe pruritis.
Instruct patient/family in methods to decrease itching: soothing massages, avoidance of extra covers, and use of clean white gloves at night.	Helps prevent patient from scratching during the night and reduces the tendency to scratch.
Provide attention-diverting activity.	May refocus concentration in order to decrease scratching.

NIC: *Skin Surveillance*

Discharge or Maintenance Evaluation

- Patient will exhibit no evidence of skin breakdown.
- Patient will be able to use discussed methods to avoid scratching.

- Patient will have no complications from lack of skin integrity.
- Patient/family will be able to accurately verbalize understanding of need to avoid scratching and to use methods to accomplish this.

RISK FOR INJURY

Related to: hemorrhage, altered clotting factors, esophageal varices, portal hypertension

Defining Characteristics: bleeding, exsanguinations, decreased hemoglobin and hematocrit, decreased prothrombin, decreased fibrinogen, decreased clotting factors VIII, IX, and X, vitamin K malabsorption, thromboplastin release

Outcome Criteria

✔ Patient will exhibit no evidence of abnormal bleeding.

NOC: *Risk Detection*

INTERVENTIONS	RATIONALES
Monitor all bodily secretions for presence of blood; test stools and drainage for guaiac.	GI bleeding may occur from altered clotting factors and changes that occur with cirrhosis and liver diseases.
Observe for bleeding from patient's puncture sites, presence of hematomas or petechiae, or bruising.	May indicate a form of disseminated intravascular coagulation as a result of altered clotting factors.
Monitor vital signs and hemodynamic parameters. Avoid rectal thermometers if possible.	Changes in vital signs may indicate loss of circulating blood volume. Vasculature in rectum may be susceptible to rupture.
Insert nasogastric tube gently and lavage as ordered.	Esophageal vasculature may be susceptible to rupture. Removal of blood from the stomach decreases synthesis to ammonia.
Administer vitamins as ordered.	Vitamin K facilitates synthesis of prothrombin and coagulation only if liver is functional. Vitamin C may reduce the potential for GI bleeding and facilitates the healing process.

INTERVENTIONS	RATIONALES
Administer stool softeners as ordered.	Prevents straining to pass stool which may result in rupture of vasculature or increase in intra-abdominal pressures.
Monitor lab work for CBC and clotting studies.	Helps to identify blood loss or impending DIC.
Instruct patient/family regarding potential for bleeding disorders.	Promotes knowledge and facilitates understanding of gravity of patient's illness.
Instruct patient/family regarding need for supplemental vitamins.	Vitamin K facilitates coagulation, which may be impaired by liver failure.

NIC: *Bleeding Precautions*

Discharge or Maintenance Evaluation

- Patient will be stable with no active bleeding.
- Patient will have lab work within normal limits.
- Patient will not exhibit any hemorrhagic complications from invasive lines/tube placement.
- Patient/family will be able to accurately verbalize understanding of need for supplemental vitamins and potential for bleeding dyscrasias.

DEATH ANXIETY

Related to: terminal illness, liver failure, recurrent ascites

Defining Characteristics: concern over the effect of one's death on their family, powerlessness over disease process, fear of loss of mental and physical abilities while dying, fear of pain while dying, fear of delayed death, negative death images, loss of control over one's own mortality, fear of premature death preventing accomplishments of important goals in life, concern over being the cause of other's suffering and grief, fear of leaving one's family alone after death, concern over spiritual matters, meeting one's Creator, or feeling doubtful about the existence of God

Outcome Criteria

✔ Patient will be able to experience dying with dignity.

✔ Patient will be able to address concerns with family, friends, and ministers to facilitate feelings of comfort and peace.

NOC: *Dignified Dying*

INTERVENTIONS	RATIONALES
Assess patient's level of understanding of disease process, predicted length of time left until dying, and understanding of issues related to the death process.	Provides information to use as a baseline for establishing a plan of care. Identifies patient's knowledge and facilitates education regarding misperceptions.
Assess whether patient desires someone to be present at his bedside all the time.	Some patients who are approaching death desire the presence of another person, but do not want to inconvenience them or have to "entertain" that person.
Provide comfort measures, such as bathing, massage, repositioning, oral care, and so forth if patient desires.	Provides comfort, but some patients prefer being left alone and not bothered unless they specifically ask for something.
Spend time with patient as he or she desires and be willing to listen actively.	Helps to foster open discussions and shows readiness to discuss spiritual aspects of death and dying.
If patient has a special prayer or poem that he or she especially likes and that is of comfort to patient, recite this to patient if requested.	Shows support for patient's spiritual needs and conveys a caring and accepting attitude.
Provide physical touch and support, unless patient finds this disturbing.	As patient begins to let go of life, they sometimes desire less tactile stimulation.

INTERVENTIONS	RATIONALES
Do not leave patient alone unless requested.	Patients frequently want someone to be in the room with them as they are afraid of dying alone. Others want no one in the room and this is their process of letting go.
Instruct family members regarding the need to discuss and resolve issues that are important to them and to the patient.	Family members may need assistance in providing support to the patient who needs their encouragement.
Instruct family members that it is acceptable for them to discuss the patient's dying, to be able to touch him, to verbalize feelings, and so forth.	Allows for opportunity to support patient and have therapeutic interaction.
Contact patient's minister or rabbi as he desires.	Demonstrates your respect for patient's beliefs and provides expert spiritual care.

NIC: *Dying Care*

Discharge or Maintenance Criteria

- Patient will be able to discuss death and dying, and make contact with family members.
- Patient will experience peace and have less anxiety.
- Patient will be able to make decisions regarding own care in the dying process.
- Patient will be able to access spiritual counselor for comfort and care.

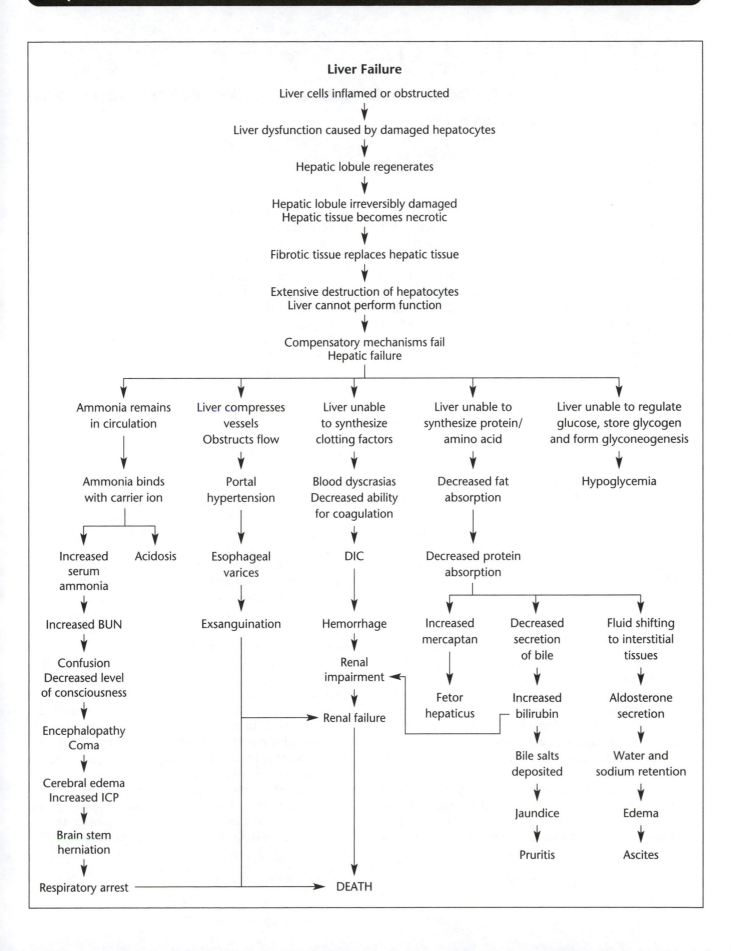

CHAPTER 4.9

MALNUTRITION

The elderly represent one of the largest demographic groups at risk for malnutrition, and poor nutrition is common in this age group. Age-related influences on nutrition include abnormalities in the mouth or dental factors, reduced metabolic rates, decreased caloric content, decreased energy levels, sensory and motor deficits, chronic diseases, isolation, depression, anxiety, grief, and the effect of medications. The results of poor nutrition in the aged help predispose them to injury, infection, bowel problems, ineffective coping, fluid and electrolyte imbalances, skin and mucosal impairment, as well as pressure sores, hip fractures, and infections.

The Food Guide Pyramid is known as a graphic description of the dietary recommendations for different food groupings developed by the U.S. Department of Agriculture, and most currently revised in 2000. It has been based on the dietary needs of healthy younger individuals, and has not taken into account the needs of the elderly population who have special dietary needs. A modified food pyramid has been developed that identifies the special requirements of people over the age of 70, but the U.S.D.A. has not adopted it. This customized food pyramid takes into account the decreased energy requirement of the elderly patient, but accentuates their need for water, fiber, and nutrient-dense foods. In addition, there is a definite likelihood built in that the elderly will more than likely require supplementation of calcium and vitamins, such as D and B_{12}.

The maintenance of a positive nitrogen balance is best facilitated by increased protein requirements in the elderly. Impaired mobility, surgery, fractures, sepsis, pressure ulcer development, and immunosuppression are conditions that are best served by increasing the amount of dietary protein. In the elderly population, protein needs may not be met because of the expense of the usual sources for protein (meat, fish, poultry, and milk), their limited incomes, and some foods may be tiring to chew, if

dentition is a problem. Preparation of these foods is another factor that may impair the elderly obtaining their required amounts of protein, caused, in part, by functional limitations.

For many years, a low-fat diet has been the standard recommendation, but it may not always be the best one for the elderly. Underweight elderly patients may profit from a higher fat intake because of the potential for inclusive nutrition consumption. Unless the patient has a specific dietary restriction correlated to a specific disease process, stringent limitation on fat may not be prudent.

Vitamin and mineral requirements in the elderly are frequently deficient, especially B-complex vitamins, vitamin C, vitamin D, zinc, magnesium, and calcium. The intake of these vitamins in food may be impaired, as well as physiologic illnesses or injuries placing a demand on these nutrients, leading to deficiencies. Vitamin D, in particular, is of concern, especially with patients who are homebound or are in long-term care facilities. Although foods can replace vitamin D, natural sunlight is important for synthesis of vitamin D, and patients who rarely go outside in the sun are susceptible to deficiency, which can lead to bone loss and impaired immunity.

Risk factors that have been identified for poor nutritional intake in the elderly include: inadequate food intake, social isolation, disability, disease processes, dependence on others, poverty, multiple medication usage, and advancing age. Malnutrition may be insidious and develop over a long period of time, and contribute to impairment of an already-compromised immune system. Elderly patients with protein calorie malnutrition cannot correct this deficiency by oral intake alone, and may require aggressive nutritional therapy.

Drugs that may impair dietary balance include digoxin, diuretics, NSAIDs, sulfasalazine, phenytoin, bile acid sequestrants, and cancer chemotherapy drugs. Alcoholism worsens anorexia and compromises nutrient intake by replacing calories with empty nutrition.

The goals to reverse malnutrition in the elderly include relaxing restrictions, when feasible, increasing nutrient-rich foods, and modifying consistencies of food to ensure adequate consumption in those patients who have dysphagia and/or poor dentition. Enteral or parenteral nutrition may be required to achieve a positive nitrogen balance and to minimize feeding intolerance.

MEDICAL CARE

Laboratory: CBC to identify infection, anemia, or other disease process, and lowered hemoglobin and hematocrit may indicate poor intake and nutritional deficiencies; lymphocyte count indicates immune function and is decreased with malnutrition; electrolyte profiles used to evaluate imbalance and efficacy of replacement therapy; drug toxicity levels used to identify therapeutic versus toxic drug levels as a result of dietary interactions; lipid profiles used to identify cholesterol, triglyceride, and lipid levels related to nutritional intake, with a low cholesterol level indicating impaired nutritional status; vitamin levels used to identify deficiencies; serum albumin used and considered the most reliable marker of nutritional status; renal profiles used to identify concurrent renal dysfunction and increased BUN and sodium may be present with nutritional deficiencies; albumin, prealbumin, and protein levels may be low indicating nutritional impairment and malnutrition

Dietary requirements: water (at least 6–8 glasses/day) is the most important item, followed by fiber, and nutrient-rich foods, whole grains, fruits and vegetables, protein, fats, oils, and sweets, and complex carbohydrates

Vitamin/mineral supplementation: used to replace vitamins and mineral deficiencies that cannot be restored by oral intake of specific food groups

Enteral/parenteral nutrition: may be required if patient cannot absorb nutrients through the gut, or if adequate nutrition cannot be gained in other ways; in order for enteral nutrition to be effective, the patient's gut must be functional or else other complications may ensue

COMMON NURSING DIAGNOSES

IMBALANCED NUTRITION: LESS THAN BODY REQUIREMENTS (see COPD)

Related to: aging, nausea, vomiting, inability to ingest food, increased metabolism caused by disease process, decreased level of consciousness, inability to absorb nutrients because of biologic or psychological factors, poverty, isolation, medications

Defining Characteristics: actual inadequate food intake, altered taste, altered smell sensation, weight loss, body weight 20% or more under ideal for height and frame, anorexia, absent bowel sounds, decreased peristalsis, muscle mass loss, decreased muscle tone, changes in bowel habits, nausea, vomiting, abdominal distention, lack of interest in food, abdominal pain or discomfort, depression, anxiety, social isolation, changes in mental status, weakness, lack of interest in food, poor dentition, dysphagia, chronic illness, decreased albumin and prealbumin levels, decreased protein levels

IMBALANCED NUTRITION: MORE THAN BODY REQUIREMENTS (see GERD)

Related to: decreased physical activity, excessive intake in relationship to metabolic need of high caloric foods, decreased metabolic rate

Defining Characteristics: body weight 10% or more over ideal weight, triceps skin-fold measurement more than 15 mm in men and 25 mm in women, eating in response to social situations, sedentary activity level, decreased metabolic rate, eating in response to cues other than hunger, pairing food with other activities, eating in response to ulcerative conditions to improve pain

INEFFECTIVE TISSUE PERFUSION: CARDIOPULMONARY, CEREBRAL, GASTROINTESTINAL, PERIPHERAL, RENAL (see CAD)

Related to: reduced oxygen supply, atherosclerotic lesions, hypoperfusion, hypovolemia, coexisting disease processes, age-related vascular structure changes, inactivity

Defining Characteristics: vital sign changes, delayed capillary refill time, dyspnea, nasal flaring, use of accessory muscles, increased work of breathing, tachypnea, bradypnea, changes in mental status, weakness, paralysis, behavioral changes, abdominal distention, ileus, hypoactive or absent bowel sounds, nausea, vomiting, edema, weak or absent peripheral pulses, skin temperature changes, skin color changes, decreased peripheral tactile sensation, hematuria, oliguria, anuria, increased BUN and creatinine, reduced circulation and transport of nutrients, reduced absorption and transport of nutrients from the intestines, weight loss

RISK FOR INFECTION (see TB)

Related to: malnutrition, risk factors that threaten physical well-being, crowded living conditions, presence of HIV infection, presence of chronic illnesses, nutritional status, immunocompromise, polypharmacy

Defining Characteristics: exposure to pathogens, inadequate nutrients reaching tissues to maintain integrity, fever, cough, lung consolidation, abscesses, sputum production, anorexia, weight loss, fatigue, dementia, confusion, neurologic deficits, dyspnea, dysphagia, elevated white blood cell count

DISTURBED BODY IMAGE (see PACEMAKERS)

Related to: changes in physical appearance related to age or disease, chronic disease process, emaciation, obesity

Defining Characteristics: fear of rejection, fear of reaction from others, negative feelings about body, refusal to participate in care, refusal to look at self, withdrawal from social contacts, withdrawal from family, depression, verbal response to actual change in body structure

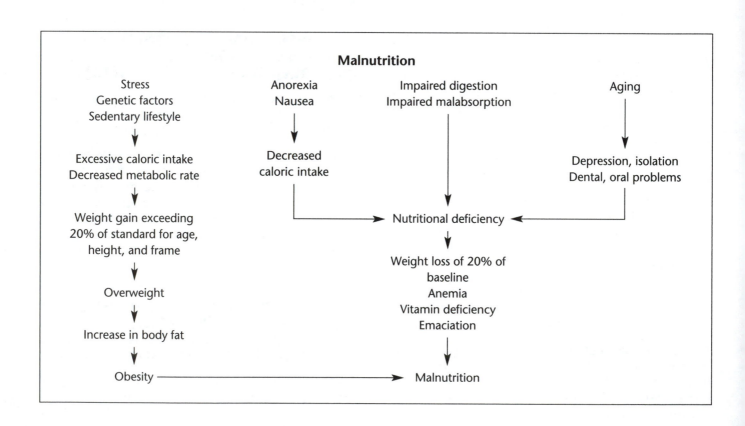

Malnutrition

Stress
Genetic factors
Sedentary lifestyle
↓
Excessive caloric intake
Decreased metabolic rate
↓
Weight gain exceeding
20% of standard for age,
height, and frame
↓
Overweight
↓
Increase in body fat
↓
Obesity ──────────────────────────────→ Malnutrition

Anorexia
Nausea
↓
Decreased
caloric intake ──────→ Nutritional deficiency

Impaired digestion
Impaired malabsorption
↓
Nutritional deficiency
↓
Weight loss of 20% of
baseline
Anemia
Vitamin deficiency
Emaciation
↓

Aging
↓
Depression, isolation
Dental, oral problems
←────── Nutritional deficiency

UNIT 5

GENITOURINARY SYSTEM

CHAPTER 5.1

INTERSTITIAL CYSTITIS

Interstitial cystitis, or Hunner's ulcer, is a chronic, noninfectious disorder involving inflammation and irritation of the bladder resulting from damaged tissue between the lining and the muscular wall of the bladder. With a cystoscopic examination, the bladder wall is noted to have a unifocal or multifocal infiltration of mucosal ulcerations and inflammation with scarring, pinpoint areas of bleeding, or a wedge-shaped eroded area in the bladder wall (Hunner's ulcer). This results in contraction of the smooth muscle, decreased urinary capacity, and symptoms of dysuria and hematuria. The underlying origin is unknown, but many have theorized that it is part of an autoimmune disorder or allergic disorder, caused by radiation therapy, or caused by treatment with medications that can cause cystitis.

This disease presents with similar symptoms of a urinary tract infection: pain and pressure to the bladder and pelvic region, dysuria, urinary frequency, and hematuria. Pain increases as the bladder fills and is relieved when it is empty, but frequently there is the sensation of incomplete emptying.

The goal of treatment is aimed at supportive care until a definitive treatment is found. Often bladder dilatations and instillation of a silver nitrate solution help temporarily. Dimethyl sulfoxide (DMSO) is also used as an instilled solution and its anti-inflammatory action affords some relief. Currently several other drugs are being tested for use to treat this condition.

Avoidance of certain foods that stimulate the bladder, such as caffeine, chocolate, carbonated beverages, fruits, fruit juices, tomatoes, brewer's yeast, and artificial sweeteners, have been found to help prevent exacerbations of this disease.

If conservative treatment is not successful, laser treatment or surgery may be required, and these modalities have not been remarkably successful so far in alleviating the symptoms.

MEDICAL CARE

Laboratory: CBC used to rule out infective process; urinary cytology used to rule out carcinoma in situ of the bladder that can mimic symptoms of interstitial cystitis

Radiography: IVP may be used to identify any structural reasons for condition or to observe for obstruction of flow from kidneys

Cystoscopy: used to diagnose condition after the bladder is distended with fluid; biopsy of the bladder can be done to evaluate for bladder cancer

Cystometrogram: used to identify contractions in the bladder by measuring changes in pressures; if contractions begin before the bladder reaches normal capacity of fluid, interstitial cystitis can be diagnosed

Surgery: used when all other methods have failed; replacement of the bladder with a pouch made out of part of the colon, or an iliostomy may be performed after cystectomy

COMMON NURSING DIAGNOSES

 ### DISTURBED SLEEP PATTERN (see HEART FAILURE)

Related to: internal factors from interstitial cystitis, nocturia

Defining Characteristics: interrupted sleep, fatigue, lethargy, irritability, disorientation, complaints of not feeling rested, insomnia, sleeplessness, loss of libido, nocturia, urinary frequency, urinary urgency, urinary retention, dysuria, pelvic pain, bladder pain

ADDITIONAL NURSING DIAGNOSES

ACUTE PAIN

Related to: bladder pain, dysuria, urinary frequency, inflammation and ulceration in bladder

Defining Characteristics: verbalization of pain and discomfort, suprapubic pain, flank pain, dysuria, hematuria, urinary frequency, lack of infectious process, inflammation, Hunner's ulcerations

Outcome Criteria

✔ Patient will have pain relieved or controlled to his or her satisfaction.

✔ Patient will exhibit no complications from treatments required.

NOC: *Pain Control*

INTERVENTIONS	RATIONALES
Evaluate patient and assess for severity of pain, site of pain, dysuria, or hematuria.	May indicate exacerbation of interstitial cystitis. Pain results from the bladder being in spasm.
Administer analgesics as ordered.	Controls pain by interfering with CNS pathways.
Position with support of pillows.	May promote comfort and prevents pressure to painful areas.
Assist with bladder instillations as warranted.	Instillations of silver nitrate or DMSO, or other solutions, may be required to temporarily relieve the pain.
Instruct patient regarding taking warm sitz baths, or application of heat to the perineal area. Patient should avoid harsh soaps, bath oils, bubble baths, vaginal deodorants, and so forth.	Measures help to promote comfort and relief from dysuria. Use of soaps and oils may irritate sensitive perineal tissues and change the pH of perineum, which may predispose the patient to infection or inflammation.
Instruct patient regarding remaining in close proximity to bathroom.	Prevents dribbling accidents from dysuria and urgency.

NIC: *Pain Management*

Discharge or Maintenance Evaluation

■ Patient will be able to verbalize that pain is controlled.

■ Patient will exhibit decreased need for the use of analgesics.

■ Patient will tolerate bladder instillation procedures without complications.

■ Patient will refrain from using harsh chemicals, bubble baths, and so forth, to prevent exacerbations of condition.

IMPAIRED URINARY ELIMINATION

Related to: interstitial cystitis, Hunner's ulceration, changes in urinary function

Defining Characteristics: bladder pain, suprapubic pain, dysuria, hematuria, urinary frequency, incomplete bladder emptying, nocturia, urgency

Outcome Criteria

✔ Patient will exhibit ability to manage urinary elimination problem.

✔ Patient will be able to have increased understanding of treatment, and will maintain continence.

NOC: *Urinary Elimination*

INTERVENTIONS	RATIONALES
Assess patient for incontinence, urinary frequency, retention, hematuria, or for presence of urinary infection symptoms.	Symptoms may result from infection or interstitial cystitis exacerbation.
Assess patient for changes in urinary patterns.	Reflects the result of interstitial cystitis, but may also indicate a coexisting urinary tract infection.
Obtain urine specimen as ordered.	Urinalysis and/or culture may identify the presence of an infection if specimen is cloudy, foul smelling, contains pus, mucus, or blood, or if patient has dysuria.
Administer antimicrobials as indicated if culture is positive.	Provides treatment to eradicate causative organism if infection is present.

(continues)

(continued)

INTERVENTIONS	RATIONALES
If patient has an indwelling catheter, maintain patency by avoidance of kinks in tubing, daily cleansing of meatal site and perineal area, maintaining closed system, keeping collection bag below the level of the bladder, utilizing aseptic technique to obtain specimen, and changing catheter at specified intervals.	Treats or prevents infection caused by catheter and/or direct pathway to bladder.
Provide access to bathroom or commode for patient.	Urgency and frequency may cause incontinence and embarrass patient.
Encourage fluids of at least 2 L/day, avoiding fruit juices, carbonated beverages, chocolate, and caffeine.	Provides hydration, dilutes urine, and prevents further exacerbation of interstitial cystitis.
Instruct patient regarding avoidance of bath oils, bubble bath, and harsh chemicals to perineal area.	Helps to prevent irritation and inflammation to perineal area.
Instruct patient to empty bladder completely and frequently, and to urinate when the urge is present.	Prevents urinary stasis, which may predispose patient to a urinary tract infection.
Prepare patient for surgical intervention if required.	Cystectomy or urinary diversion may be required, and preparation helps patient and family to cope with changes in function and appearance.

NIC: *Urinary Elimination Management*

Discharge or Maintenance Evaluation

- Patient will be compliant with fluid hydration measures, and avoidance of substances that may exacerbate condition.
- Patient will be able to manage urinary elimination problem.
- Patient will be able to maintain urinary continence.
- Patient will be able to accurately verbalize understanding of all instructions given.
- Patient will be able to discuss complications, treatments, adjustments to lifestyle, and will be able to accept consequences of urinary diversion surgery.

FUNCTIONAL URINARY INCONTINENCE

Related to: interstitial cystitis, sensory, cognitive, or mobility deficits

Defining Characteristics: urge to void or bladder contractions strong enough to result in loss of urine before reaching commode or bathroom, lack of caretaker availability or interest, decreased bladder size and capacity, urgency, frequency, incontinent episodes, inability to find and reach commode or bathroom in time, lack of awareness, memory, poor bladder control, unpredictable passage of urine

Outcome Criteria

✔ Patient will maintain continence of urine as long as possible, and have a decreased incidence of incontinent episodes.

NOC: *Urinary Continence*

INTERVENTIONS	RATIONALES
Assess patient's physical and cognitive capabilities, voiding pattern, ability to sense that bladder is full and communicate desire to void, urgency or frequency, amount and time of day of fluid intake.	Provides information about reasons for incontinence and establishes baselines as goals for continence.
Assess for presence of chronic disease or procedures that may contribute to incontinence.	Mental and physical disorders may prevent finding and using bathroom or walking to facility.
Evaluate medication use, such as diuretics, sedatives, psychotropics.	May reduce sensation to urinate or cause large amounts of urine to be excreted.
Remind patient to use bathroom q 2 hours and assist to sit or stand and to adjust clothing if necessary. Keep call light within reach.	Cognitive deficits causing forgetfulness are common and patient may need reminding to respond to urge for elimination.
Provide privacy for urinary elimination; have bedpan or commode within easy access.	Privacy is important to elderly clients and will promote continence.
Schedule for toileting q 2h during day and q 4h during night, at times identified in urinary pattern assessment.	Promotes bladder training to prevent incontinence.

INTERVENTIONS	RATIONALES
Lengthen time periods for voiding as continence progresses.	Allows patient longer intervals between voidings.
Promote fluid intake of at least 2 L/day (8–10 glasses).	Dilutes urine and prevents concentration of urine which is irritating to bladder.
Reduce fluid intake 3 hours before bedtime; limit caffeine-containing beverages.	Prevents nocturia.
Provide pads or waterproof underwear; utilize aids such as condom catheter or female continence pouch.	Protects clothing and prevents embarrassment of soiled clothes. Serves as temporary measure to manage incontinence until bladder control is regained.
Insert indwelling catheter as a last resort.	Incontinence that becomes impossible to control may require continuous drainage by indwelling catheter.
Instruct patient in Kegel exercises.	Strengthens pelvic and perineal muscles to enhance control of urgency.
Instruct patient/family in modification of patient's environment with use of handrails, elevated toilet seat in bathroom, and commode within easy access.	Promotes continence by adjustments that facilitate use of bathroom.

INTERVENTIONS	RATIONALES
Instruct patient and assist to plan toileting schedule and use of aids to control incontinence.	Promotes independence and continence.
Instruct patient/family in skin care with mild soap, warm water, and drying well with soft cloth after each incontinence episode.	Prevents skin irritation and breakdown.

NIC: *Urinary Habit Training*

Discharge or Maintenance Evaluation

- Patient will have improved urinary continence with reduced incontinent episodes.
- Patient will be able to utilize toilet, commode, or bedpan with or without assistance.
- Patient will be compliant with urinary training program.
- Patient will achieve total continence of urine.
- Patient/family will be able to accurately verbalize and demonstrate understanding of instructions given to promote continence.
- Patient will exhibit no signs or symptoms of skin breakdown from incontinence.

Interstitial Cystitis

Theoretical causes
(Collagen diseases, autoimmune diseases, allergic manifestation, radiation therapy, drugs)

↓

Inflammation and irritation to bladder

↓

Mucosal ulceration

↓

Erosion into the bladder wall (Hunner's ulcer)

↓

Pinpoint areas of hemorrhage in bladder

↓

Scarring of the bladder wall

↓

Contraction of smooth muscle

↓

Decreased urinary capacity

↓

Frequency, urgency, retention
Dysuria
Hematuria
Bladder/suprapubic pain

Urinary Incontinence

Aging

| Dementia Confusion | Decreased bladder muscle tone and weakness of pelvic muscles and urethral sphincter Prostatectomy Urinary tract infection | Reduced bladder size and capacity Bladder overdistention and retention Bladder irritation and spasms (infection) Indwelling catheter CNS depressant drugs | Sensory, cognitive or mobility deficits Neurologic dysfunction Neuropathy affecting awareness of bladder fullness Spinal cord nerve injury/disease |

Dementia
Confusion

↓

Unaware of need
to urinate
Inability to make
effort to urinate

↓

Psychological
incontinence

Decreased bladder muscle
tone and weakness of
pelvic muscles and
urethral sphincter
Prostatectomy
Urinary tract infection

↓

Bladder pressure exceeds
maximal urethral
pressure in absence
of detrusor activity

↓

Increased intra-abdominal
pressure

↓

Activity causing pressure
on bladder (coughing,
laughing, lifting,
climbing stairs)

↓

Stress incontinence

Reduced bladder size
and capacity
Bladder overdistention
and retention
Bladder irritation and
spasms (infection)
Indwelling catheter
CNS depressant drugs

↓

Strong desire to urinate

↓

Inability to reach
bathroom on time

↓

Urge incontinence
Overflow incontinence

Sensory, cognitive or
mobility deficits
Neurologic dysfunction
Neuropathy affecting
awareness of bladder
fullness
Spinal cord nerve
injury/disease

↓

Absence of sensation
and desire to urinate
Unpredictable urination
Unawareness of
incontinence
Constant flow of urine
Loss of urine before
reaching bathroom

↓

Functional incontinence
Total incontinence

CHAPTER 5.2

MENOPAUSE

Menopause, also known as the "change of life," occurs when the loss of ovarian function results in the permanent termination of menstrual periods. The transitional period leading up to this irreversible event is called the climacteric and is characterized by the decline in the number of ovarian follicles, which also become less responsive to gonadotropic hormonal stimulation, and by the decrease of estrogen production by the ovaries until there is not enough to cause the endometrium to grow and shed. At menopause, estrogen is secreted by the adrenal glands and to some degree by fatty tissue that converts androgens into estrogen. This may explain why heavier women have relatively fewer menopausal symptoms.

The average age at which menopause occurs is around 50, and as today's woman's average life span is in the upper 70s, approximately one-third of her life occurs after menopause. This fact has focused more attention on changes that occur as a result of menopause.

Early signs and symptoms of menopause, or perimenopause, include irregular menses, mood changes, hot flashes, insomnia, fatigue, and headache. Later indicators include dry skin, breast changes, dyspareunia, decreased pelvic muscle tone, cystitis, vaginitis, urinary incontinence, and genital atrophy. For approximately ten years after menopause, bone loss increases, and osteoporosis becomes a common occurrence and may result in pathologic fractures.

Atherosclerosis increases at menopause, most probably because of the decrease in estrogen levels, which increases cholesterol levels. Estrogen replacement may protect patients against atherosclerosis by increasing vasodilation, preventing platelet aggregation, slowing lipoprotein oxidation, lowering homocysteine levels, and reducing smooth muscle proliferation.

Treatment for menopause is symptomatic. Estrogen replacement therapy is the most advantageous treatment for symptoms, but some women are unable to take the drug, and it has some adverse effects and inherent risks, so it is not suitable for all patients.

MEDICAL CARE

Laboratory: serum follicle-stimulating hormone levels are elevated in menopause; serum estradiol not diagnostic as decreases are noted during menses; cultures of vaginal drainage may be used to identify atrophic vaginitis or potential for diabetes; glucose levels used to identify potential dysfunction; lipid profiles used to identify potential for CAD; estrogen levels used to identify decrease noted with menopause; Pap smears used to evaluate cervix and rule out potential neoplasms; thyroid profiles used to identify dysfunction

Endometrial biopsy: used to evaluate vaginal tissue and atypical lesions to rule out cancer

Estrogen replacement therapy (ERT): 17 beta-estradiol/norgestimate (Ortho-Prefest), estradiol cypionate or valerate (Alora, Climara, Estrace, Fempatch, Depo-Estradiol, Depogen, Clinagen, Menaval), estradiol/norethindrone acetate (Combipatch), conjugated estrogens (Premarin), estropipate (Ogen, Eortho-Est), ethinyl estradiol and desogestrel (Desogen, Ortho-Cept), ethinyl estradiol and norethindrone acetate (Loestrin), ethinyl estradiol and norgestimate (Ortho-Cyclen), levonorgestrel (Norplant), medroxy-progesterone acetate (Amen, Curretab, Cycrin, Depo-Provera, Provera), and norethindrone (Micronor, Aygestin); used alone or in conjunction with a progestin to relieve hot flashes, prevent osteoporosis, and reduce atherosclerosis and CAD risk; estrogens can cause nausea, mastalgia, headache, mood changes, endometrial hyperplasia, and increased risk of endometrial, ovarian, and breast cancers, cholelithiasis, and thromboembolic disease

COMMON NURSING DIAGNOSES

 ### DISTURBED SLEEP PATTERN (see HEART FAILURE)

Related to: menopausal symptoms, insomnia, psychological stress, headache

Defining Characteristics: hot flashes, interrupted sleep, insomnia, nervousness, anxiety, depression, emotional mood swings, decreased REM sleep

 ### SEXUAL DYSFUNCTION (see SEXUAL DISORDERS)

Related to: changes in body structure and function from decreased estrogen secretion

Defining Characteristics: thin, dry vaginal mucosa, dyspareunia, slight bleeding during intercourse, verbalization of problems with sexual function, avoidance of engaging in sexual intercourse, need for confirmation of desirability, decreased vaginal lubrication

 ### RISK FOR INJURY (see FRACTURES)

Related to: menopause, perimenopause, abnormal bone density, estrogen level decrease, osteoporosis, fractures

Defining Characteristics: osteoporosis, bone loss, decreased bone density, brittle bones, overproduction of interleukin-6, increased bone resorption, hyperthyroidism, Paget's disease, pathologic fractures usually of the vertebrae or Colles' fractures

ADDITIONAL NURSING DIAGNOSES

 ### STRESS URINARY INCONTINENCE

Related to: aging changes, such as degenerative changes in pelvic musculature and structural supports, atrophic vaginitis, uterine prolapse, urinary incontinence

Defining Characteristics: urinary urgency, urinary frequency, reports of dribbling with increased abdominal pressure, cough, or sneezing

Outcome Criteria

✔ Patient will be able to resume normal activities and maintain continence of urine.

NOC: *Urinary Continence*

INTERVENTIONS	RATIONALES
Assess patient for incontinence associated with coughing, laughing, sneezing, or lifting heavy objects.	Increased intra-abdominal pressure causes involuntary loss of urine when the pelvic support organs are weakened by aging, catheter use, vaginal childbirth, or with menopause.
Evaluate and discuss patient's understanding of incontinence and disease process.	Provides information to establish a baseline for teaching and for the plan of care. Many patients are hesitant to discuss incontinence, believing it to have a stigma attached to it. A nonjudgmental attitude may assist patient to be less embarrassed and discuss the problem openly.
Identify patient's current medications and evaluate regimen for drugs that could contribute to incontinence.	Diuretics, CNS depressants and anticholinergics may all cause urinary incontinence and may require medication alteration or change.
Provide patient with pads or leak-proof undergarments as appropriate.	Prevents patient embarrassment and wetting of clothing.
Administer estrogens as ordered.	Estrogen loss during menopause affects the muscles that help maintain continence of urine. During perimenopause, the patient's well-vascularized urethral mucosa is lost, resulting in loss of resistance to urinary flow and causing incontinence.
Instruct patient regarding potential reasons for urinary dribbling and incontinence.	Menopausal changes can result in urinary incontinence, as can physiologic changes involved with aging.
Instruct patient in performance of Kegel exercises.	Exercises help strengthen perineal musculature and improve sphincter tone and control over urine loss.

(continues)

(continued)

INTERVENTIONS	RATIONALES
Instruct patient to contract perineal muscles before coughing or sneezing to avoid or decrease incontinence.	Helps prevent increased intra-abdominal pressure, which promotes urine loss.

NIC: *Urinary Incontinence Care*

Discharge or Maintenance Evaluation

■ Patient will have an absence or reduction in urinary incontinence.

■ Patient will be able to perform exercises according to plan.

■ Patient will be able to prevent incontinence episodes associated with coughing, sneezing, or laughing.

RISK FOR INFECTION

Related to: inadequate primary defenses caused by aging or chronic illness, menopause, traumatized tissues, change in pH of secretions

Defining Characteristics: change to alkaline secretions in vagina, decreased estrogen level secretion, thinning of vaginal mucosa, atrophy of vaginal mucosa

Outcome Criteria

✔ Patient will have an absence of vaginal discomfort and/or infection.

NOC: *Risk Detection*

INTERVENTIONS	RATIONALES
Assess patient's vagina and genitalia for itching, burning, pain, lack of secretions, or foul-smelling secretions.	Changes associated with aging predispose patient to easily traumatized mucosa and susceptibility to atrophic vaginitis.
Administer estrogen cream by vaginal applicator or suppository as ordered.	Provides estrogen replacement and moisture to vagina to treat atrophic vaginitis.
Obtain vaginal smear for culture. Administer antimicrobial if culture is positive.	Identifies infectious organism, if present, and allows for eradication of causative organism.

INTERVENTIONS	RATIONALES
Instruct patient to apply water soluble lubricant to genitalia and vagina prn.	Treats dryness.
Instruct patient to avoid tight girdles or other tight clothing and to wear cotton underwear.	Irritates genitalia. Cotton is more porous and prevents dampness, resulting in less risk of infection.
Instruct to cleanse perineum frequently; wash genitalia from front to back.	Promotes comfort and prevents introduction of microorganisms.
Inform patient to avoid use of douches, sprays, or irritating soaps.	Prevents alteration in pH of vagina and irritation of genitalia.
Recommend yearly gynecologic checks and Pap smear.	Identifies presence of cancer and ensures gynecologic health.

NIC: *Infection Protection*

Discharge or Maintenance Evaluation

■ Patient will correctly administer estrogen therapy.

■ Patient will be able to verbalize increased comfort and absence of symptoms of infection.

■ Patient will be able to demonstrate appropriate health practices with genitalia and perineal care.

■ Patient will exhibit no evidence of vaginal infection or tissue trauma.

■ Patient will comply with all instructions to decrease potential for infection.

SITUATIONAL LOW SELF-ESTEEM

Related to: biophysical factors, loss of reproductive capability, hormonal changes

Defining Characteristics: self-negating verbalizations, loss of self-worth, expressions of guilt, depression, boredom, anxiety, insomnia, hot flashes, nervousness, change in self-perception of role

Outcome Criteria

✔ Patient will express feelings of reduced frustration, anxiety, nervousness and enhanced feeling of self-worth during adjustment to menopause.

NOC: *Self-Esteem*

INTERVENTIONS	RATIONALES
Assess patient's expressions of negative feelings, uselessness, self-worth, chronic anxiety or depression, and general complaints about present status in life.	Menopause creates more difficulty for women who feel that child-bearing is the main reason for existence and self-worth. Loss of reproductive ability then results in deeper emotional consequences.
Encourage expression of feelings in a nonjudgmental environment.	Provides venting of concerns and reduces anxiety.
Inform patient that feelings and symptoms caused by decrease in hormone secretion are not unusual.	Promotes understanding of problem for resolution and/or acceptance.
Suggest referral to counseling for chronic anxiety or depression if patient does not improve.	Prevents prolonged depression and permanent emotional disability.

NIC: *Self-Esteem Enhancement*

Discharge or Maintenance Evaluation

- Patient will express improved self-esteem and self-worth.
- Patient will have reduced anxiety and nervousness.
- Patient will be able to discuss concerns and develop a trusting relationship with caregiver.
- Patient will be able to verbalize adjustment to menopause and associated changes.
- Patient will be able to access resources for counseling to improve chronic anxiety or depression.
- Patient will exhibit improvement in comfort with hot flashes controlled and sleep pattern returned to normal.

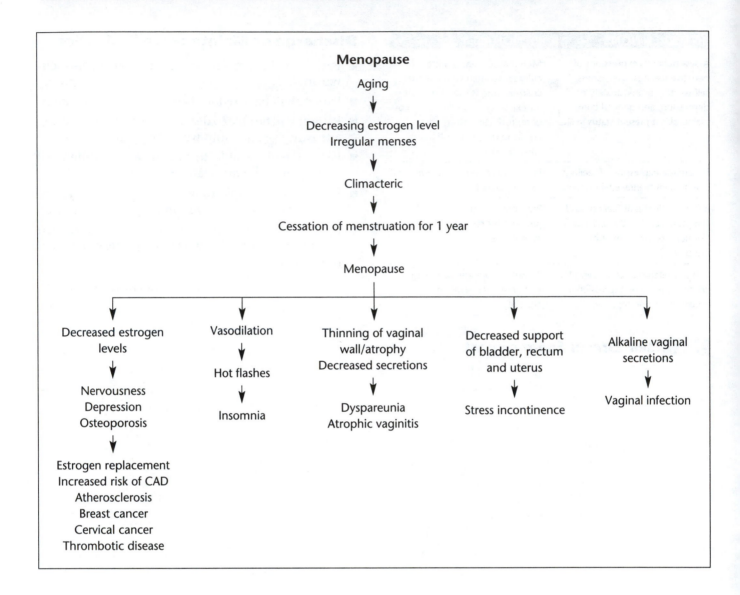

CHAPTER 5.3

BENIGN PROSTATIC HYPERTROPHY

Benign prostatic hypertrophy (BPH), or benign prostatic hyperplasia, occurs commonly in males, with approximately half of all men having some degree of the disease at age 50, and 80% of men age 80 or more. BPH results in a narrowing of the urethral opening as it connects to the prostate. This reduction in lumen size causes an obstruction to the outlet. Further obstruction is created by the mediation of alpha-adrenergic receptors with prostatic smooth muscle tone. The prostate becomes enlarged and results in urinary hesitancy, decreased urinary stream, intermittency, and a feeling of incomplete bladder emptying. Nocturia and urinary frequency occur as the bladder becomes more and more irritated.

Digital rectal examination of the elderly patient may expose either focal or uniform enlargement of the prostate. Areas of induration may correspond to malignant growth of the prostate. The estimated volume of the prostate should not guide treatment because the size estimated may not correlate with the symptoms of the need for treatment. The symptoms that are created by BPH can also be associated with other disorders, such as bladder outlet obstruction, urethral stricture, bladder calculi, and neoplasm of the bladder or prostate. These diagnoses should be excluded prior to treatment for BPH.

Treatment focuses on symptomatic relief, or if a urinary tract infection develops, on antimicrobial therapy. Initial therapy is begun with the use of drug treatment, but if the patient presents with severe urinary retention, surgery may be appropriate as the initial management. Surgery is usually recommended if renal insufficiency, recurrent retention, calculi, gross hematuria, or recurrent urinary infections occur.

Other treatment options that are less invasive include balloon dilation, laser tissue destruction, placement of intraurethral stents, and microwave hyperthermia. These are still investigational.

MEDICAL CARE

Laboratory: urinalysis used to identify infection and presence of hematuria; urine cultures used to identify causative pathogen in the case of urinary tract infection to direct antimicrobial therapy; prostate-specific antigen (PSA) used to identify prostate cancer, but is usually elevated in BPH also; renal profiles used to identify dysfunction; BUN and creatinine usually elevated in patients with BPH who have high postvoid residuals and renal impairment; CBC used to evaluate blood volume and hydration; electrolyte profiles used to identify imbalances

Radiography: IVP used to identify prostate enlargement and effect on renal function if an obstruction is present; abdominal X-rays used to show urinary tract calculi

Ultrasonography: may be used to identify prostate size, prostate volume, and to assess bladder and upper urinary tract changes

Urodynamic testing: used to identify maximum urinary flow rate, peak flow rate, and urethral obstruction to urine flow; peak flow rates less than 10 cc/sec indicate intravesical obstruction

Cystoscopy: used when the diagnosis is unclear and when patients are being evaluated for more invasive or newer procedures; reveals amount of enlargement and obstruction by prostate and presence of small areas of hemorrhage

Medical management: alpha-adrenergic blockers, such as doxazosin mesylate (Cardura), fenoldopam mesylate (Corlopam), labetalol hydrochloride (Normodyne, Trandate), phentolamine mesylate (Regitine), prazosin hydrochloride (Minipress), tamsulosin hydrochloride (Flomax), and terazosin hydrochloride (Hytrin), used to act on the peripheral vasculature to help decrease obstructive symptoms by blocking the receptors of smooth muscle at the bladder neck and decrease the outlet resistance; these drugs do have cardiovascular side effects, especially hypotension; 5-alpha-reductase inhibitors, such as finasteride (Propecia, Proscar) impede the change of testosterone to dihydrotestosterone and minimize prostate size, reducing obstruction and the prominent obstructive symptoms; this drug has also been shown to reduce PSA levels by half

Antimicrobials: used in the treatment of urinary tract infections to eradicate the causative organism

Surgery: remains the treatment of choice for symptomatic BPH and provides the most consistently immediate improvement; transurethral resection of the prostate (TURP) is less dangerous than open prostatectomy but does require anesthesia in an inpatient locale; open prostatectomy is best for patients with prostates >100 grams; transurethral incision of the prostate (TUIP) is best for patients with prostates <30 grams in size and who have an obstruction located at the neck of the bladder

Other invasive treatments: ablation therapy using microwaves, radiofrequency, and ultrasound waves destroy prostatic tissue; a stent can be positioned inside the prostatic urethral opening to facilitate keeping the urethra open and has been used in elderly men who cannot undergo anesthetic complications

COMMON NURSING DIAGNOSES

DISTURBED SLEEP PATTERNS (see HEART FAILURE)

Related to: internal factors from BPH, enlarged prostate, nocturia

Defining Characteristics: interrupted sleep, fatigue, lethargy, irritability, disorientation, complaints of not feeling rested, insomnia, sleeplessness, loss of libido, nocturia, urinary frequency, urinary urgency, urinary retention, dysuria, pelvic pain, bladder pain

SEXUAL DYSFUNCTION (see SEXUAL DISORDERS)

Related to: changes in body structure and function from urethral obstruction, biopsychosocial alteration of sexuality from altered body structures, prostatectomy, medications

Defining Characteristics: verbalization of problems with sexual function, avoidance of engaging in sex-

ual intercourse, need for confirmation of desirability, actual or perceived limitation imposed by BPH, anxiety

RISK FOR INFECTION (see MENOPAUSE)

Related to: inadequate primary defenses, stasis of body fluids, invasive procedures, indwelling catheters, medications, physiologic changes related to aging

Defining Characteristics: increased temperature, cloudy urine, foul-smelling urine, positive urine cultures, frequency, dysuria, burning, pelvic pain, hematuria

ADDITIONAL NURSING DIAGNOSES

URINARY RETENTION

Related to: obstruction to urinary flow, enlarged prostate compressing on urethra, medications, aging

Defining Characteristics: bladder distention, small, frequent voiding, dribbling, residual urine, overflow incontinence, nocturia, urgency, sensation of bladder fullness, sensation of inadequate bladder emptying, dysuria, pelvic pain

Outcome Criteria

✔ Patient will achieve or maintain adequate urinary flow and output.

NOC: *Urinary Elimination*

INTERVENTIONS	RATIONALES
Monitor I&O every 2–4 hours. Monitor patient for urinary frequency, urgency, dribbling, and bladder distention by palpation.	Incomplete voluntary control over one's bladder function and the decreased bladder capacity may cause frequency and nocturia, which is further compromised when an enlarged prostate compresses the urethra. Intake and output data provides information regarding fluid status and imbalances.
Encourage fluids of at least 2 L/day, unless contraindicated. Decrease intake prior to bedtime.	Prevents dehydration and urinary bladder infection. Decreasing fluids just prior to bedtime may prevent nocturia and disturbance of patient's sleep.

INTERVENTIONS	RATIONALES
Prepare and catheterize patient if unable to void, or if residual urine check is ordered. Use aseptic technique.	May need a retention catheter inserted if patient is unable to urinate based on presence of obstruction. Residual volume may be desired to evaluate voiding pattern and retention of urine. Aseptic technique prevents risks of infection.
Administer medications as ordered.	Alpha-adrenergic blockers or 5-alpha-reductase inhibitors help improve symptoms; alpha blockers decrease obstructive symptoms by acting on smooth muscle at the bladder neck and decreasing outlet resistance, but may cause hypotension if the dosage is not titrated over several weeks; the 5-alpha-reductase inhibitor, finasteride, hinders the conversion of testosterone to dihydrotestosterone to decrease the size of the prostate and improve the obstructive symptoms.
Instruct patient to void as soon as the urge is felt.	Reduces urinary stasis and retention, which can result in infection.
Instruct patient to avoid caffeine and alcoholic beverages.	Increases prostatic obstructive symptoms.
Instruct patient to continue to see physician for follow-up checks to evaluate prostate and diagnose symptoms, if present.	Provides early identification for prompt treatment of prostatic conditions and complications.
Instruct patient regarding need to maintain fluid hydration of at least 8 glasses of fluid per day regardless of symptoms.	Reduction in fluid intake does not reduce symptoms and may predispose patient to urinary infection.
Instruct patient/family to make themselves aware of location of bathrooms when away from home, to have patient void before leaving home, and to make frequent stops to allow for patient to void.	Provides for immediate voiding when needed and prevents embarrassment of dribbling and wetting clothing.

NIC: *Urinary Retention Care*

Discharge or Maintenance Evaluation

- Patient will exhibit a decrease in the frequency and urgency of urination and have less nocturia.
- Patient will have complete emptying or improvement in emptying of bladder.

- Patient will maintain fluid hydration status.
- Patient will have adequate urinary flow established.
- Patient/family will be able to accurately verbalize all instructions given and will be compliant with these instructions to maintain urinary flow.

DEFICIENT KNOWLEDGE

Related to: lack of information about prostatectomy

Defining Characteristics: request for information, anxiety about changes in sexual function, verbalization of the problem, anxiety about incontinence following surgery

Outcome Criteria

✔ Patient will exhibit an increase in knowledge regarding temporary postoperative changes.

NOC: *Knowledge: Treatment Procedures*

INTERVENTIONS	RATIONALES
Assess presence of patient's anxiety, concern about results of surgery, and effect on lifestyle and body image.	Impending surgery causes anxiety about sexual functioning and incontinence problems.
Instruct patient that postoperative incontinence is temporary and tapers off within 6 months.	Incontinence may be caused by trauma to bladder sphincter during surgery, or an indwelling catheter which reduces muscle tone.
Instruct patient in pelvic muscle strengthening exercises to be performed for 10 minutes 4 times/day; practice starting and stopping during urination.	Improves muscle tone and strength to control incontinence when stress of increased intra-abdominal pressure is present.
Suggest use of pads or leak-proof underwear.	Prevents wetting of clothing and embarrassment.
Suggest refraining from sexual intercourse for 3–6 weeks after surgery.	Permits tissue healing.
Instruct patient of retrograde ejaculation during intercourse with transurethral prostatectomy.	Prevents alarm at change in urine after intercourse and absence of semen during ejaculation.
Instruct patient about alternative sexual methods, if impotency is expected following prostatectomy.	Provides information to allay anxiety.

NIC: *Teaching: Disease Process*

Discharge or Maintenance Evaluation

■ Patient will verbalize reduced anxiety.

■ Patient will be able to verbalize understanding of consequences of surgery, possible resolution of symptoms, and potential complications.

■ Patient will exhibit no sexual complications following surgery.

Benign Prostatic Hypertrophy

Aging

Sexual hormone imbalance
Enlargement of prostate
Nodules in periurethral region

Compression of urethra

Partial or complete obstruction of urine flow

Decreased stream
Difficulty in voiding
Urinary retention and overdistention
Frequency, nocturia
Overflow incontinence

Destructive changes in bladder wall

Herniation/diverticula of bladder wall

Stasis of urine

Urinary tract infection
Hydronephrosis

CHAPTER 5.4

SEXUAL DISORDERS

Sexual interest and activity continue throughout life and provide physiologic and psychologic outlets and satisfaction for the elderly patient. The intimacy of touching, closeness, and sexual intercourse are expressions of sexuality that are very important to an older adult, and may be altered by declining health and energy, privacy, loss of a partner, medications, chronic illness, or problems of the reproductive system. Regardless of the cause, a change in sexual pattern or function results in anxiety, concern with failure, and dissatisfaction with sexual intercourse, which ultimately affects the patient's self-esteem, identify, and role performance.

In men, testosterone production and metabolic clearance decrease with age. These changes affect libido, energy, memory, and muscle strength. Testosterone influences the incidence of nocturnal erections. Aging is correlated with the decrease in sperm quality and quantity, but spermatogenesis does not stop completely.

The most common dysfunction in men is erectile dysfunction, or impotence, which is the inability to achieve and maintain an erection adequate to have satisfactory sexual intercourse at least half the time. The incidence of erectile dysfunction, ED, is almost 95% among men 70 years of age and older who have other underlying medical diseases (Beers & Berkow, 2000). Causes of ED include neurologic, endocrine, and vascular disorders, abnormalities of the structure of the penis, side effects from medications, and psychologic dysfunction.

Treatment for ED consists mainly of drug therapy, but other measures have been utilized with varying degrees of success. Constriction rings decrease venous outflow at the base of the penis and are useful in men who can achieve an erection but are not able to sustain them. Vacuum tumescent devices increase engorgement by the creation of negative pressure in order to draw blood into the penis. Penile prostheses or implants may be used when ED does not respond to any other treatment. Penile revascularization surgery is experimental and without high success rates for long-term assistance.

Sexual dysfunction in women includes decreased libido, sexual arousal disorder, and dyspareunia. A decrease in sexual drive is testosterone-dependent, and causes include increased prolactin, decreased estrogen, and the use of alcohol, drugs, anticonvulsants, and chemotherapy agents.

Sexual arousal disorder occurs when there is a persistent inability to achieve or to maintain sexual excitement until the completion of sexual activity. Causes include the use of anticholinergic drugs, tricyclic antidepressants, and chemotherapy agents, as well as a decrease in estrogen, a decrease in vaginal lubrication, and decreased elasticity of tissues related to the aging process.

Dyspareunia is intercourse that is painful, and occurs in approximately one-third of all women over the age of 65. Causes include inadequate vaginal lubrication, irritation and dryness of the genitalia, vulvovaginitis, episiotomy scars, improper angle of entry, anorectal dysfunction, and prolapsed uterus. Treatment of the underlying cause is the preferred method of management.

MEDICAL CARE

Laboratory: testosterone levels used to identify bioavailable amounts of the hormone that may affect libido; prolactin levels used to identify elevations that may result in decreased libido for women; estrogen levels used to identify decreases that may result in decreased libido in women; CBC used to identify anemia, infection, or other cause that may contribute to dysfunction; glucose and thyroid profiles used to identify dysfunction that may contribute to sexual dysfunction

Drug therapy: estrogen (17 beta-estradiol/ norgestimate [Ortho-Prefest], estradiol cypionate or valerate [Alora, Climara, Estrace, Fempatch, Depo-Estradiol, Depogen, Clinagen, Menaval], estradiol/norethindrone acetate [Combipatch], conjugated estrogens [Premarin], estropipate [Ogen, Eortho-Est], ethinyl estradiol and desogestrel [Desogen, Ortho-Cept], ethinyl estradiol and norethindrone acetate [Loestrin], ethinyl estradiol and norgestimate [Ortho-Cyclen], levonorgestrel [Norplant], medroxy-progesterone acetate [Amen, Curretab, Cycrin, Depo-Provera, Provera], and norethindrone [Micronor, Aygestin]); used alone or in conjunction with a progestin to relieve dyspareunia and prevent atrophic vaginitis, hot flashes, prevent osteoporosis, and reduce atherosclerosis and CAD risk; estrogens can cause nausea, mastalgia, headache, mood changes, endometrial hyperplasia, and increased risk of endometrial, ovarian, and breast cancers, cholelithiasis, and thromboembolic disease; oral erectile agents, such as sildenafil (Viagra), used for men to achieve and maintain erection by decreasing the action of phosphodiesterase type 5 which is responsible for the degradation of cyclic guanosine monophosphate in the corpus cavernosum and allows more blood flow into the area to have improved sexual activity; sildenafil should not be utilized by patients who are also concurrently taking nitrates because of the potential for life-threatening cardiac events

Nonpharmacologic measures: constriction rings used by men who can achieve erection but are unable to sustain them; vacuum tumescent devices used to increase penile engorgement

Surgery: penile prostheses or implants may be helpful when ED is not responsive to any other therapy; penile revascularization surgery, which is comparatively experimental, may be performed but has not been noted to have high success rates

NURSING DIAGNOSES

SEXUAL DYSFUNCTION

Related to: biopsychosocial alterations of sexuality, misinformation or lack of knowledge, lack of privacy, lack of significant other, impaired relationship with significant other, altered body structure or function, drugs, surgery, disease process, radiation

Defining Characteristics: verbalization of the problem, change in sexual behavior or activities, alterations in achieving perceived sex role, actual or perceived limitation imposed by disease or therapy, alterations in achieving sexual satisfaction, inability to achieve desired satisfaction, alteration in relationship with significant other, change in interest in self and others, impotence, dyspareunia, erectile dysfunction, decreased libido

Outcome Criteria

✔ Patient will have satisfying sexual function.

NOC: *Sexual Functioning*

INTERVENTIONS	RATIONALES
Assess patient's sexual interest, desire, affect of health status on sexuality, and psychosocial factors affecting sexual function.	Age-related sexual changes do not alter the need for sexual closeness and companionship, however, chronic illness, drugs, fear of inability to perform, lack of or an impaired relationship with partner, cultural beliefs, lack of privacy, or disinterest in sex do alter sexual function.
Assess presence of impotence, dyspareunia, feelings of inadequacy, or fear of sexual function and failure.	Changes related to aging, such as slower arousal time, reduced rigidity of erection, reduced lubrication of the vagina, and atrophy of vaginal lining, resulting in painful intercourse, may be responsible for the sexual problems. Chronic illnesses compromise sexual functioning by causing physiologic changes and fear of recurrence of symptoms.
Include partner in discussion, if appropriate.	May be embarrassed to have partner present or even approach the subject. Patient may be more comfortable discussing the subject alone.
Discuss past sexual experiences and practices, interest and satisfaction, and medications taken for control of chronic diseases that affect sexual function.	Provides individual needs regarding sexual behavior based on history.
Discuss importance of maintaining sexual functioning by intercourse or masturbation.	Maintains interest and sexual function.
Encourage to vary positions during intercourse, especially in patients with arthritis, dyspnea, COPD, and post-myocardial infarction.	Pain and dyspnea may be exacerbated during exertion and a more passive position may promote participation in safe sexual activity.

INTERVENTIONS	RATIONALES
Provide privacy.	Some elderly live with family members or in long-term facilities and may lack the privacy needed because of attitudes about aging and sex.
Provide pain medication, bronchodilators, oxygen, or vasodilators, as appropriate before sexual intercourse.	Promotes comfort, and prevents pain or dyspnea during activity as pulse, BP, and O₂ consumption increase.
Use exercise and pain tolerance and changes in VS caused by activity as guidelines for a progressive sexual activity plan based on physical limits.	Provides baselines to promote sexual activity without symptoms that create fear or interfere with sexual activity.
Correct any misinformation about effects of sexual activity; inform patient that correct information assists to identify fears, concerns and remedy sexual dysfunction.	Fear of precipitating angina episode, heart attack, dyspnea from COPD, of injury to inflamed joints is usually caused by lack of correct information.
Instruct patient of age-related physical changes, and male/female reproductive system anatomy and physiology.	Provides information to promote understanding of sexual functioning.
Inform patient to avoid sexual activity if environmental temperature is excessively hot or cold, after eating large meal, or if anxious, angry, or fatigued.	Has a negative effect on sexual ability and activity.
If partner has died, instruct on importance of continuing sexual activity.	A loss of sexual functioning may occur with prolonged abstinence.
Instruct patient of erectile or ejaculation changes related to disease or surgery, retrograde ejaculation causing a cloudy appearance to the urine, impotence from erectile or ejaculation failure, and effect of fear on libido.	Reduces anxiety and fear of impotence. Changes may be noted following transurethral prostatectomy, caused by incomplete closure of bladder sphincter, circulatory impairment in diabetes, or atherosclerosis affecting blood flow and interfering with ability to achieve an erection.
Instruct patient of effect of drugs on sexual performance. Suggest discussion with physician about problem.	The changing, elimination, or adjustments in doses of medications may prevent or reduce impotence.
Use charts to demonstrate position variations for arthritic, stroke, COPD, MI, and angina patients. Instruct in use of medications, and when to cease activity and rest.	More dependent, passive positions permits intercourse without producing symptoms that interfere with performance.

INTERVENTIONS	RATIONALES
Instruct female patient to use water-soluble lubricant during intercourse.	Lubricates vagina to prevent pain and irritation during intercourse from thinning, dry mucosa.
Instruct patient of penile implant possibility and to discuss with physician.	Treatment is used for impotence caused by stroke or surgery that does not respond to therapy.
Instruct female with catheter to tape to thigh or abdomen; male to hold catheter in place with condom and tape tubing to abdomen. Catheter should be disconnected from tubing and clamped.	Stabilizes catheter and prevents injury to the urethra. Backflow is prevented by clamp.
If incontinent of feces, instruct to administer enema before intercourse.	Decreases possibility of fecal incontinence during intercourse.
Instruct to void before and after intercourse.	Clears meatus of infectious organisms that may cause bladder infection.
Suggest sexual or psychological therapy, if appropriate.	Anxiety and reduced self-esteem resulting from altered sexuality are common problems that can be helped by counseling.
If sexual dysfunction is a result of cognitive functioning, inform family of reduced sex interest and inappropriate sexual behaviors.	Promotes understanding of antisocial sexual behavior as dementia progresses and prevents embarrassment to family.

NIC: *Sexual Counseling*

Discharge or Maintenance Evaluation

- Patient will be able to verbalize understanding of sexuality changes associated with aging.
- Patient will be able to verbalize understanding of difficulties and limitations of sexual experience and discuss possible reasons for them.
- Vital signs will be within baseline ranges after intercourse, and patient will have no complications from activity.
- Patient will achieve satisfaction with alterations in sexual patterns and positions within physical limitations.
- Patient will have reduced anxiety and fear in contemplation of sexual intercourse.
- Patient will return to previous sexual patterns as a result of rehabilitation.
- Patient will be free of pain during intercourse.

■ Family will be able to verbalize understanding and demonstrate use of measures taken to reduce inappropriate sexual behavior by mentally incapacitated elderly patients.

■ Patient will express reduced anxiety as sexual activity improves.

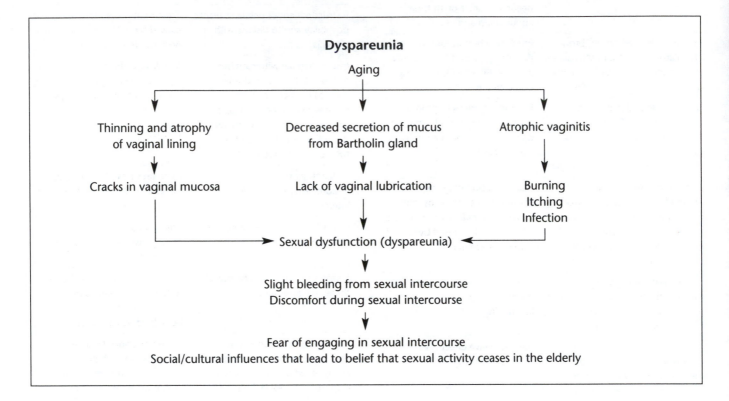

Dyspareunia

Aging

Thinning and atrophy of vaginal lining

Decreased secretion of mucus from Bartholin gland

Atrophic vaginitis

Cracks in vaginal mucosa

Lack of vaginal lubrication

Burning
Itching
Infection

Sexual dysfunction (dyspareunia)

Slight bleeding from sexual intercourse
Discomfort during sexual intercourse

Fear of engaging in sexual intercourse
Social/cultural influences that lead to belief that sexual activity ceases in the elderly

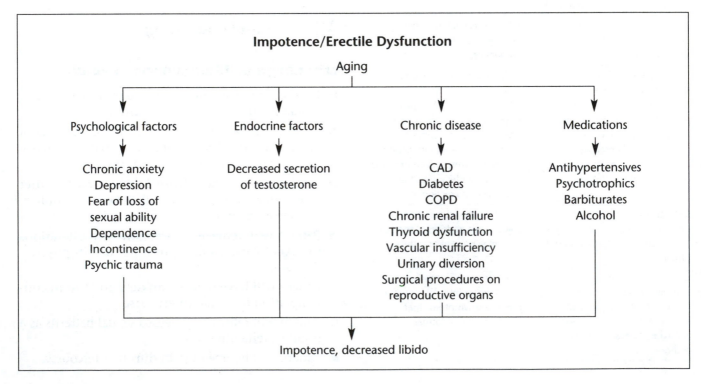

Impotence/Erectile Dysfunction

Aging

Psychological factors

Endocrine factors

Chronic disease

Medications

Chronic anxiety
Depression
Fear of loss of
sexual ability
Dependence
Incontinence
Psychic trauma

Decreased secretion of testosterone

CAD
Diabetes
COPD
Chronic renal failure
Thyroid dysfunction
Vascular insufficiency
Urinary diversion
Surgical procedures on reproductive organs

Antihypertensives
Psychotrophics
Barbiturates
Alcohol

Impotence, decreased libido

CHAPTER 5.5

URINARY TRACT INFECTIONS

Urinary tract infections, or UTIs, are commonplace among the elderly, but diagnosis may be difficult because of atypical presenting symptoms. A lower tract infection (cystitis) will frequently lead to an upper tract infection (pyelonephritis) when bacteria travel up the ureters and cause inflammation and infection in the renal pelvis. In the male patient, the cause is bladder neck obstruction, and in the female patient, the cause is frequently contamination from bowel excreta via the urethra from improper cleansing.

Risk factors that are common in the elderly patient for UTIs include indwelling catheter use, atrophic urethritis, atrophic vaginitis, cancer of the prostate, BPH, bacterial prostatitis, calculi, renal and perinephric abscesses, urinary diversion procedures, and urethral strictures. The incidence of UTI increases with age. The most common organism that results in urinary infection is *Escherichia coli*, and *Klebsiella*, especially *Klebsiella pneumoniae*, is the second most common pathogen. Nosocomial UTIs usually yield positive cultures for *Serratia*, *Enterobacter*, *Citrobacter*, *Acinetobacter*, and *Pseudomonas* species.

Uterine prolapse, urolithiasis, and neoplasms in the GU tract and uterus produce a higher incidence of recurrent and complex infections. Bacteria multiply in stationary urine found in the bladder and establish bacteriuria. Untreated and undiagnosed, this bacteriuria can develop into full-blown urosepsis, which has a high morbidity rate among the elderly because of their immunocompromised status.

Many elderly patients are asymptomatic, but the most frequent symptoms include dysuria, frequency, sudden incontinence, flank pain, and fever. Treatment of UTI involves antimicrobials that are specific to the organism identified as the causative pathogen. In the case of urosepsis, second- and third-generation antibiotics are initially used in addition to ampicillin. Maintenance of fluid hydration and perfusion is essential.

MEDICAL CARE

Laboratory: CBC used to identify infective process, with shift to the left on differential indicating an acute infection; urinalysis and culture done to identify presence of urinary infection and to isolate the causative pathogen in order to administer the most effective antimicrobial; nitrite test used for quick identification of bacteriuria, but does not demonstrate infections caused by *Pseudomonas*, *Staphylococci*, or *Enterococci*; antimicrobial drug levels used to identify therapeutic versus toxic levels; electrolyte profiles used to evaluate imbalances; renal profiles used to identify worsening renal status and dysfunction

Radiography: KUB X-rays used to show obstruction or other abnormality leading to UTI; IVP may be done to identify urinary obstruction or deformity of the kidneys, as well as any urine residual

CT scan: used to identify structural abnormalities

Ultrasonography: used to identify abnormalities and urinary reflux

Antimicrobials: used to eradicate causative organisms, usually by inhibiting growth or by interfering with protein synthesis of the cell wall structure; frequently used drugs include: nitrofurantoin (Macrobid, Macrodantin), trimethoprim (Trimpex, Proloprim), aztreonam (Azactam), first-generation cephalosporins (cefadroxil [Duricef], cefazolin sodium [Ancef, Kefzol, Zolicef], cephalexin hydrochloride [Keftab, Biocef, Keflex], or cephradine [Velosef], cefuroxime [Ceftin, Kefurox, Zinacef], trimethoprim-sulfamethoxazole [Bactrim, Bethaprim, Comoxol, Septra, Sulfatrim], and levofloxacin [Levaquin]), second–generation cephalosporins (cefaclor [Ceclor], cefonicid sodium [Monocid], cefotetan disodium [Cefotan], cefoxitin sodim [Mefoxin], cefprozil [Cefzil], cefuroxime axetil or sodium [Ceftin, Kefurox, Zinacef], and loracarbef

[Lorabid]), and third-generation cephalosporins (cefdinir [Omnicef], cefixime [Suprax], cefoperazone sodium [Cefobid], cefotaxime sodium [Claforan], cefpodoxime proxetil [Vantin], ceftazidime [Ceptaz, Fortaz, Tazicef, Tazidime], ceftibuten [Cedax], ceftizoxime sodium [Cefizox] or ceftriaxone sodium [Rocephin], ceftazidime [Ceptaz, Fortaz, Tazicef, Tazidime] in addition to an aminoglycoside, such as tobramycin (Nebcin, Tobrax) or amikacin (Amikin), or an antipseudomonal penicillin (mezlocillin sodium [Mezlin], piperacillin sodium [Pipracil], or ticarcillin disodium [Ticar])

Urinary analgesics: flavoxate hydrochloride (Urispas), oxybutynin chloride (Ditropan), and phenazopyridine hydrochloride (Pyridium, Urogesic, Viridium, Baridium, Phenazodine) used to relieve pain, burning, frequency, and urgency by soothing the inflamed urinary tract mucosa

COMMON NURSING DIAGNOSES

 ### IMBALANCED NUTRITION: LESS THAN BODY REQUIREMENTS (see COPD)

Related to: inability to ingest food because of biological factors from acute infectious process of pyelonephritis

Defining Characteristics: nausea, vomiting, anorexia

 ### ACUTE PAIN (see INTERSTITIAL CYSTITIS)

Related to: bladder pain, dysuria, urinary frequency, inflammation in bladder, infection, urosepsis

Defining Characteristics: verbalization of pain and discomfort, suprapubic pain, flank pain, dysuria, hematuria, urinary frequency, inflammation, urgency

 ### HYPERTHERMIA (see INFLUENZA)

Related to: urinary tract or kidney infection, exposure to infection, alterations in fluid and electrolyte balance

Defining Characteristics: fever, warm, flushed skin, tachycardia, tachypnea, dry mucous membranes, dehydration, oliguria, seizures, changes in mental

status, increased BUN and creatinine, electrolyte imbalances, cloudy urine, increased white blood cell count, positive nitrite test, positive cultures

 ### IMPAIRED URINARY ELIMINATION (see INTERSTITIAL CYSTITIS)

Related to: renal infection, bladder infection, use of indwelling catheter, changes in urinary function

Defining Characteristics: bladder pain, suprapubic pain, dysuria, hematuria, urinary frequency, incomplete bladder emptying, nocturia, urgency, presence of indwelling catheter, cloudy urine, concentrated urine, oliguria

ADDITIONAL NURSING DIAGNOSES

 ### RISK FOR INFECTION

Related to: bladder outlet obstruction, BPH, urinary retention

Defining Characteristics: increased WBC count with shift to the left on differential, cloudy urine, sediment in urine, dysuria, frequency of urination, urinary retention, hematuria, presence of indwelling catheters, incontinence, flank pain, pelvic pain, fever

Outcome Criteria

✔ Patient will be free of urinary tract infection and will be able to prevent recurrence.

NOC: *Risk Detection*

INTERVENTIONS	RATIONALES
Assess patient for signs and symptoms of urinary tract dysfunction.	UTIs become more common with age because of frequent use of invasive catheters and procedures, as well as physiologic changes in the immune system of the elderly. Patients may complain of back or pelvic pain, abrupt onset of frequency of urination or incontinence, or hematuria.
Monitor vital signs every 2–4 hours and prn. Notify physician for significant changes in status.	Increased temperature, pulse, respiration, and blood pressure may indicate the presence of infection and possible sepsis.

INTERVENTIONS	RATIONALES
Identify potential cause for infective process, and remove cause if possible.	Bacteria thrive in stagnant urine, so if patient has tendencies toward urinary retention, this may preclude the incidence of infection. Narrowing of the bladder outlet, especially in men, may increase the amount of UTIs because of retention. Foreign bodies, such as catheters, promote infection and bacterial growth.
Obtain UA and urine culture and sensitivity as ordered.	Provides for identification of infection as well as causative organism and antimicrobials that organism is sensitive to in order to eradicate it.
Administer antimicrobials as ordered.	Eradicates causative organism to cure bladder infection.
Ensure that proper handwashing is done by all personnel who come in contact with patient.	Helps to prevent further infection or spread of bacteria.
Use Standard Precautions with all patients.	Wearing gloves helps protect personnel while providing direct care to patient by protecting them from bacteria.
Monitor lab work, especially CBC.	WBC should decrease with the use of antimicrobials. If it does not, or if the WBC actually increases, it may indicate a superinfection or lack of antimicrobials' ability to eradicate the causative organism.
Instruct patient/family regarding the need for good handwashing and demonstrate proper procedure.	Hands should be washed for at least 15 seconds, using brisk rubbing motions with plenty of soap and water. Hands should be dried and then the paper towel used to turn the faucets off.

INTERVENTIONS	RATIONALES
Instruct patient/family to notify nurse or physician for episodes of diarrhea.	May be caused from the particular antimicrobial agent and may require changing drugs to prevent dehydration. Loose stools may also indicate the presence of *Clostridium difficile* bacterium.
Instruct patient/family to use disposable tissues and bags for expectorations.	Helps to prevent spread of bacteria.
Instruct patient/family to cleanse perineum from front to back.	Prevents the spread of fecal material into the urinary meatus, which may result in infection.
Instruct patient/family regarding need for protective isolation as warranted.	Patient may be immunocompromised and helps to protect patient from environmental pathogens.

NIC: *Infection Protection*

Discharge or Maintenance Evaluation

- Patient will exhibit no signs or symptoms of urinary infection.
- Urine will be clear, pale yellow, and patient will be free of pain and dysuria.
- Patient/family will be able to accurately verbalize understanding of infection control procedures, such as good handwashing, disposal of contaminated secretions, and so forth.
- Patient/family will be able to prevent recurrence of infection.

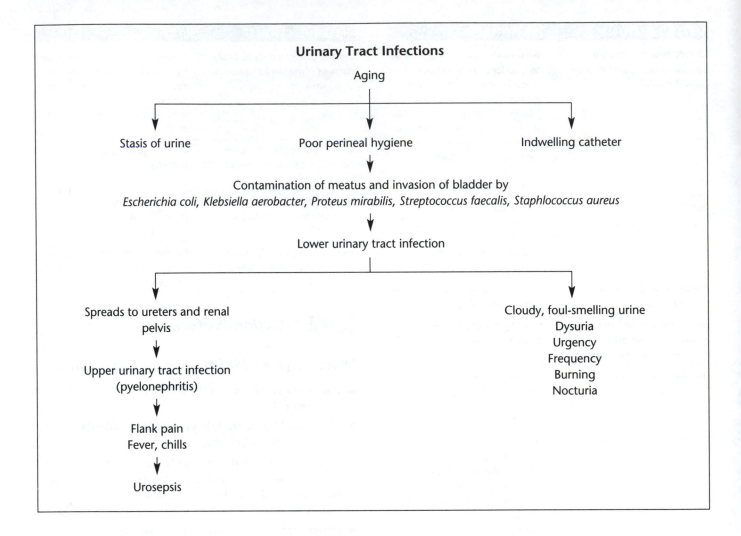

Urinary Tract Infections

Aging

Stasis of urine   Poor perineal hygiene   Indwelling catheter

Contamination of meatus and invasion of bladder by
Escherichia coli, Klebsiella aerobacter, Proteus mirabilis, Streptococcus faecalis, Staphlococcus aureus

Lower urinary tract infection

Spreads to ureters and renal
pelvis

Upper urinary tract infection
(pyelonephritis)

Flank pain
Fever, chills

Urosepsis

Cloudy, foul-smelling urine
Dysuria
Urgency
Frequency
Burning
Nocturia

CHAPTER 5.6

CHRONIC RENAL FAILURE

Chronic renal failure, or CRF, is a progressive renal condition that results from a variety of pathologic developments and leads to the insufficiency of the renal system to maintain regulatory and excretory function. This usually culminates in end-stage renal disease and depends upon the number of nephrons lost. The prognosis in the elderly patient depends upon the cause of the insufficiency or failure and can be poor if the kidney parenchyma is involved. If obstruction or a reversible disease entity is present, prognosis is somewhat improved. The renal impairment that results from dehydration, malnutrition, anemia, electrolyte imbalances, infection and fever usually leads to a buildup of uremic toxins that can affect the function of all body organs.

Milder forms of chronic renal failure can present with fewer symptoms. As waste products accumulate in the blood, uremia develops, and causes nausea, vomiting, abdominal pain, headache, diarrhea, weight loss, fatigue, weakness, dizziness, blurry vision, muscle fasciculations, decreased mentation, seizures, and coma. Jaundice, hypertension, GI bleeding, and itching may result, and complications can lead to heart failure and pericarditis.

Causes that result in chronic renal failure that are more prevalent in the elderly patient population than in the general population include chronic urinary tract infections, prostatic hypertrophy leading to hydronephrosis, hypertension, diabetes, atherosclerosis, carcinoma, and long-term use of nonsteroidal anti-inflammatory drugs and analgesics.

Sometimes the progression of the disease can be slowed by modifying the patient's lifestyle and addressing the medical conditions of the patient, such as dietary restriction of protein, salt, and potassium, use of antihypertensive drugs to control blood pressure, maintaining tight control of diabetes and glucose levels, and prevention of the abuse of analgesics. Dialysis, either hemodialysis or peritoneal dialysis, is the usual treatment for patients who are unable to biologically remove toxins from their own bodies. Currently, renal transplantation, although very selective, is being used in persons older than 60 years of age. It is controversial, however, because of the reluctance in donating an organ that is in high demand but in low supply to a person with a limited life expectancy, as well as increased comorbidities from chronic illnesses.

There are four phases of chronic renal failure defined by the amount of nephron loss (Grif, 1998). A 50% loss indicates that the renal reserve is decreased, with mildly reduced kidney function, but basically the patient is without significant problems. Phase 2 involves a 75% nephron loss and indicates renal insufficiency, with mild azotemia, anemia, and the ability to concentrate urine is slightly decreased. Phase 3 involves a 90% nephron loss and indicates end-stage renal disease, where kidney function has become so deteriorated that the patient will require artificial support via dialysis or transplantation to continue life. Phase 4 is the uremic syndrome in which the body's organs are failing as a result of the toxins that have built up from the uremic waste products.

Complications associated with renal failure include electrolyte imbalances, fluid imbalances, and anemia, which may require more vigorous treatment in the elderly patient because of existing coronary disease. Blood and blood product transfusions and the use of erythropoietin (EPO) are used to treat this anemia in end-stage renal dysfunction. Although treatment may be costly, it is usually reassuring to the patient that Medicare pays for this treatment.

MEDICAL CARE

Laboratory: CBC used to identify presence of infections, anemia, and to evaluate efficacy of treatment for each; electrolyte profiles used to identify imbalances that are caused from renal failure, most often sodium, potassium, phosphorus, and calcium imbalances; renal profiles used to identify improvement or worsening of renal dysfunction with BUN and creatinine levels; 24-hour creatinine clearance urine testing used to evaluate the amount of creatinine that is cleared during this period of time to identify the severity of the dysfunction; decreases of 10–50 ml/min is usually associated with renal insufficiency, whereas a value of 10–15 ml/min usually indicates end stage renal failure; urinalysis done to evaluate for specific gravity changes, proteinuria, glycosuria, hematuria, and osmolality; albumin levels used to identify nutritional status; urine cultures used to detect the presence of infection and identify the causative organism; serum creatinine used to identify the relationship between creatinine and glomerular filtration rate to identify the decrease in renal reserve; lipid profiles used to identify presence of increased triglycerides, and risk for atherosclerosis; glucose tolerance testing used to identify the presence of carbohydrate intolerance; uric acid levels to identify presence of gout

Radiography: KUB X-rays used to identify size, shape, and placement of kidneys, ureters, and bladder; chest X-rays used to identify cardiac silhouette, pericardial effusions, pleural effusions, infiltrates, and consolidations that may result as a complication of renal failure; X-rays of the skull, hands and feet identify the potential for uremic neuropathy and bone disease

Intravenous pyelogram (IVP): used to identify degree of renal function, size of kidneys, obstruction, or scarring

CT scan: renal CT may be done to identify renal blood flow and glomerular and tubular function

Ultrasonography: used to identify obstruction or masses

Renal biopsy: may be done to establish the diagnosis, to determine presence of carcinoma, or identify reversible etiology

Diuretics: chlorthalidone (Hygroton, Thalitone), hydrochlorothiazide (Esidrix, Ezide, HydroDiuril, Microzide, Oretic), indapamide (Lozol), and metolazone (Mykrox, Zaroxolyn) are thiazide-acting diuretics that increase sodium and water excretion by inhibiting reabsorption of sodium in the cortical diluting site of the ascending loop of Henle, or inhibit sodium and chloride reabsorption in the distal segment of the nephron; amiloride hydrochloride (Amiloride, Midamor), spironolactone (Aldactone), and triamterene (Dyrenium) are potassium-sparing diuretics that inhibit sodium reabsorption and potas-

sium and hydrogen excretion by action on the distal tubules; both promote diuresis and elimination of acebutolol hydrochloride sodium; used to relieve edema

ACE inhibitors: benazepril hydrochloride (Lotensin), candesartan cilexetil (Atacand), captopril (Capoten), enalapril (Vasotec), eprosartan mesylate (Teveten), fosinopril sodium (Monopril), irbesartan (Avapro), losartan potassium (Cozaar), moexipril hydrochloride (Univasc), perindopril erbumine (Aceon), quinapril hydrochloride (Accupril), ramipril (Altace), telmisartan (Micardis), trandolapril (Mavik), and valsartan (Diovan) used to prevent the conversion of angiotensin I to angiotensin II by inhibiting the angiotensin converting enzyme (ACE) to enable the decrease in vasoconstriction, preload, and afterload; angiotensin II receptor blockers inhibit angiotensin II at the end-organ receptor level and tend to have less incidence of coughing; these drugs used to lower blood pressure as well as to decrease the rate of advancement of nondiabetic related renal dysfunction

Antihypertensives: vasodilators (hydralazine [Apresoline], minoxidil [Loniten], and nitroprusside sodium [Nitropress]) are used to relax smooth muscle in the arterioles that help to reduce peripheral resistance; beta-adrenergic blockers: ([Sectral], atenolol [Tenormin], betaxolol [Kerlone], bisoprolol fumarate [Zebeta], carteolol hydrochloride [Cartrol], carvedilol [Coreg], metoprolol [Lopressor], nadolol [Corgard], penbutolol [Levatol], pindolol [Visken], propranolol [Inderal], and timolol maleate [Blocadren]) used to decrease blood pressure by inhibiting the impulse through the sympathetic pathways and to decrease cardiac output, sympathetic stimulation, and renin secretion by the kidneys; alpha-adrenergic blockers: (doxazosin mesylate [Cardura], fenoldopam mesylate [Corlopam], labetalol hydrochloride [Normodyne, Trandate], phentolamine mesylate [Regitine], prazosin hydrochloride [Minipress], and terazosin hydrochloride [Hytrin]) used to reduce blood pressure by acting on the peripheral vasculature to generate vasodilatory action and to decrease peripheral vascular resistance; calcium channel blockers: (diltiazem [Cardizem], felodipine [Plendil], isradipine [DynaCirc], nicardipine [Cardene], nifedipine [Procardia], nisoldipine [Sular], and verapamil [Calan, Isoptin]) used to reduce blood pressure by inhibition of calcium ion influx across the smooth muscle and cardiac cells which reduces arteriolar resistance; these drugs may be required if reduction of the extracellular fluid does not control blood pressure in renal failure patients

Antacids: aluminum carbonate (Basaljel), aluminum hydroxide (AleternaGEL, Amphojel, Dialume), calcium carbonate (Alka-Mints, Amitone, Chooz, Dicarbosil, Maalox, Rolaids, Tums), magaldrate (Lowsium, Riopan), and magnesium oxide (Mag-Ox, Maox, Uro-Mag) used to help neutralize gastric acid and to bind to dietary phosphates to reduce hyperphosphatemia

Cation exchange resin: sodium polystyrene sulfonate (Kaexalate) assists in the removal of potassium by exchanging sodium for potassium primarily in the large intestine

Antipruritics: cyproheptadine hydrochloride (Periactin), diphenhydramine hydrochloride (Benadryl, Banophen, Beldin), fexofenadine hydrochloride (Allegra), hydroxyzine embonate, hydrochlorid, or pamoate (Atarax, Anx, Vistaril), loratadine (Claritin), and promethazine hydrochloride (Pentazine, Phenergan, Prothazine) used for supportive care with severe pruritis seen with elderly uremic patients; most drugs should be used with caution in the elderly because of sedation effect and other CNS adverse effects

Transfusions: blood and blood products used to treat anemia that results as a consequence of renal failure

Erythropoietin (EPO): used for anemia caused by renal failure or reduced endogenous EPO production; helps to correct hemostatic dysfunction with uremia; helps to reduce the amount of transfusions the patient must receive by stimulating red blood cell production

Vitamin and mineral supplementation: based on laboratory values, may be used to supplement a restrictive diet, to provide lacking nutrient substances, and to help prevent and treat secondary hyperparathyroidism that can occur in chronic renal insufficiency

Dietary management: restriction of protein, sodium and fat may improve the longevity of the renal failure patient; protein places an increased burden on the already-impaired kidneys; sodium may be restricted to help stem fluid expansion, and lowering cholesterol and triglyceride levels helps to decrease the deterioration seen in renal failure

Surgical interventions: may be required for placement of AV fistula/graft for dialysis or for placement of abdominal catheter in order to use peritoneal dialysis; transplantation is being used more frequently in people over the age of 60, but criteria is very selective because of the lack of sufficient organ donors

COMMON NURSING DIAGNOSES

IMBALANCED NUTRITION: LESS THAN BODY REQUIREMENTS (see LIVER FAILURE)

Related to: inability to ingest foods because of dietary protein, sodium, and potassium restrictions

Defining Characteristics: anorexia, weight loss, altered taste sensation, lack of interest in eating, inadequate food intake, nausea, vomiting, accumulation of nitrogen wastes

RISK FOR IMPAIRED SKIN INTEGRITY (see PERIPHERAL VASCULAR DISEASE)

Related to: external factors of immobility, excretion of urea, internal factor of altered nutritional status from malnutrition, changes in the skin from the aging process, pressure on skin surfaces, intermittent claudication, alteration in arterial and venous circulation, alterations in tissue perfusion, renal failure

Defining Characteristics: thin, dry skin on extremities, redness to pressure areas, edema, ulcerations or lesions to extremities, dermatitis, decreased or absent pulses, disruption of skin surface, excoriation of skin, pruritis, scratching, uremic frost on skin, emaciation, pale, sallow color

DISTURBED THOUGHT PROCESSES (see ANEMIA)

Related to: renal failure, electrolyte imbalances, uremic encephalopathy, anemia

Defining Characteristics: increased BUN and creatinine, mental status changes, decreasing level of consciousness, lethargy, memory deficit, asterixis, delirium, seizures, coma, anemia, decreased hemoglobin and hematocrit

SEXUAL DYSFUNCTION (see SEXUAL DISORDERS)

Related to: changes in body structure and function from renal failure

Defining Characteristics: verbalization of problems with sexual function, avoidance of engaging in sexual intercourse, need for confirmation of desirability, impotence, loss of libido

CONSTIPATION
(see HEART FAILURE)

Related to: renal failure, lack of adequate intake from fluid restrictions, less than adequate physical activity caused by weakness and changes related to aging

Defining Characteristics: passage of hard, formed stool, decreased bowel sounds, inability to evacuate stool, abdominal pain, abdominal distention, ileus, absent bowel sounds, nausea, vomiting, frequency of stool less than normal, less than usual amount of stool, palpable mass, feelings of rectal fullness, inability to ingest bulk-containing foods, flatulence, fluid restriction, dietary restrictions

INEFFECTIVE COPING
(see DEPRESSION)

Related to: depression, lack of coping skills, loss of independence, limitations on lifestyle, chronic renal failure, chronic illnesses

Defining Characteristics: verbalizations of inability to cope, inappropriate coping strategies, social withdrawal, irritability, inability to ask for help, fatigue, poor concentration, decreased problem-solving ability, worry, anxiety, poor self-esteem

ACTIVITY INTOLERANCE
(see CAD)

Related to: fatigue, weakness, renal failure, physiologic changes associated with the aging process, chronic illness, hypoxia, hypoxemia, increased metabolic demand, anemia

Defining Characteristics: verbalizations of fatigue or weakness, dyspnea, decreased oxygen saturation levels with movement or activity, increased heart rate and blood pressure with movement or activity, feelings of tiredness, weakness, decreased hemoglobin and hematocrit, decreased oxygen-carrying capability, increased oxygen consumption needs, uremia, inability to maintain usual routines of daily living

ADDITIONAL NURSING DIAGNOSES

 EXCESS FLUID VOLUME

Related to: compromised regulatory mechanisms from renal insufficiency, end stage renal disease

Defining Characteristics: interstitial edema, generalized edema, weight gain, oliguria, anuria, azotemia, hypertension, sodium retention, increased filling pressures, dyspnea, adventitious breath sounds, cardiac gallops, intake greater than urinary output, increased blood pressure, jugular vein distention, increased pulmonary congestion on x-ray, decreased hemoglobin and hematocrit, increased BUN and creatinine levels, decreased specific gravity less than 1.015

Outcome Criteria

✔ Patient will have equivalent intake and output, with no edema, and will be able to maintain his specific dry weight.

NOC: *Fluid Balance*

INTERVENTIONS	RATIONALES
Assess patient for renal function, urine amount, color, clarity, and intake and output.	Provides information as to patient's current status and amount of excessive fluid.
Determine patient's specific renal cause of fluid excess.	Allows for identification of source to provide for appropriate treatment method. If sodium is retained, blood volume expansion may be secondary to this electrolyte imbalance. Increased capillary permeability and the potential for decreases in plasma proteins may result in changes in oncotic pressures leading to fluid overload.
Measure I&O q 2–4 hours, and notify physician if imbalances are significant.	Provides for accurate comparison of patient's fluid status without the use of hemodynamics. Continued outputs that are less than intake will result in fluid overload, and potential cardiovascular complications, such as heart failure and dysrhythmias.
Weigh patient every day, at same time, on same scale, if at all possible.	Helps to provide data to correlate with I&O, and allows for consistency of information by utilization of same scale. An increase in weight of 1 pound correlates to approximately 500 cc of fluid. The patient's "dry weight," or the weight that should be maintained with the use of therapies, such as dialysis, gives all caregivers a goal at which to aim.

INTERVENTIONS	RATIONALES
Maintain patient's dietary restrictions, including fluid restrictions. Post signs and remove water pitcher from room.	Sodium intake will be restricted to help avoid retention of fluid, and protein will be limited to 0.3–0.7 grams of protein/kg of body weight to reduce the workload on the kidneys. Restriction of fats also helps to slow the deterioration of renal dysfunction.
Administer diuretics as ordered.	Osmotic diuretics cause water in excess of the sodium content to be excreted, but may cause fluid and electrolyte imbalances. Loop diuretics are potent drugs that act on the ascending loop of Henle to block the reabsorption of sodium and increase potassium excretion. These drugs can cause volume depletion, alkalosis, and hypokalemia. Thiazide diuretics inhibit sodium from being reabsorbed and increase the excretion of potassium, but may result in hypercalcemia. The potassium-sparing diuretics inhibit aldosterone in the renin-angiotensin-aldosterone cascade, and increase the secretion of sodium into the distal tubule and thus increase the reabsorption of potassium. Side effects can include hyperkalemia, hyponatremia, headache, urticaria, and nausea.
Administer antihypertensives as ordered.	If hypertension is one of patient's diagnoses, these drugs may decrease the potential for complications, such as stroke or MI.
Monitor vital signs q 2h, and prn. Notify physician for significant changes.	Diuresis may result in hypotension from dehydration and result in circulatory collapse.
Auscultate lung fields at least q 4h, and prn. Notify physician for changes in breath sounds, especially crackles (rales) or new adventitious breath sounds.	May indicate pulmonary edema with resultant cardiovascular compromise.
Observe patient and assess for degree of edema to extremities and periphery.	As fluid increases within the interstitial spaces, edema will occur from fluid shifting and changes in oncotic pressures. Pitting edema is usually only seen if there is more than a 5–10 pound fluid gain.

INTERVENTIONS	RATIONALES
Monitor lab work for BUN, creatinine, and electrolyte levels.	Aggressive diuresis may result in electrolyte imbalances. As renal function declines, BUN and creatinine will rise.
Assess patient for signs that hemodialysis is indicated.	Increased BUN and creatinine levels despite usual conservative treatment measures, such as reducing fluids, sodium, potassium, and protein, or when medication in chronic renal failure patients no longer is able to maintain renal status are indications for the use of hemodialysis.
Assess patient for contraindications for types of dialysis.	Hemodialysis may be contraindicated if patient is hemodynamically unstable with rapid changes in fluid volume status, if their cardiovascular condition is unstable, or if the patient is unable to tolerate heparinization. Peritoneal dialysis, which is usually the second option, may be contraindicated if the patient has peritonitis, bleeding disorders, recent abdominal surgery, or abdominal adhesions.
Prepare patient for and assist with hemodialysis procedure as warranted.	Some facilities have nurses who specialize in dialysis care. Dialysis removes the toxins from the systemic circulation by osmosis, diffusion, and convection or ultrafiltration.
Administer heparin as ordered prior to and during the procedure as ordered.	Anticoagulation is performed to keep the blood anticoagulated within the machine to prevent clotting of the semipermeable membrane that filters out the toxic wastes.
If AV fistula is utilized to administer hemodialysis, auscultate and palpate area for bruit and thrill at least q 4h.	Identifies patency of the shunt. Loss of bruit or thrill must be reported immediately and may require surgical intervention, including declotting or revision of the shunt, or possible replacement. Blood pressure readings, lab draws, and IV insertion should never be done on the same arm as the AV graft to minimize potential for clotting and impairment of circulation.

(continues)

(continued)

INTERVENTIONS	RATIONALES
Prepare for and assist with beginning peritoneal dialysis, as warranted.	Peritoneal dialysis may be the preferred method for patients who are too hemodynamically unstable to tolerate rapid removal of fluid and toxins. It utilizes diffusion and osmosis by instilling a dialysate solution (its contents based upon the patient's condition and lab values) into the peritoneal cavity, allowing it to remain for a determined length of time, and then allowing it to drain out. The solution is usually made up of a glucose solution, heparin, potassium chloride, insulin, lidocaine and/or antibiotics.
Weigh patient before and after procedure.	Helps to identify amount of fluid removed from patient; 500 cc fluid approximates 1 pound of weight loss.
Observe the fluid that is drained out from patient and notify physician for significant abnormalities.	Typically, a normal drainage should be clear and pale yellow in color. If solution is cloudy, it indicates an infective process or the potential for peritonitis. If the solution is brown, it may indicate a bowel perforation, and an amber color may indicate a bladder perforation. Some blood noted in the solution may be normal, but if the bleeding continues after the fourth exchange, it may indicate that the patient has a uremic coagulopathy, and the physician should be notified.
Monitor vital signs during procedure, especially during the draining phase.	Changes in vital signs or cardiac rhythm may indicate impending shock, hypoglycemic reaction, or fluid excess.
Observe peritoneal catheter site for signs or symptoms of infection, and perform wound care with dressing changes after each treatment and prn.	Catheter provides direct access to peritoneal cavity for bacterial invasion and aseptic wound care helps to decrease the potential for wound infection.
Monitor lab work for abnormalities.	Renal failure patients normally have abnormal electrolytes due to decreased glomerular filtration and impaired function, especially with potassium and sodium. Drug toxicity may occur

INTERVENTIONS	RATIONALES
	even if the patient is taking an appropriate dosage of medication because of the lack of renal clearance.
Instruct patient/family regarding the need for and particular type of dialysis to be performed.	Promotes knowledge of disease process, need for therapy, and facilitates compliance.
Instruct patient in care of AV fistula or peritoneal catheter.	Provides for reduction of infection and for prompt recognition of potential problems that may require emergent medical attention.
Instruct patient/family regarding dietary restrictions and fluid restrictions.	Patient may be manipulative and try to obtain more fluid that he is allowed. Discussion of the risks involved regarding potential complications such as fluid overload and heart failure may help to facilitate compliance.
Instruct patient/family to weigh each day, at same time, and on same scale, and to report changes in weight >2 lbs/day or 5 lbs/week.	Increases in weight this dramatically usually indicate fluid gain and allows for prompt recognition in order to change medical regimen to prevent complications.

NIC: *Hypervolemia Management*

NIC: *Hemodialysis Therapy*

NIC: *Peritoneal Dialysis Therapy*

Discharge or Maintenance Evaluation

- Patient will be free of edema.
- Patient will achieve and be able to maintain dry weight.
- Patient will exhibit no signs or symptoms of complications from access portals for dialysis procedures.
- Patient will suffer no complications from dialysis procedures.
- Patient will achieve diuresis of sufficient amount to return to dry weight.
- Patient will have stable vital signs, and have no adventitious breath sounds to auscultation.
- Patient will be compliant with dietary and fluid restrictions.
- Patient/family will be able to accurately verbalize understanding of need for specific type of dialysis procedures.

■ Patient/family will be able to accurately verbalize signs and symptoms of which to notify physician.

IMPAIRED GAS EXCHANGE

Related to: metabolic acidosis as a result of the kidney being unable to excrete hydrogen ions

Defining Characteristics: pH <7.35, HCO_3 level <22 mEq/L, decreased blood pressure, decreased level of consciousness, Kussmaul's respirations, headache, dysrhythmias, seizures, coma, osteomalacia

Outcome Criteria

✔ Patient will have stable, normalized ABGs, and dialysis will be able to control acidosis.

NOC: *Respiratory Status: Gas Exchange*

INTERVENTIONS	RATIONALES
Assess blood gases and identify type of acid–base problem, and treat as warranted.	Metabolic acidosis occurs when acids accumulate and a high anion gap occurs, such as in diabetic ketoacidosis, drug poisoning with salicylates, antifreeze, alcohol, or paraldehyde, with hypoperfusion states, like shock and sepsis, and with uremia and renal failure. Treatment involves management of the underlying problem, correction of the renal failure state, and/or the administration of sodium bicarbonate. Metabolic disturbances in acid–base management usually result in compensation by the lungs, but this requires time. If the patient is ventilated, hyperventilation will decrease the $PaCO_2$, and help to compensate for the acidosis.
Assist with/prepare patient for dialysis.	Dialysis is successful in treatment of metabolic acidosis by removal of toxic waste products and free acids that accumulate. The acetate or lactate found in dialysis baths is absorbed into the patient's body and converted to bicarbonate, or the physician can order specific bicarbonate bath solution so that the patient does not have to provide the conversion to bicarbonate from acetate or lactate.

INTERVENTIONS	RATIONALES
Administer sodium bicarbonate PO as ordered.	May be required for long-term control in the chronic renal failure patient to neutralize excess acid and restore the patient's buffering ability. Excessive bicarbonate may cause a rebound alkalosis.
Monitor vital signs, especially respiratory status q 2–4 hours, and prn. Notify physician of abnormalities. Pulse oximetry should be used, if available, and physician notified if oxygen saturation is <90%.	With metabolic acidosis, the lungs attempt to compensate for the increased acid, but eventually tire out, resulting in Kussmaul's respirations, which are slow, deep respirations. As fluid accumulates, the renal patient may have complaints of dyspnea as heart failure, pulmonary edema, and anemia also interact with the kidney dysfunction.
Instruct patient/family regarding the acid–base imbalance, why this happens, and methods for controlling this condition.	Facilitates patient knowledge, and may increase compliance with long-term use of bicarbonate as ordered.
Instruct patient to notify nurse or physician if patient suffers with symptoms, such as headache, dyspnea, or changes in mentation.	May indicate worsening metabolic acidosis. Prompt notification allows for timely interventions.

NIC: *Acid–Base Management: Metabolic Acidosis*

Discharge or Maintenance Evaluation

■ Patient will have normalized ABGs, including pH and bicarbonate level.

■ Patient will have stable vital signs, with no respiratory difficulty.

■ Patient will not suffer any complication from the administration of sodium bicarbonate.

■ Patient will not exhibit any signs or symptoms of complications from dialysis.

■ Dialysis will normalize acid–base disturbance in a timely manner.

■ Patient will have no signs or symptoms of metabolic acidosis.

RISK FOR INJURY

Related to: electrolyte imbalances, renal insufficiency and failure, abnormal hemoglobin and hematocrit, thrombocytopenia, leukopenia, infection, anemia

Defining Characteristics: decreased hemoglobin and hematocrit, altered coagulation, thrombocytopenia, leukopenia, sodium, potassium, chloride and phosphorus imbalances, decreased calcium level, fluid retention, edema, fever, infection, immunosuppression, inability of kidneys to excrete potassium and sodium, resorption of calcium by the bone, anemia

Outcome Criteria

✔ Patient will have electrolyte imbalances corrected and maintained, with the absence of respiratory dysfunction, urinary infection, or bleeding tendency.

NOC: *Symptom Control*

INTERVENTIONS	RATIONALES
Assess patient for weakness, flaccidity of muscles, abdominal cramping with diarrhea, and irregular pulse.	Indicates hyperkalemia as renal tubular function decreases. Electrolyte balance is more easily disturbed, and imbalances are more difficult to reverse in the elderly. Sodium, potassium, and chloride are major influences in maintaining electrolyte balance.
Assess patient for lethargy, weakness, restlessness, or increased tendon reflexes.	Indicates hypernatremia as nephrons lose ability to filter sodium.
Assess patient for muscle cramping, numbness in fingers and toes, and mentation changes.	Indicates hypocalcemia as the kidneys become unable to metabolize vitamin D that is needed for calcium absorption and resorption of calcium by bones.
Assess patient for muscle cramping or paresthesias.	Indicates hyperphosphatemia as kidneys are unable to excrete phosphate.
Assess patient for hematemesis, ecchymosis, and prolonged bleeding from mucous membranes or injection sites.	Altered platelet function and coagulation levels result in bleeding tendencies, especially of gastrointestinal tract and skin.
Monitor lab work for CBC, especially hemoglobin, hematocrit, and number of red blood cells, and other chemistry profiles for dysfunction.	Anemia is a result of decreased erythropoietin by the kidneys affecting the production of red blood cells by the bone marrow. Nutritional deficiencies and electrolyte disturbances can also contribute to anemia and dysfunction.

INTERVENTIONS	RATIONALES
Restrict sodium, potassium, and protein intake with diet to ordered amounts.	Reduction in renal function results in sodium and potassium retention that mandates a reduction in dietary consumption of these nutrients.
Avoid invasive procedures if possible.	Prevents introduction of microorganisms and trauma causing prolonged bleeding.
Perform handwashing and sterile technique for all procedures.	Prevents infections in immunosuppressed condition.
Provide oral care with soft brush, gentle brushing and mouthwash, and use electric razor prn.	Prevents trauma to skin and mucous membranes that may cause bleeding.
Cleanse perineal area after each elimination, wiping from front to back in females.	Prevents infection caused by bowel excreta contamination.
Instruct patient/family to avoid contact with people with infections.	Reduces the potential for infection.
Instruct patient to avoid blowing nose hard, straining at defecation, or performing Valsalva-type maneuvers.	Avoidance of increasing pressures decreases the potential for bleeding.
Instruct patient/family to avoid use of aspirin or aspirin-containing products.	Aspirin decreases platelet aggregation, which can result in bleeding.
Instruct patient regarding the need to use a soft toothbrush or toothette applicator to perform oral care.	Reduces potential for oral tissue injury and bleeding.
Instruct patient/family to ensure pathways are clear, to use assistive aids when necessary, avoid rushing, and have proper lighting.	Reduces the potential for falls and injury that could worsen because of tendency for bleeding.
Instruct patient/family regarding avoidance of foods that contain salt and potassium, especially in hidden sources, such as tomatoes, prepared meats, and monosodium glutamate.	Provides knowledge to facilitate compliance with dietary restrictions.
Instruct patient/family regarding the need to include dairy products in diet.	Calcium-rich foods should be encouraged to replace deficiencies and help prevent osteoporosis from calcium resorption into bones. If patient is also taking bicarbonate routinely, the addition of calcium products at the same time may promote hypercalcemia and should be avoided.

INTERVENTIONS	RATIONALES
Instruct patient/family to notify physician or nurse of changes in breathing, cough with sputum, especially yellow or green in color, or cloudy, foul-smelling urine.	Indicates respiratory or urinary tract infection.

NIC: Risk Identification

Discharge or Maintenance Evaluation

- Patient/family will be able to accurately verbalize understanding of the need to avoid potentially infectious persons.
- Patient/family will be able to accurately verbalize understanding of the need to avoid Valsalva's maneuvers and to avoid potential bleeding problems.
- Patient/family will be able to accurately verbalize and demonstrate understanding of maintenance of safe environment.
- Patient/family will be able to accurately verbalize and demonstrate compliance with dietary restrictions and inclusion of dietary sources of calcium.
- Patient will be free of any infective process.
- Patient/family will be able to accurately verbalize understanding of symptoms to report to physician or nurse indicating infection or bleeding problem.

DEFICIENT KNOWLEDGE

Related to: lack of exposure to information about renal dialysis, renal failure, or anemia

Defining Characteristics: verbalization of the problem, request for information, presence of preventable complications

Outcome Criteria

✔ Patient will exhibit an appropriate knowledge of dialysis procedures to clear body of metabolic wastes, understanding of renal failure, and the association of anemia complications.

NOC: Knowledge: Treatment Regimen

INTERVENTIONS	RATIONALES
Assess patient's knowledge of disease, reason for and procedure for dialysis prescribed (peritoneal or hemodialysis), and knowledge of anemia.	Provides information for teaching plan without repetition to promote understanding and compliance of medical regimen.
Provide explanations and information in clear and simple language that is understandable. Provide limited amounts of information over periods of time rather than large amounts at one sitting.	Reduces potential for noncompliance of medical regimen related to decreased cognitive ability to understand.
Include caregiver/family in all teaching.	Promotes understanding of disease for family so support can be provided.
Allow patient/family to have exposure to supplies and equipment used in dialysis.	Promotes understanding of procedures to allay anxiety and fear of unknown.
Instruct patient/family of importance of adhering to having laboratory tests, keeping appointments with physician, and dialysis schedule. Instruct patient/family that the government (Medicare) pays for treatments and procedures related to dialysis for patients who have renal failure.	Helps promote patient's and family's understanding of long-term requirements in order to prolong the patient's state of wellness. Hemodialysis may be performed three times/week, and is prescribed when the patient's condition is not able to be managed by any other conservative method.

NIC: Treatment: Disease Process

Discharge or Maintenance Evaluation

- Patient/family will be able to accurately verbalize understanding of need for dialysis, dialysis procedure, and potential benefits.
- Patient/family will be compliant with maintaining dialysis and lab work schedules.
- Patient/family will be able to access resources to ensure that the government will pay for dialysis services and treatments related to chronic renal failure.

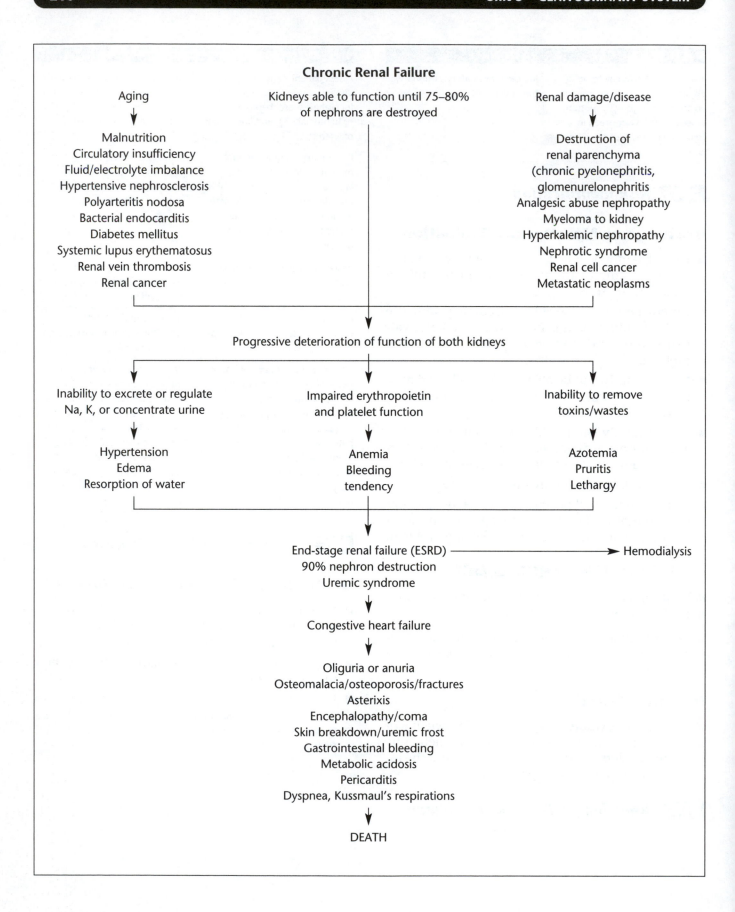

Chronic Renal Failure

Aging

Kidneys able to function until 75–80%
of nephrons are destroyed

Renal damage/disease

Malnutrition
Circulatory insufficiency
Fluid/electrolyte imbalance
Hypertensive nephrosclerosis
Polyarteritis nodosa
Bacterial endocarditis
Diabetes mellitus
Systemic lupus erythematosus
Renal vein thrombosis
Renal cancer

Destruction of
renal parenchyma
(chronic pyelonephritis,
glomenurelonephritis
Analgesic abuse nephropathy
Myeloma to kidney
Hyperkalemic nephropathy
Nephrotic syndrome
Renal cell cancer
Metastatic neoplasms

Progressive deterioration of function of both kidneys

Inability to excrete or regulate
Na, K, or concentrate urine

Impaired erythropoietin
and platelet function

Inability to remove
toxins/wastes

Hypertension
Edema
Resorption of water

Anemia
Bleeding
tendency

Azotemia
Pruritis
Lethargy

End-stage renal failure (ESRD) ⟶ Hemodialysis
90% nephron destruction
Uremic syndrome

Congestive heart failure

Oliguria or anuria
Osteomalacia/osteoporosis/fractures
Asterixis
Encephalopathy/coma
Skin breakdown/uremic frost
Gastrointestinal bleeding
Metabolic acidosis
Pericarditis
Dyspnea, Kussmaul's respirations

DEATH

UNIT 6

OPHTHALMOLOGIC SYSTEM

CHAPTER 6.1

CATARACTS

A cataract is a lens opacity that diminishes visual acuity. After age 40, the lens that is normally clear begins to have ill-defined densities. Oxidative damage to the proteins that are found in the lens reduces the solubility and ultimately results in insoluble opacities.

Cataracts are classified by their location within the lens. Nuclear cataracts are found in the center portion of the lens and cortical cataracts are noted more peripherally. Idiopathic posterior subcapsular cataracts occur at a younger age and most likely have a genetic foundation, or form as a complication from corticosteroid use. Cataracts are one of the primary causes of blindness today, but advances in surgical techniques can restore vision in most cases.

The classic symptoms of all cataracts are painless, with initial blurring of vision, and advancing to loss of sight. Photophobia and night blindness are frequently concurrently noted. Vision is also complicated by difficulty seeing in bright light and glare because the cataract distributes light in a refractory fashion, with a clear halo encircling lights.

A condition known as second sight occurs when lens opacification first begins. Visual acuity is unaffected, but the refractive index and power of the lens increases and can partially compensate for the loss in accommodation and temporarily corrects presbyopia. In the elderly person, early lens changes may allow them to read without the use of glasses.

The goal of treatment is to improve visual function, and surgical intervention is usually the option of choice. The lens is removed through an incision in the outer area of the cornea and an artificial plastic lens is implanted. It used to be considered the standard of care for the cataract "to mature" prior to surgery, but this is rarely done today. If the patient can perform their desired activities, surgery is delayed, but if the patient is not able to perform work, drive a car, watch television, or do other enjoyable activities, surgery is considered a valid option.

Complications are rare, but can include expulsive choroidal hemorrhage causing blindness, faulty wound closure with aqueous humor leakage, iris prolapse into the corneal wound, and intractable secondary glaucoma.

There is currently no known way to absolutely prevent the occurrence of cataracts as they occur as an age-related change. Prevention of excessive ultraviolet exposure may preclude additional eye damage, and diabetics who maintain close control of their blood glucose levels also have favorable results.

MEDICAL CARE

Ophthalmology examination: used to identify cataract formation by visualization of the opacity; identifies visual acuity in normal light and with glare, visual accommodation, and the presence of other complications from chronic illnesses

Surgery: cataract extraction with intraocular lens implantation is the treatment of choice

NURSING DIAGNOSES

DISTURBED SENSORY PERCEPTION: VISUAL

Related to: cataracts, poor visual acuity, changes in the eyes caused by the aging process

Defining Characteristics: visual distortions, loss of vision, diminished visual acuity, photophobia, night blindness, myopia, presbyopia, accommodation changes, changes in usual response to stimuli, presence of cataract

Outcome Criteria

✔ Patient will regain optimal vision possible and will adapt to permanent visual changes.

 Vision Compensation Behavior

INTERVENTIONS	RATIONALES
Assess patient's ability to see and perform activities.	Provides baseline for determination of changes affecting the patient's visual acuity.
Encourage patient to see ophthalmologist at least yearly.	Monitors for progressive visual loss or complications. Decreases in visual acuity can increase confusion in the elderly patient.
Provide sufficient lighting for patient to carry out activities.	Elderly patients over the age of 60 need twice as much light for close tasks as a person 20 years old.
Provide lighting that avoids glare on surfaces of walls, reading materials, and so forth.	Elderly patient's eyes are more sensitive to glare and cataracts diffuse the glare so that patient has more difficulty with vision.
Provide night light for patient's room and ensure lighting is adequate for patient's needs	Elderly patient's eyes require longer accommodation time to changes in lighting levels. Provision of adequate lighting helps to prevent injury.
Prepare patient for cataract surgery as warranted.	Provides knowledge, and facilitates compliance with regimen.
Instruct patient regarding normal age-related visual changes, cataracts, and methods of dealing with visual acuity changes.	Helps to increase the patient's understanding of visual changes and to make informed choices about options. As the patient ages, the lens becomes more dense and has less elasticity, so accommodation is decreased. Presbyopia is an age-related change that begins in people who are in their 40s and progresses. Visual acuity changes occur as the eye becomes more hyperopic as a result of neurologic changes in the visual pathways of the brain. The ability to distinguish fine details decreases because of loss of neurons in the visual pathways in the brain. Vitreous humor changes related to aging occur and consist of haziness, vertical flashing lights, lines, spots, or clusters of moving dots. The ability to differentiate colors also decreases with age because the cones that are responsible for color vision decline in sensitivity. In patients over the age of 60, the lens may

INTERVENTIONS	RATIONALES
	become yellowed from age, which results in blue objects appearing gray. Visual field decreases by approximately 1–3 inches per decade after 50.
Provide large print objects and visual aids for teaching.	Assists patient to see larger print, and promotes sense of independence.
If surgery is planned, instruct patient/family regarding procedure, postprocedure care, and need for follow-up with physician. Instruct about complications and emergency signs and symptoms (flashing lights with a loss of vision, a "veil" falling over visual field, loss of vision in a specific portion of the visual field, etc.) of which to notify physician.	Prepares patient for what to expect, facilitates compliance, and provides instruction about potential problems to lessen anxiety.

NIC: *Communication Enhancement: Visual Deficit*

Discharge or Maintenance Evaluation

- Patient will be able to verbalize understanding of visual loss and disease of eyes.
- Patient will be able to regain vision to the maximum possible extent with surgical procedure.
- Patient will be able to deal with potential for permanent visual loss.
- Patient will maintain a safe environment with no injury noted.
- Patient will be able to use adaptive devices to compensate for visual loss.
- Patient will be compliant with instructions given, and will be able to notify physician for emergency symptoms.

RISK FOR INJURY

Related to: cataracts, decreased vision, night blindness, aging changes in eye

Defining Characteristics: confusion, presence of cataracts, decreased visual acuity, photophobia, night blindness, changes in vision, floaters, night blindness, inability to tolerate glare

Outcome Criteria

✔ Patient will be free of injury and will be able to perform activities within parameters of sensory limitations.

NOC: *Safety Status: Physical Injury*

INTERVENTIONS	RATIONALES
Assess patient for degree of visual impairment.	Increases awareness of problem, and identifies severity to allow for establishment of a plan of care.
Ensure room environment is safe with adequate lighting and furniture moved toward the walls. Remove all rugs, and objects that could be hazardous.	Provides for a safe environment to reduce potential for injury.
Keep patient's glasses and call bell within easy reach.	Provides for assistance for patient and for optimal visual acuity.
Instruct patient/family regarding need for maintaining safe environment.	Reduced visual acuity puts patient at risk for injury.

INTERVENTIONS	RATIONALES
Instruct patient/family regarding safe lighting. Patient should wear sunglasses to reduce glare. Advise family to use contrasting bright colors in household furnishings.	These techniques enhance visual discrimination and reduce potential for injury.

NIC: *Security Enhancement*

Discharge or Maintenance Evaluation

■ Patient will be able to be free of injury.

■ Patient/family will be able to modify environment to ensure safety.

■ Patient will be able to perform self-care activities within limitations of visual disturbance.

■ Patient/family will be able to accurately verbalize and understand need to minimize potential for injury.

Cataracts

Aging

Lens thickens and becomes opacified
because of oxidative damage to lens proteins

Decreased accommodation for near vision
Lens with increased opacity

Refraction decreased
Decreased peripheral vision
Decreased night vision
Blurred vision

Progressive visual loss

Withdrawal, social isolation
Disorientation

CHAPTER 6.2

GLAUCOMA

Glaucoma is a term that encompasses a collection of eye disorders which involve an increase in the fluid pressure within the eye. This increase in intraocular pressure can result in irreversible damage to the optic nerve and visual loss, and glaucoma accounts for approximately 10% of all cases of blindness in the United States. Increased intraocular pressure, IOP, can occur as a result of increased production of aqueous fluid or impairment of outflow of this fluid. If the blood pressure within the optic nerve surpasses the IOP, the nerve will be able to receive sufficient nutrition.

Narrow-angle glaucoma is the only type of the disease that can be cured. The anterior chamber of the eye is extremely shallow and becomes even shallower with age as the lens continues to thicken and move the iris forward. When the pupil margin of the iris presses against the lens, it prevents the aqueous humor from entering the anterior chamber and the fluid pushes the middle of the iris forward which prevents access to the trabecular area of the outflow channels. IOP increases to levels of 50–60 mm Hg in a matter of hours (normal ranges are 11–21 mm Hg). Signs of this type of glaucoma include redness in the eye, pain in or around the eye, severe headache, nausea, vomiting, blurred vision, and/or visualization of halos around lights. Treatment of this narrow-angle glaucoma is an emergency, and must be dealt within 72 hours or vision may be irreversibly lost. Eye drops and administration of acetazolamide is required as an emergency treatment until surgical intervention can be performed.

Open-angle glaucoma is found in approximately 80% of patients who have this disease, but this type is asymptomatic until the later stages. In this form of the disease, the drainage angle is not blocked, and the exact site of the strain against outflow is unidentified, but thought to be in the cells lining the canal of Schlemm in the sclera. Loss of peripheral vision develops slowly and may be unnoticed by the patient until the disease is advanced. IOP is usually more than 21 mm Hg, but can be normal and still high enough in a specific patient to create a resistance to the aqueous humor outflow. Optic atrophy, with pallor and cupping of the nerve head, are seen and indicate advanced disease. If the patient has no visual field defect in the presence of increased IOP, the diagnosis is called ocular hypertension and requires no treatment. Open-angle glaucoma cannot be cured but can be controlled with drug therapy to reduce IOP. If pharmacologic therapy is not sufficient for a patient, surgery involving laser trabeculoplasty or other procedures may be required.

MEDICAL CARE

Mydriatics: atropine sulfate (Atropisol, Isopto Atropine), cyclopentolate hydrochloride (Cyclogyl, Pentolair, AK-Pentolate), epinephrine hydrochloride or borate (Epifrin, Glaucon, Epinal), homatropine hydrobromide (Isopto Homatropine, Minims), phenylephrine hydrochloride (AK-Dilate, AK-Nefrin, Mydfrin, Phenoptic, Prefrin) and scopolamine hydrobromide (Isopto Hyoscine) are eye drops used to produce dilation of the pupils by blocking the responses of the iris and ciliary muscles to cholinergic stimulation and decreased intraocular pressures

Miotics: acetylcholine chloride (Miochol-E), carbachol (Miostate, Carboptic, Isopto Carbachol), echothiophate iodide (Phospholine Iodide), and pilocarpine hydrochloride or nitrate (Ocusert, Adsorbocarpine, Akarpine, Isopto Carpine, Pilocar, Pilagan) are eye drops used to reduce IOP by facilitating outflow and reducing the production of aqueous humor

Osmotic diuretics: acetazolamide (Diamox, Dazamide) and mannitol (Osmitrol) used for emergency treatment in narrow-angle closure to break the attack by decreasing fluid and IOP

Other IOP decreasing drugs: apraclonidine hydrochloride (Iopidine), betaxolol hydrochloride (Betoptic), brimonidine tartrate (Alphagan), carteolol hydrochloride (Ocupress), dorzolamide hydrochloride (Trusopt), emedastine difumarate (Emadine), ketotifen fumarate (Zaditor), latanoprost (Xalatan), levobunolol hydrochloride (Betagan, AKBeta), metipranolol hydrochloride (OptiPranolol), and timolol maleate (Betimol, Timoptic) are adrenergic blockers that reduce aqueous production and decrease IOP

Tonometry: used to identify intraocular pressure

Perimetry: used to identify peripheral vision and visual field acuity

Surgery: iridectomy used to establish a channel to help equalize the pressure of the aqueous humor on both sides in narrow-angle glaucoma; laser trabeculoplasty or filtration procedures may be required for open-angle glaucoma

COMMON NURSING DIAGNOSES

DISTURBED SENSORY PERCEPTION: VISUAL (see CATARACTS)

Related to: presence of glaucoma, increased intraocular pressure, eye pain, obstruction of outflow of aqueous humor

Defining Characteristics: increased intraocular pressure greater than 21 mm Hg, optic nerve damage, decreased visual acuity, visualization of halos around lights, redness of eyes, pain in or around the eye, headaches, nausea, vomiting, blurred vision, tenderness to eye, eye feels firmer than the other eye, loss of visual field, loss of peripheral vision, ocular hypertension, presence of ocular tumors, secondary glaucoma

RISK FOR INJURY (see CATARACTS)

Related to: glaucoma, decreased vision, physiologic changes to eyes related to aging, decreased peripheral vision

Defining Characteristics: presence of glaucoma, decreased visual acuity, decreased visual fields, decreased peripheral vision, confusion

ADDITIONAL NURSING DIAGNOSES

 ### DEFICIENT KNOWLEDGE

Related to: lack of information about glaucoma, lack of understanding about age-related visual changes

Defining Characteristics: verbalized lack of knowledge, questions concerning care, lack of attention to eye problems, development of preventable complications, blindness, difficulty seeing and learning information

Outcome Criteria

✔ Patient will be able to understand disease process and methods of treatment to be utilized, so as to exhibit no preventable complications.

NOC: *Knowledge: Disease Process*

INTERVENTIONS	RATIONALES
Assess patient's visual abilities and their understanding of glaucoma.	Helps to establish a baseline from which to guide establishing a plan of care for instruction. Patient's visual abilities may require specific individualized teaching aids, such as large letters, contrasting colors, or verbal, taped instructions.
Ascertain what type of glaucoma patient has been diagnosed with, and discuss causes and concerns patient may have.	Narrow-angle glaucoma is responsible for approximately 10% of all cases but is the only type that can be cured. Open-angle glaucoma occurs in approximately 80% of all patients and causes a gradual loss of sight unless treated. Although this type of glaucoma cannot be cured, it can be controlled with medications.
Determine if patient has other disease processes that may contribute to glaucoma problem, and discuss with patient.	Hypertension and diabetes can cause retinal changes because of problems with vascularity resulting from the disease. These patients should have annual dilated eye examinations to assess for underlying symptomatology and pathology. If patient suffers from uveitis, inflammatory cells and debris are prone to obstruct the outflow channels and lead to secondary glaucoma.

INTERVENTIONS	RATIONALES
Administer medications as ordered, and inform patient/family of appropriate method of instilling eye drops.	Midriatics, myopics, or adrenergic blockers may be ordered. The correct number of drops ordered should be instilled into an opened eye, with the head held back, and with the eye looking upward. Once the medication has been instilled, the eye may be closed, and the patient should rotate the eye in a circular motion to disseminate the mediation. Any excess may be dabbed with a tissue from the corner of the eye.
Instruct patient/family in importance of keeping appointments with ophthalmologist.	Regular and routine examinations must be performed at specified intervals to identify any further developments or problems, and to identify efficacy of prescribed treatment.
Instruct patient/family in visual aids that may be used.	If patient has declining visual acuity, he may require reading glasses, bifocals, magnifying glass, large print books, and so forth.
Instruct patient/family in signs and symptoms of glaucoma.	Open-angle glaucoma is asymptomatic until the later stages. A gradual loss of the visual field and peripheral vision frequently is not noticed by patients until the disease is advanced. IOP can be within normal ranges, although it usually is above 21 mm Hg. Unless the patient is treated with drugs to reduce the IOP, irreversible optic nerve damage may occur and peripheral vision may be lost forever. Narrow-angle glaucoma usually shows symptoms in one eye only, although the other eye also has a shallow anterior chamber. There is a rapid increase in the IOP, redness and pain to the eye, and severe headache are signs of

INTERVENTIONS	RATIONALES
	this emergency problem. Treatment must be given within 72 hours or vision may be lost. This is the only type of glaucoma that can be cured. Secondary glaucoma occurs with the presence of a concurrent disease process, such as diabetes mellitus, hypertension, or uveitis. Symptoms include reddened eyes, an uncomfortable feeling in the eyes, and decreased visual acuity, but patients can be asymptomatic. Treatment of this type of glaucoma involves treatment of the cause of the obstruction of the outflow channels, drugs to reduce the IOP, and/or surgery to create a new outflow path.
Instruct patient on medications, use, side effects, and symptoms to report to physician.	Mydriatics are used to dilate the pupil and block the responses of the iris and ciliary muscle to cholinergic stimulation to decrease IOP. Miotics are used to decrease IOP by increasing the outflow and reducing the production of aqueous humor.

NIC: *Teaching: Disease Process*

Discharge or Maintenance Evaluation

- Patient will be able to identify which type of glaucoma has been diagnosed and appropriate treatment for the disease.
- Patient/family will be able to administer medications correctly.
- Patient will not exhibit increased IOP because of lack of medical attention or lack of compliance with prescribed regimen.
- Patient will suffer no further loss of vision.
- Patient will be able to use visual aids to assist with activities if needed.

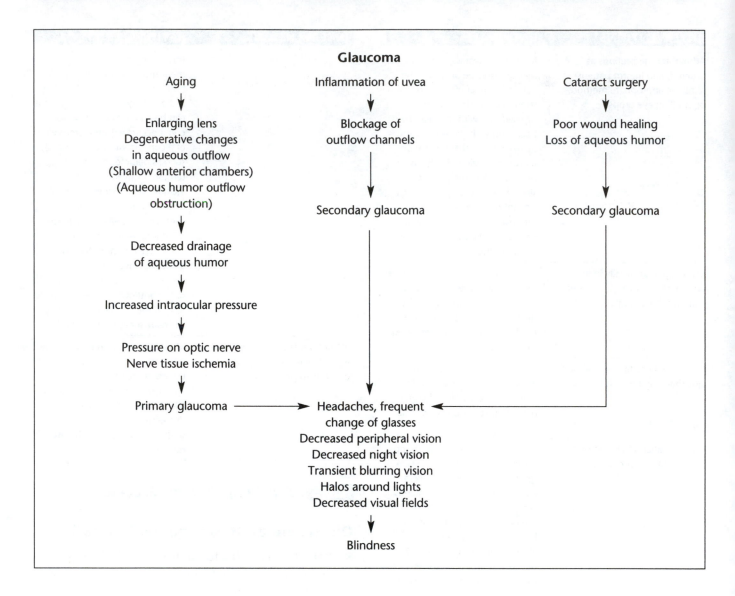

Glaucoma

Aging	Inflammation of uvea	Cataract surgery
↓	↓	↓
Enlarging lens Degenerative changes in aqueous outflow (Shallow anterior chambers) (Aqueous humor outflow obstruction)	Blockage of outflow channels	Poor wound healing Loss of aqueous humor
↓	↓	↓
Decreased drainage of aqueous humor	Secondary glaucoma	Secondary glaucoma

Aging path continues:

Decreased drainage of aqueous humor
↓
Increased intraocular pressure
↓
Pressure on optic nerve
Nerve tissue ischemia
↓
Primary glaucoma ⟶ Headaches, frequent
change of glasses
Decreased peripheral vision
Decreased night vision
Transient blurring vision
Halos around lights
Decreased visual fields
↓
Blindness

CHAPTER 6.3

MACULAR DEGENERATION

Macular degeneration is a progressive eye disease in which the central portion of the retina gradually deteriorates. The retinal pigment epithelium lies directly beneath the retina and these cells nourish the retina and photoreceptor cells that contain the visual pigments. Aging causes this membrane complex to become sclerotic, allowing fluid or blood leakage beneath the retinal pigment epithelium as well as between this epithelium and the retina. Scarring intrudes on the ability of the cells to nourish the retina and leads to their demise and a loss of central vision. This is called the wet type of macular degeneration.

The dry type of age-related macular degeneration occurs when the retinal pigment epithelium and the overlying photoreceptor cells disintegrate and reduce central visual acuity. If there is no other type of eye damage, the peripheral vision remains intact.

Initial symptoms of the disease include distortion of lines or irregular patches of dim vision moving across the visual field, and progressing to blurring of vision in the center portion of the visual field. Sometimes a blind spot may develop, straight lines may appear curvy, colors fade, and objects may look larger or smaller than normal.

Treatment of this disease involves supportive lifestyle changes to adapt to the decrease in vision, unless the degeneration is new and caused by abnormal blood vasculature, then laser surgery can sometimes slow or halt the deterioration by sealing off the leaking vessels. Reversal of damage that has already occurred is not possible.

MEDICAL CARE

Fluorescein angiography: used to identify changes and dysfunction within ocular vasculature and with optic nerves

Amsler grid: a grid of fine bisecting lines used by patients to observe visual distortion

Surgery: laser surgery may be helpful for the wet type of macular degeneration if done early; if the procedure is done later, only approximately 20% of patients will have any improvement in visual function

NURSING DIAGNOSES

DISTURBED SENSORY PERCEPTION: VISUAL (see CATARACTS)

Related to: macular degeneration, presence of drusen, loss of central vision, age-related ocular changes

Defining Characteristics: distortion of central vision, straight lines appear distorted, objects appear smaller or larger than normal, distortion of vision noted on grid, drusen, legal blindness, subretinal edema, retinal bleeding

RISK FOR INJURY (see CATARACTS)

Related to: macular degeneration, decreased vision, aging, decreased central vision

Defining Characteristics: presence of drusen, decreased visual acuity, decreased visual fields, decreased central vision, retinal changes, retinal hemorrhage, visual distortion, confusion

Macular Degeneration

Aging/senile degeneration

Decreased nourishment of macular area by choroid
New vessel development
Vessels leak blood/fluid
Fibrous scarring causes photoreceptor death

Detachment of macular area

Loss of function of light sensitive cones

Distortion of lines/central vision

Loss of central vision
Unimpaired peripheral vision

Difficulty seeing at long distances
Difficulty in doing close work, reading
Difficulty in distinguishing colors
Difficulty in seeing faces clearly

Blindness

UNIT 7
HEMATOLOGIC SYSTEM

7.1 Anemia

CHAPTER 7.1

ANEMIA

Anemia is a condition in which the red blood cell count, hemoglobin, and hematocrit are decreased. This decrease results in a decrease in the oxygen-carrying capability and causes tissue hypoxia. As the body tries to compensate, blood is shifted from areas that have a plentiful amount in tissues that have low oxygen requirements to those areas that require higher oxygen concentrations, such as the heart and the brain.

There are several types of anemia: those that are caused by decreased red blood cell production, those that are caused by blood loss, and the hemolytic anemia caused from G6PD deficiency, autoimmunity, or physical causes.

Microcytic, or iron deficiency anemia, is the most common type seen in the elderly patient, and develops when the transportation of iron by transferrin is insufficient to meet requirements of the erythropoietic cells. It is frequently caused by an inadequate intake of iron in the diet, gastrectomy, or other reason for malabsorption in the elderly, or from normal or abnormal bleeding.

Macrocytic, or megaloblastic, anemia occurs because of a deficiency in vitamin B_{12} or folic acid. Pernicious anemia is a type of megaloblastic anemia, in which the absence of vitamin B_{12}, as well as a lack of the intrinsic factor is noted. It is also seen commonly in the elderly because of an absence of the secretion of the protein by the gastric mucosa that is needed to absorb vitamin B_{12}. This type of anemia is also known as pernicious anemia. It may occur if patients have an inadequate diet without foods rich in vitamin B_{12}, if the patient has had stomach surgery, has a congenital abnormality, or other acquired defect that interferes with production of the intrinsic factor.

Normocytic, or aplastic anemia, is caused from the failure of the bone marrow to produce red blood cells, or destruction of bone marrow by either chemical or physical means. This can occur as a result of chemotherapy, or from disease states, such as myeloma, myelofibrosis, or hemolysis.

Autoimmune anemia is an acquired condition that involves premature erythrocyte destruction from the person's own immune system.

Hemolytic anemia results when erythrocyte destruction is increased and cells have a shortened life span. This type of anemia increases in incidence with age, and elderly patients are prone to drug-induced hemolysis because they take multiple medications. All hemolytic anemias require treatment with folic acid, because this vitamin is utilized with increased bone marrow production of erythrocytes.

Sickle cell anemia is an inherited condition in which hemoglobin S is present in the blood, resulting in sickle-shaped cells, and abnormal hemolyzation that obstructs capillary flow. The abnormality can lead to excruciating pain and chronic organ damage, and is most common in people of African descent.

Thalassemia is a group of inherited anemias that result from faulty production of alpha or beta-hemoglobin polypeptides. This causes a decreased rate of production of hemoglobin by the bone marrow and abnormal-appearing blood cells, and results in facial deformities, growth retardation, fragility of bones, and usually, early death, commonly from heart failure.

Anemia can occur as the direct result of prosthetic heart valves or extracorporeal circulation and the destruction of red blood cells by these entities. Anemia can also be precipitated by toxic substance exposure or chronic disease processes, such as uremia or chronic liver disease. In the elderly patient, chronic renal failure, hypothyroidism, malignancies, hypertension, and eating disorders can predispose them to the development of anemia.

Because anemia is a sign of other disease states, it is vital to identify the type of anemia in order to diagnose the inherent problem. Symptoms of anemia include severe fatigue and weakness, shortness of breath, chest pain, peripheral edema, mental changes, depression, pallor, and dizziness.

Treatment is based upon the type of anemia noted. Iron-deficiency anemia is treated with oral or

IV iron supplementation, and pernicious anemia is treated with life-long vitamin B_{12} supplementation. Sickle-cell anemia or thalassemia may require packed red blood cell transfusions at regular intervals, and surgery may be required if the anemia is caused by a loss of blood from the GI tract.

MEDICAL CARE

Laboratory: CBC is used to differentiate the type of anemia—RBCs are reduced; hemoglobin is decreased with mild decrease considered 10–14 g/dl, moderate 6–10 g/dl, and severe below 6 g/dl; hematocrit is decreased; MCH and MCHC variable dependent on type of anemia; MCV 80–100 fL w/ normocytic, greater than 100 fL with macrocytic, and less than 80 fL with microcytic; platelet count usually decreased, but may be elevated after hemorrhage; RDW increased in iron-depletion anemia, B_{12} level and folate decreased; serum iron and TIBC may be decreased; stool guaiac may be positive if blood loss is from the GI tract; transferrin levels used to identify the ratio of serum iron to total iron-binding capacity, and used to indicate iron deficiency; ferritin levels used to reflect bone marrow iron stores but can be inaccurate if infection, inflammation, or liver disease is present; hemoglobin electrophoresis used to identify changes in minor hemoglobins; liver profiles used to identify dysfunction that can contribute to anemia; thyroid profiles used to identify hypothyroidism which can cause a normocytic anemia; albumin levels used to identify malnutrition as a source for anemia; cold and warm agglutinins and complement levels used to identify idiopathic autoimmune hemolysis that may cause hemolytic anemia; direct and indirect Coombs' test used to identify drug-binding to the RBCs in drug-induced hemolysis; serum vitamin levels used to identify deficiencies; *Helicobacter pylori* testing to identify infection that may cause macrocytic anemia; homocysteine levels used to identify folate deficiency anemia; drug levels used to identify therapeutic versus toxic levels; Schilling test used to identify amounts of B_{12} excreted in the urine; blood typing and cross-matching used to prepare transfusion of blood and blood products

Radiography: chest X-rays used to detect pulmonary or cardiac complications; upper and lower gastrointestinal series may be done to identify active or current bleeding

Bone marrow aspiration/biopsy: used to determine type of anemia or neoplastic disease

Bone marrow transplantation: may be required for severe aplastic anemia

Blood transfusions: may be required to replace blood volume if patient has hemorrhage or in sickle-cell anemia

Vitamin/mineral supplementation: may be required to replace iron in iron-deficiency anemia, and B_{12} in pernicious anemia

Surgery: may be required to control bleeding if this is the cause of the decreased hemoglobin and hematocrit

Genetic counseling: used for patients who may want children if one or both partners have sickle-cell anemia or thalassemia, or if hereditary factors are involved with anemia

COMMON NURSING DIAGNOSES

INEFFECTIVE TISSUE PERFUSION: CARDIOPULMONARY, CEREBRAL, GASTROINTESTINAL, PERIPHERAL, RENAL (see CAD)

Related to: anemia, lack of blood supply, reduced oxygen supply, hypoperfusion, hypovolemia, dysrhythmias, valvular heart disease, coexisting disease processes, age-related vascular structure changes, inactivity

Defining Characteristics: pallor, confusion, chest pain, conduction disturbances, dysrhythmias, vital sign changes, ECG changes, delayed capillary refill time, chest retractions, dyspnea, nasal flaring, use of accessory muscles, increased work of breathing, tachypnea, bradypnea, changes in mental status, weakness, paralysis, behavioral changes, abdominal distention, ileus, hypoactive or absent bowel sounds, nausea, vomiting, edema, weak or absent peripheral pulses, skin temperature changes, skin color changes, decreased peripheral tactile sensation, hematuria, oliguria, anuria, increased BUN and creatinine, decreased hemoglobin and hematocrit, alterations in absorption of vitamins and minerals, presence of hemoglobin S, abnormal arterial blood gases, abnormal oxygen saturation

RISK FOR DEFICIENT FLUID VOLUME (see HTN)

Related to: bleeding, anemia, lack of adequate blood volume

Defining Characteristics: hypotension, tachycardia, decreased skin turgor, weakness, decreased urinary output, pallor, diaphoresis, decreased capillary refill, mental changes, restlessness, decreased filling pressures, hemorrhage, confusion, dysrhythmias

IMBALANCED NUTRITION: LESS THAN BODY REQUIREMENTS (see COPD)

Related to: anemia, inability to absorb nutrients that are required for red blood cell production, inability to absorb and utilize vitamin B$_{12}$, nausea, vomiting, gastrointestinal bleeding, increased metabolism due to disease process, decreased level of consciousness, inability to absorb nutrients because of biologic or psychological factors

Defining Characteristics: actual inadequate food intake, weight loss, body weight 20% or more under ideal for height and frame, anorexia, absent bowel sounds, decreased peristalsis, muscle mass loss, decreased muscle tone, changes in bowel habits, nausea, vomiting, abdominal distention, lack of interest in food, abdominal pain or discomfort, sore, inflamed buckle cavity, depression, anxiety, social isolation, changes in mental status, fatigue from work of breathing, weakness, activity intolerance, gastrointestinal bleeding

ACTIVITY INTOLERANCE (see CAD)

Related to: reduced oxygen-carrying capability of blood, anemia, fatigue, hypoxia, hypoxemia, aging

Defining Characteristics: lethargy, fatigue, dyspnea, decreased oxygen saturation levels with movement or activity, increased heart rate and blood pressure with movement or activity, feelings of tiredness, weakness, chest pain, palpitations, tachycardia, tachypnea, hypertension

ADDITIONAL NURSING DIAGNOSES

INEFFECTIVE PROTECTION

Related to: abnormal blood profile, anemia

Defining Characteristics: tissue hypoxia, weakness, malnutrition, inability to produce intrinsic factor

Outcome Criteria

✔ Patient will have a reduced potential for hypoxia, infection, or immunocompromise.

NOC: *Infection Status*

INTERVENTIONS	RATIONALES
Assess presence of patient's activity intolerance, fatigue, and weakness.	May be the result of anemia.
Administer whole blood or packed red cells as ordered.	Replaces needed RBCs to carry oxygen to the cells.
Administer iron preparation or vitamin B$_{12}$ IM or IV.	Iron replacement treats iron-deficiency and B$_{12}$ is used for pernicious anemia.
Offer diet with high iron/folic acid content and high protein inclusions, as warranted.	Provides iron that is necessary for hemoglobin synthesis.
Instruct patient to comply with B$_{12}$ injections and that these must be continued monthly throughout life.	Treatment for pernicious anemia must be life-long.
Instruct patient to eat meals that include green, leafy vegetables, eggs, dried fruits, meat, legumes, and whole grains.	Foods rich in iron are required to supply body need to prevent recurrence of anemia. (1 mg iron is absorbed from 10–20 mg of iron ingested with 5–10% actually absorbed.)

NIC: *Blood Products Administration*

Discharge or Maintenance Evaluation

■ Patient will achieve and maintain adequate iron intake by dietary sources or by supplementation.

■ Patient will exhibit no complications from blood product transfusions.

■ Patient will be compliant with dietary measures to increase vitamin and mineral supplies.

■ Patient will be compliant with obtaining vitamin B$_{12}$ injections to prevent complications and adverse effects.

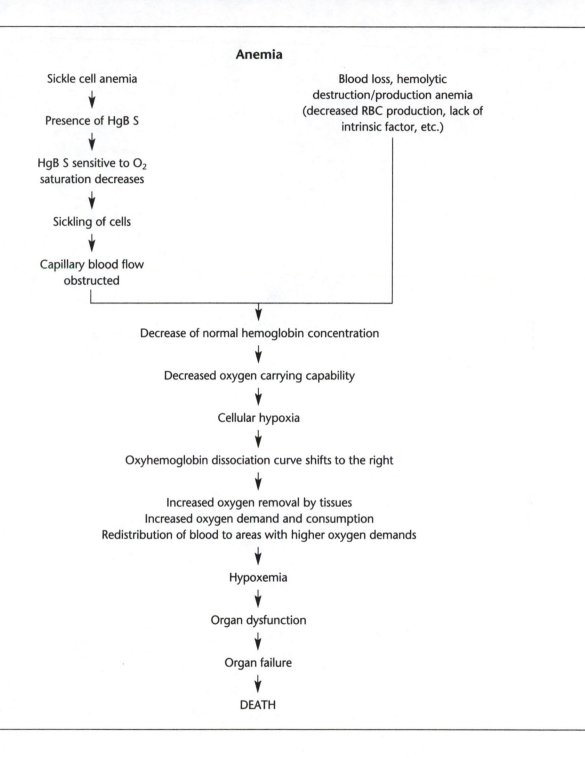

Anemia

Sickle cell anemia

↓

Presence of HgB S

↓

HgB S sensitive to O$_2$
saturation decreases

↓

Sickling of cells

↓

Capillary blood flow
obstructed

Blood loss, hemolytic
destruction/production anemia
(decreased RBC production, lack of
intrinsic factor, etc.)

↓

Decrease of normal hemoglobin concentration

↓

Decreased oxygen carrying capability

↓

Cellular hypoxia

↓

Oxyhemoglobin dissociation curve shifts to the right

↓

Increased oxygen removal by tissues
Increased oxygen demand and consumption
Redistribution of blood to areas with higher oxygen demands

↓

Hypoxemia

↓

Organ dysfunction

↓

Organ failure

↓

DEATH

UNIT 8
ENDOCRINE SYSTEM

CHAPTER 8.1

DIABETES MELLITUS

Diabetes mellitus, DM, is a condition that is distinguished by hyperglycemia that results from an impairment of insulin action and/or secretion. Insulin removes glucose from the blood and converts it for storage in the body cells, and assists in the metabolism of carbohydrates, proteins, and fats.

In type I diabetes, which is known as juvenile diabetes and insulin dependent diabetes mellitus (IDDM), the pancreas does not produce sufficient insulin, and patients who have this type must receive injections of insulin regularly for life. Control of the patient's blood glucose level is done by adherence to a diet, maintenance of regular exercise, and adjustment of insulin dosages based on frequent measurement of serum glucose throughout the day.

People who develop diabetes as adults have type II, or non-insulin-dependent diabetes mellitus (NIDDM), in which the body's requirements for insulin are greater than normal in order to achieve normal blood glucose levels. Cells within the body may not react appropriately to the insulin that is received. Control of the glucose levels in this type of diabetes is done by controlling weight and using dietary management. If diet and weight control are not effective, oral hypoglycemics and the oral antidiabetic drug, metformin, may help to manage glucose concentrations.

Hyperglycemia, characterized by fasting glucose levels above 125 mg/dl or postprandial levels greater than 200 mg/dl, may be a consequence of diabetes, and also a cause of further impairment in glucose tolerance because hyperglycemia reduces insulin sensitivity and glucose uptake, and increases glucose production.

Diabetes can be caused by other endocrine disorders that are associated with either peripheral or hepatic insulin resistance, such as Cushing's syndrome, pheochromocytoma, and primary hyperaldosteronism.

Diabetes typically presents with polyuria, polydipsia, glucosuria, weight loss, blurred vision, fatigue, nausea, recurrent infections, or dehydration. Type I patients can also present with diabetic ketoacidosis, and type II patients can exhibit symptomatic nonketotic hyperglycemic hyperosmolar coma, or hyperosmolar hyperglycemic state, as it is now known.

Hyperglycemia increases the risks of atherosclerosis, stroke, coronary artery disease, claudication, skin breakdown, retinopathy, neuropathies, and infections, and can affect all body systems.

MEDICAL CARE

Laboratory: glucose levels used to identify diagnosis and dysfunction; oral glucose tolerance testing used to help diagnose the type II diabetic; glycosylated hemoglobin (Hb A_{1c}) used to estimate the average blood glucose level over a period of 1–3 months; fructosamine level used as an indirect test of glucose control over the past 1–3 weeks; lipid profiles used to identify risk for atherosclerosis; renal profiles used to identify dysfunction; urinalysis used to identify infection and the presence of glucose and ketones; electrolytes used to identify imbalances, serum insulin levels used to identify improper utilization of insulin or presence of insulin resistance; CBC used to identify infection, anemia, or dehydration that may occur with DKA; osmolality used to identify changes in serum or urine

Electrocardiogram: used to identify heart rhythm, changes in conduction, potential dysrhythmias, and ischemic changes

Ophthalmology exam: essential because of the potential for diabetic retinopathy

Diet: specific nutrition that is aimed at decreasing variances in timing, portion sizes, and composition of nutrients to enhance the insulin and other medications that are being used; total daily caloric intake and proportions of carbohydrates, protein, and fats must be incorporated in an individualized plan

Antihyperglycemic drugs: oral hypoglycemics (glimepiride [Amaryl], and pioglitazone hydrochloride [Actos]) used only for type II DM with single or combination therapy; biguanides (metformin [Glucophage]) used to decrease glucose production by the liver and may increase insulin sensitivity; alpha-glucosidase inhibitors (acarbose [Precose] and miglitol [Glyset]) may be used for patients with mild hyperglycemia, and works by inhibiting the hydrolysis of oligosaccharides and monosaccharides that delay carbohydrate digestion and absorption; thiazolidinediones (rosiglitazone maleate [Avandia] and troglitazone [Rezulin]) used to increase insulin sensitivity in skeletal muscle and suppress glucose output from the liver; sulfonylureas (acetohexamide [Acetohexamide], chlorpropamide [Chlorpropamide, Diabenese], glipizide [Glucotrol], glyburide [DiaBeta, Glynase PresTab, Micronase], tolbutamide [Orinase, Tolbutamide]) used to decrease glucose levels by stimulating insulin secretion, improve peripheral and liver insulin sensitivity, and potentiate the action of antidiuretic hormone; meglitinides (repaglinide [Prandin]) used to stimulate insulin release by closing potassium channels and thus opening the calcium channels to increase insulin secretion to lower blood-glucose levels

Insulin: human insulin preferred because is it less antigenic than animal-derived types, but insulin antibody levels develop in patients who use this type of insulin; insulins classified as short-acting, intermediate-acting, or long-acting, and mixtures of different insulin types are often given as a single injection; treatment usually begun with a bedtime dose of NPH insulin, and later the total dose may be divided so that half the dose is administered prior to breakfast, one-fourth prior to dinner, and one-fourth at bedtime; insulin—regular, crystalline zinc: Humulin-R, Novolin R, Regular Iletin I, Regular Iletin II, Regular Purified Pork Insulin; insulin—lispro: Humalog; isophane insulin suspension—neutral protamine Hagedorn, NPH: Humulin N, Iletin II, Novolin N, NPH insulin, NPH Purified Pork; isophane insuline suspension with insulin injection: Humulin 50/50, Humulin 70/30, Novolin 70/30; insuline zinc suspension—lente: Humulin L, Lente Iletin II, Lente Insulin, Lente Purified Pork Insulin, Novolin L; insulin zinc suspension, extended—ultralente: Humulin-U, Ultralente Insulin; insulin

aspart—rDNA origin: NovoLog; insulin glargine—rDNA origin: Lantus

Glucagon: Glucagon used to increase blood glucose level in cases of hypoglycemia by raising the depolymerization of glycogen in the liver to glucose; IV administration has immediate onset

COMMON NURSING DIAGNOSES

INEFFECTIVE TISSUE PERFUSION: CARDIOPULMONARY, CEREBRAL, GASTROINTESTINAL, PERIPHERAL, RENAL (see CAD)

Related to: interruption of arterial flow from macroangiopathies and microangiopathies, reduced oxygen supply, atherosclerotic lesions, hypoperfusion, hypovolemia, dysrhythmias, coexisting disease processes, age-related vascular structure changes

Defining Characteristics: vasoconstriction, hypotension, tachycardia, tachypnea, carotid bruits, chest pain, conduction disturbances, dysrhythmias, ECG changes, delayed capillary refill time, chest retractions, dyspnea, nasal flaring, use of accessory muscles, increased work of breathing, changes in mental status, weakness, behavioral changes, abdominal distention, ileus, hypoactive or absent bowel sounds, nausea, vomiting, edema, weak or absent peripheral pulses, skin temperature changes, skin color changes, decreased peripheral tactile sensation, oliguria, retinopathy, nephropathy, abnormal renal profiles, dermopathy, hair loss, dependent rubor, gangrene

DISTURBED SENSORY PERCEPTION: VISUAL, TACTILE, KINESTHETIC (see CATARACTS, ALZHEIMER'S DISEASE)

Related to: alteration in sensory reception, transmission, and or integration of neurologic deficit from neuropathy; altered status of sense organ from retinopathy, diabetes, medications, physiologic changes related to aging

Defining Characteristics: decreased visual acuity, glaucoma, cataract formation, retinopathy, retinal hemorrhages, pain and paresthesias to extremities, tingling, burning, itching sensations, loss of sensitivity to touch, temperature changes to skin, numbness, intermittent claudication, decreased or absent peripheral pulses

SEXUAL DYSFUNCTION (see SEXUAL DISORDERS)

Related to: changes in body structure and function from diabetes process, neuropathy affecting autonomic nervous system

Defining Characteristics: verbalization of problems with sexual function, avoidance of engaging in sexual intercourse, need for confirmation of desirability, impotence, inability to achieve desired satisfaction

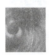
RISK FOR IMPAIRED SKIN INTEGRITY (see PERIPHERAL VASCULAR DISEASE)

Related to: diabetic process, altered pigmentation from microangiopathy, skin changes related to the aging process, pressure on skin surfaces, bed rest, immobility, intermittent claudication, alteration in arterial and venous circulation, alterations in tissue perfusion

Defining Characteristics: brown spots on lower extremities, thin, dry skin on extremities, redness to pressure areas, edema, ulcerations or lesions to extremities, dermatitis, pigmentation to legs, mottling, cyanosis, pallor, decreased or absent pulses, warmth to area, disruption of skin surface, excoriation of skin, decreased tactile sensation, necrosis to skin on legs

FUNCTIONAL URINARY INCONTINENCE (see INTERSTITIAL CYSTITIS)

Related to: diabetic neuropathy affecting the autonomic nervous system, aging process

Defining Characteristics: decreased awareness of bladder fullness, urinary retention, infrequent voiding, difficulty voiding, nocturia, incontinence, weak stream of urine, dysuria

IMBALANCED NUTRITION: MORE THAN BODY REQUIREMENTS (see GERD)

Related to: excessive intake in relationship to metabolic needs, obesity, decreased insulin receptors in skeletal muscle and fat cells, insulin resistance, decreased physical activity, decreased metabolic rate

Defining Characteristics: body weight 10% or more over ideal weight, triceps skin-fold measurement more than 15 mm in men and 25 mm in women, eating in response to social situations, dysfunctional eating patterns, eating in response to cues other than hunger, pairing food with other activities, sedentary lifestyle, lack of control of hyperglycemia

RISK FOR INFECTION (see UTI)

Related to: diabetes, chronic glycosuria, inadequate primary defenses, stasis of body fluids, medications, physiologic changes related to the aging process

Defining Characteristics: increased temperature, cloudy urine, foul-smelling urine, positive urine cultures, frequency, dysuria, burning, pelvic pain, hematuria, skin infections, vaginal infections

ADDITIONAL NURSING DIAGNOSES

RISK FOR TRAUMA

Related to: internal factors, reduced temperature, reduced tactile sensation; neuropathic arthropathy, impaired sensory perception neuropathy

Defining Characteristics: joint dysfunction, foot drop, ulceration of leg or foot, burns or bruising of legs, slow healing, necrosis of leg/foot ulcers

Outcome Criteria

✔ Patient will have an absence of trauma, injury, falls, or other complications.

NOC: *Safety Status: Physical Injury*

INTERVENTIONS	RATIONALES
Assess patient's mobility, stability, muscle weakness, cognitive limitations, balance or gait difficulties, and factors related to disease process.	Falls are common in the elderly patient and result from weakness in muscle and skeletal support system, as well as decreased tactile and sensory status.
Assess patient's sensory deficits of visual, tactile, perceptual, and kinesthetic changes.	May contribute to falls and other trauma because of insensitivity to pain, temperature extremes, or visual acuity.
Assess patient's mentation, changes in mental status, vertigo, syncope, and penchant for wandering.	Provides information regarding potential for falls and trauma.
Evaluate patient for unexplained injuries, excessive fear, or repeated trauma.	May indicate physical abuse.

INTERVENTIONS	RATIONALES
Assess environment for safety hazards. Ensure lighting, pathways are cleared, beds are in lowest position and locked, hazardous objects out of reach, and ability to summon help within reach.	Safety hazards predispose patient to falls or serious injury. By ensuring that hazardous objects are removed, patient's environment is made safer.
Provide night light as needed and ensure that pathways are clear, and floor is dry and not slippery.	Prevents bumping into objects or stumbling and falling.
Assist with ambulation as needed.	Promotes safety and prevents falls if patient is too weak or impaired to ambulate alone.
Stay with patient if complains of faintness or dizziness.	Reduces anxiety and potential injury from fall if patient does faint.
Apply alarm system to bed or chair to alert caregivers that patient has wandered outside of safe limitations.	Provides patient the opportunity to ambulate and wander about a safe distance rather than use restraints or other confinement method, yet maintaining a safe environment.
Instruct patient/family in environmental modifications to accommodate level of functioning and awareness.	Creates a safe environment and prevents injury or trauma.
Instruct family to prevent patient from driving if not capable.	Cognitive difficulties may cause injury to patient and/or others.
Instruct patient/family regarding risk factors associated with diabetes, with falls and fractures, and with problems that affect mobility and thought processes.	Provides information to reinforce compliance in preventing injury, and promotes knowledge of disease process and complications.
Instruct patient/family regarding medication effects and side effects of medications currently being taken, and regarding potential for causing injury.	Promotes understanding of effect that medications have on well-being or that medications can predispose patient to injury and trauma.
Instruct patient/family regarding patient wearing supportive, sturdy shoes with nonskid soles.	Prevents stumbling and slipping.
Instruct patient/family regarding need for extreme caution when caring for wounds or burns caused by disease process complications.	Diabetic patients have poor wound healing that may take much longer than normal. Elderly patients usually have fragile skin that can easily be traumatized.

NIC: *Surveillance: Safety*

Discharge or Maintenance Evaluation

- Patient will have safe environment maintained with absence of safety hazards.
- Patient will have no incidence of falls or injury from dangerous objects.
- Patient will be able to ambulate and wander about in a safe environment.
- Patient/family will be able to maintain safety with medication administration and home environmental safety.
- Patient will be able to ambulate safely by self or with assistance.
- Patient/family will be able to accurately verbalize understanding of disease process as to how it affects safety within the environment.

DEFICIENT KNOWLEDGE

Related to: lack of information about disease process and care (medication, dietary and exercise regimen, testing for glucose level)

Defining Characteristics: verbalization of the problem, request for information, new diagnosis of NIDDM, conversion from NIDDM to IDDM

Outcome Criteria

✔ Patient will obtain appropriate knowledge of medical regimen prescribed to control hyperglycemia.

NOC: *Knowledge: Disease Process*

INTERVENTIONS	RATIONALES
Assess patient's knowledge of factors associated with disease, and methods to control and stabilize diabetes.	Prevents repetition of information and promotes compliance necessary to maintain normal glucose level.
Provide information and explanations in clear, simple language that is understandable. Provide limited amounts of information over time.	Encourages compliance of medical regimen according to cognitive ability and readiness to learn.
Use pictures, pamphlets, video tapes, and models in teaching.	Provides visual aids to reinforce learning.
Instruct patient of possible symptoms to report including nausea, drowsiness, lethargy, polyuria, and blood glucose of 240 mg/dL or more.	May lead to diabetic hyperglycemic coma.

(continues)

(continued)

INTERVENTIONS	RATIONALES
Instruct patient of possible hypoglycemia symptoms to report including shaky feeling, nervousness, confusion, hunger, and weakness, and to take orange juice, honey or sugar to counteract this reaction.	May lead to insulin shock.
Instruct patient to take oral hypoglycemic as ordered.	Promotes correct dosage at correct times to control NIDDM.
Instruct patient in administration of insulin; name, action, peak levels, dosage, how to store, preparation and filling syringe, rotation of sites, and procedure to inject insulin.	Ensures correct dosage to control IDDM, if able to administer own insulin.
Instruct patient and assist to develop menus for appropriate caloric amounts and food selections using American Diabetic Association guidelines. Provide sample menus and exchange lists.	Dietary management controls NIDDM and is also necessary to adjust insulin dosage.
Instruct patient not to skip meals, avoid fad diets, high sugar and carbohydrate desserts, and alcohol.	Food intake is calculated to correlate with insulin and exercise program. Alcohol inhibits gluconeogenesis.
Instruct patient in blood and urine testing using Glucometer analysis of capillary blood, obtaining samples of blood and urine for testing, and when to notify physician.	Provides glucose levels in blood and urine to determine presence of hypoglycemia, hyperglycemia, glycosuria, or ketone presence.

INTERVENTIONS	RATIONALES
Provide daily exercise/activity program. Instruct patient to avoid overactivity or strenuous activities, and to use a carbohydrate if activity is increased.	Activity is essential for optimal results of medical regimen by utilization of diet and medication.

NIC: *Teaching: Disease Process*

Discharge or Maintenance Evaluation

■ Patient will be able to accurately verbalize understanding of disease process, medications, diet requirements, and need for activity.

■ Patient will be able to accurately perform urine and blood level testing.

■ Patient will be able to accurately verbalize signs and symptoms of which to notify physician.

■ Patient will be able to verbalize understanding of complications of hypoglycemia and hyperglycemia, and appropriate actions to take.

■ Patient will achieve and maintain appropriate body weight for age, height, and frame.

■ Patient will be able to accurately verbalize understanding of dietary restrictions, menu planning, and nutrient selection.

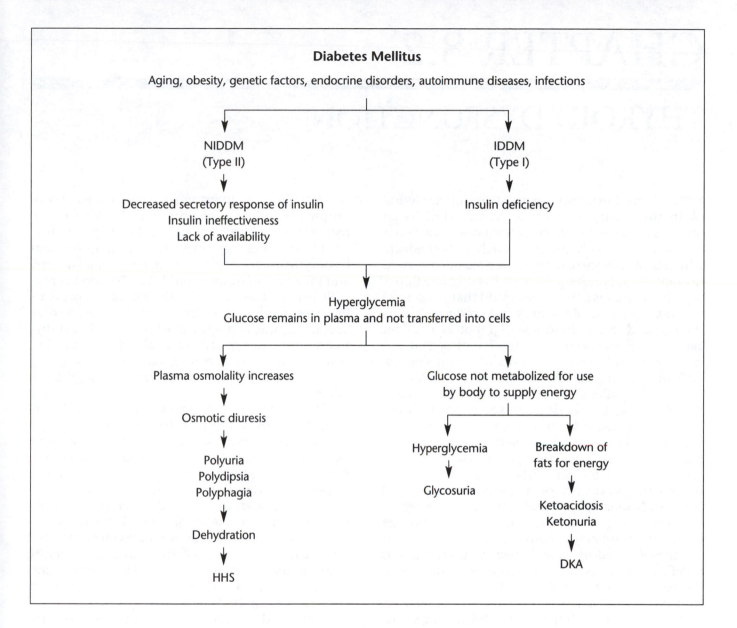

Diabetes Mellitus

Aging, obesity, genetic factors, endocrine disorders, autoimmune diseases, infections

NIDDM
(Type II)

IDDM
(Type I)

Decreased secretory response of insulin
Insulin ineffectiveness
Lack of availability

Insulin deficiency

Hyperglycemia
Glucose remains in plasma and not transferred into cells

Plasma osmolality increases

Osmotic diuresis

Polyuria
Polydipsia
Polyphagia

Dehydration

HHS

Glucose not metabolized for use
by body to supply energy

Hyperglycemia

Glycosuria

Breakdown of
fats for energy

Ketoacidosis
Ketonuria

DKA

CHAPTER 8.2

THYROID DYSFUNCTION

The thyroid dysfunctions most commonly found in the elderly are thyrotoxicosis, which is an increase in circulating thyroid hormones that causes an increase in body function, or hypothyroidism, which is an absence or decrease of circulating thyroid hormones that causes a decrease in body function.

The thyroid is a two-lobed gland that bridges the trachea at the base of the neck and produces thyroxine (T_4) and triiodothyronine (T_3), but as a patient ages, the thyroid becomes somewhat atrophied and develops fibrosis, increases in nodules, and lymphocytic infiltration. A decrease in the use of T_4 relates to the elderly patient's decrease in lean body mass. Serum T_3 and free T_3 decrease somewhat with age because of decreased pituitary secretion of thyroid-stimulating hormone (TSH) and decreased hypothalamic production of thyrotropin-releasing hormone (TRH). The average TSH level increases with age and reflects the prevalence of hypothyroidism in aged patients. Normal growth and metabolism are dependent on having correct amounts of these hormones circulating through the body.

Hypothyroidism, also known as myxedema, is a deficient level of thyroid hormone, and causes a decrease in the metabolic rate that is distinguished by weight gain, fatigue, cold intolerance, muscle cramps, and the potential for life-threatening coma. The prevalence of this disease increases with age. Causes of this disease that are most frequently seen include Hashimoto's disease (chronic autoimmune thyroiditis) which causes an inflammatory disease of the thyroid resulting in hypothyroidism, irradiation, surgical removal of the thyroid, or a nongoitrous presentation of Hashimoto's disease.

The elderly patient may present clinical symptoms that are much different from those seen in a younger population, and as such, hypothyroidism may go undiagnosed for a long period of time. Signs include confusion, anorexia, incontinence, weight loss, arthralgias, muscle aches, weakness, and decreases in mobility, all of which can be symptoms of other disorders. In myxedema coma, mental confusion can progress to stupor and on to coma, hyponatremia, hypoglycemia, and/or hypercapnia.

Treatment of hypothyroidism is most often oral levothyroxine replacement started at a small dosage, and increased as needed, until the TSH level is normalized, and then taken for the rest of the patient's life. Treatment of myxedema coma involves a more drastic therapy, involving large doses of IV levothyroxine until the patient can take the medication orally, as well as IV corticosteroids, and measures to treat hyponatremia, hypoglycemia, and respiratory failure.

Hyperthyroidism is an excess of thyroid hormone that causes in increase in the body's metabolic rate, which results in weight loss, palpitations, muscle weakness, protrusion of the eyeballs, and mood swings. Toxic goiters and toxic nodules are other causes of excessive thyroid hormone secretion.

Hyperthyroidism is found in elderly patients more frequently as a result of goiter than Graves' disease, which is a common cause in younger patients. The use of amiodarone, a cardiac drug that deposits iodine in tissues and into the circulation over a long period of time, is a frequent cause of iodine-induced hyperthyroidism in the elderly.

Signs and symptoms of hyperthyroidism are even more elusive to diagnose in the elderly than those connected with hypothyroidism. Older patients have fewer symptoms, and many of the signs can be related to other concurrent chronic illnesses. Classically, the signs in older patients are tachycardia, weight loss, and fatigue. Ocular symptoms are usually nonexistent. The most common complication in the aged is atrial fibrillation, which occurs in approximately one-fourth of the elderly population of hyperthyroid patients.

The treatment of choice for hyperthyroidism is administration of radioactive sodium iodide (^{131}I). Treatment for Graves' disease is usually antithyroid drugs and beta-blockers.

Thyroid storm, or thyrotoxicosis, is a very rare, life-threatening episode occurring with hyperthyroidism, and presents with fever, extreme tachycardia, nausea, vomiting, heart failure, and changes in mental status. This condition is considered to be an emergency, and treatment includes large dosages of propylthiouracil, propranolol, and IV glucocorticoids. Oral or IV sodium iodide can be given, but ipodate sodium is more effective in lowering the T_3 level to normal within a 24-hour period.

MEDICAL CARE

Laboratory: thyroid profiles used to identify condition; T_3 and T_4 levels identify either increased levels in hyperthyroidism or decreased levels in hypothyroidism; TSH levels increased in hypothyroidism and decreased with hyperthyroidism, and is the essential test in determining the type of thyroid dysfunction and efficacy of treatment; serum thyroid hormone levels may be done to confirm diagnosis or to establish that patient is not actually euthyroid in the presence of clinical symptomatology; triiodothyronine resin uptake (T_3RU) used to identify thyroid-binding globulin capacity which increases in hyperthyroidism and decreases in hypothyroidism; lipid profiles may be used to identify elevations in cholesterol with hypothyroidism; thyroid-stimulating immunoglobulin (TSI) used to identify Graves' disease; creatine kinase levels may be used to identify elevations with hypothyroidism; alkaline phophatase used to identify increases seen in thyroid disease; CBC used to identify the presence of infection that potentially occurs with myxedema coma or agranulocytosis that may occur with treatment of thioureas for hyperthyroidism; calcium levels used to identify imbalances that may occur after surgery if hypoparathyroidism occurs

Radiography: chest X-rays used to show heart enlargement, pulmonary vasculature, presence of infiltrates and effusions

Thyroid scan: done to evaluate thyroid function and identify any presence of nodules

Magnetic resonance imaging: MRI of the orbits may be done to visualize ophthalmopathy seen in Graves' disease; imaging is only required in severe cases or with exophthalmos that requires differentiation from orbital tumors or other disorders

Thyroid replacement: levothyroxine (T_4) (Levothroid, Levoxine, Levoxyl, or Synthroid) is the drug of choice in the treatment of hypothyroidism because of its ability to convert in the body to T_3; replaces the body's lost thyroid hormone by use of an artificial oral means, with therapy starting with a lower dosage, and gradually increasing until laboratory tests reveal euthyroid state; there are instances where the body is not able to convert T_4 to T_3, and liothyronine (T_3) (Cytomel, Triostat) may need to be added to replacement therapy; combination therapy of levothyroxine sodium and liothyronine is available as liotrix (Thyrolar); thyroid replacement (Armour Thyroid, Thyrar, or Thyroid Strong) stimulates the metabolism of all body tissues by accelerating the basal metabolic rate

Antithyroid drugs: methimazole (Tapazole), potassium iodide (Pima, Thyro-Block, SSKI, Lugol's solution), and propylthiouracil (PTU) used to block synthesis of thyroid hormones to treat hyperthyroidism; propranolol (Inderal) is the initial treatment for thyroid storm; other drugs block conversion of T_4 to T_3 within the body

Radioactive iodine (^{131}I): used to destroy overfunctioning thyroid tissue; the iodine concentrates in the thyroid and destroys the cells that concentrate it; may cause hypothyroidism several years after taking this substance

Iodinated contrast agents: ipodate sodium and iopanoic acid block conversion of T_4 to T_3 in the liver, and inhibit T_4 release; used in treatment of thyroid storm

Surgery: may be required for Graves' disease or toxic nodular goiter if drug therapy or iodine therapy has not been completely successful; thyroid vascularity is reduced by medication for approximately 10 days prior to surgery

COMMON NURSING DIAGNOSES

 ### EXCESS FLUID VOLUME (see HEART FAILURE)

Related to: compromised regulatory mechanisms from decreased thyroid hormone, hypothyroidism

Defining Characteristics: interstitial edema, face puffiness, periorbital edema, weight gain, intake more than output, pitting edema, increased blood pressure, tachycardia

DECREASED CARDIAC OUTPUT (see CAD)

Related to: alterations in contractility, changes in heart from decreased thyroid hormone, hypothyroidism, alteration in cardiac rate and rhythm, conduction defects

Defining Characteristics: ECG changes, bradycardia, hypotension, dysrhythmias, dyspnea, adventitious breath sounds, wheezing, fatigue, syncope, restlessness, cold, clammy skin, decreased peripheral pulses, jugular vein distention, skin color changes, pallor, cyanosis, edema, cardiac gallops, changes in mental status, disorientation, chest pain

 ## DISTURBED THOUGHT PROCESSES (see LIVER FAILURE)

Related to: physiologic changes from decreased thyroid hormone, hypothyroidism, mucoprotein deposits to cranial nerves, decreased blood flow to brain

Defining Characteristics: lethargy, apathy, forgetfulness, mental status changes, decreasing level of consciousness, changes in personality, inattentiveness, decreased intellectual functioning, coma

 ## RISK FOR IMPAIRED SKIN INTEGRITY (see PERIPHERAL VASCULAR DISEASE)

Related to: internal factors of altered metabolic state from decreased thyroid hormone, hypothyroidism, mucopolysaccharide deposits in subcutaneous tissues, skin changes associated with the aging process, pressure on skin surfaces, bed rest, immobility, intermittent claudication, alteration in arterial and venous circulation

Defining Characteristics: thick, dry, leathery skin, thick, brittle nails, sparse, coarse hair to head and eyebrows, ulcerations or lesions to extremities, dermatitis, pallor, decreased or absent pulses, disruption of skin surface, excoriation of skin, decreased tactile sensation, claudication, paresthesias

 ## CONSTIPATION (see HEART FAILURE)

Related to: gastrointestinal impairment from decreased thyroid hormone, hypothyroidism, immobility, less than adequate physical activity, decreased motility

Defining Characteristics: passage of hard, formed stool, decreased bowel sounds, inability to evacuate stool, abdominal pain, abdominal distention, ileus, absent bowel sounds, nausea, vomiting, frequency of stool less than normal, less than usual amount of stool, palpable mass, feelings of rectal fullness, inability to ingest bulk-containing foods, frequent bouts of constipation, impaired peristalsis, straining at stool, weakness, fatigue, confusion

 ## IMBALANCED NUTRITION: MORE THAN BODY REQUIREMENTS (see GERD)

Related to: decreased physical activity, excessive intake in relationship to metabolic need of high caloric foods, decreased metabolic rate caused from hypothyroidism

Defining Characteristics: body weight 10% or more over ideal weight, triceps skin-fold measurement more than 15 mm in men and 25 mm in women, eating in response to social situations, sedentary activity level, decreased metabolic rate, eating in response to cues other than hunger, pairing food with other activities, decreased energy, weight gain

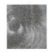 ## IMBALANCED NUTRITION: LESS THAN BODY REQUIREMENTS (see COPD)

Related to: biologic factors from increased thyroid hormone production; hyperthyroidism, inability to take in enough food, increased metabolism resulting from disease process, inability to absorb nutrients because of biologic or psychological factors

Defining Characteristics: actual inadequate food intake, weight loss in spite of appetite and adequate intake, body weight 20% or more under ideal for height and frame, anorexia, absent bowel sounds, decreased peristalsis, muscle mass loss, decreased muscle tone, changes in bowel habits, nausea, vomiting

 ## DIARRHEA (see BOWEL DISORDERS)

Related to: internal factors from increased thyroid hormone production, hyperthyroidism, increased bowel motility, infection

Defining Characteristics: frequent passage of stools, loose, liquid, or watery stools, abdominal pain, cramping, increased bowel sounds

DISTURBED SLEEP PATTERN (see ALZHEIMER'S DISEASE)

Related to: internal factors of illness from increased thyroid hormone production, hyperthyroidism, increased CNS activity, disease processes

Defining Characteristics: interrupted sleep, difficulty falling asleep, awakening early, fatigue, lethargy, irritability, disorientation, complaints of not feeling rested, insomnia, sleeplessness, sleepiness during the day, yawning, morning headache, tremor

 SEXUAL DYSFUNCTION (see SEXUAL DISORDERS)

Related to: altered body function from increased or decreased thyroid hormone production and absorption, hyperthyroidism, hypothyroidism, changes in secretions of androgens and progesterone

Defining Characteristics: verbalization of problems with sexual function, avoidance of engaging in sexual intercourse, impotence, decreased libido, inability to achieve desired satisfaction, amenorrhea, menorrhagia

ANXIETY (see CAD)

Related to: sleep deprivation, change in health status from thyroid disease, life-threatening crises, chronic nature of disease and effect on lifestyle, change in role functioning, decreased energy, exhaustion, sexual dysfunction

Defining Characteristics: fear, restlessness, muscle tension, irritability, agitation, helplessness, communication of uncertainty and apprehension, exhaustion, insomnia, impotence

 HYPERTHERMIA (see INFLUENZA, HYPERTHERMIA)

Related to: infection, increased metabolic rate, hyperthyroidism

Defining Characteristics: heat intolerance, fever, warm, flushed skin, tachycardia, tachypnea, dry mucous membranes, dehydration, oliguria

 FATIGUE (see HEART FAILURE)

Related to: decreased metabolic energy production, hypothyroidism

Defining Characteristics: verbalization of fatigue, lack of energy, inability to maintain usual routine activity, lethargy, emotionally labile, inability to achieve rest even with sleep

ACUTE PAIN (see CAD)

Related to: mucinous deposits in joints and muscles from hypothyroidism

Defining Characteristics: communication of pain, facial grimacing, restlessness, changes in pulse and blood pressure, diaphoresis, protective behavior of joints in extremities, hypoactive reflexes, decreased motor activity, decreased muscle strength

ADDITIONAL NURSING DIAGNOSES

RISK FOR INJURY

Related to: internal biochemical factor of sensory dysfunction, exophthalmos, Graves' disease

Defining Characteristics: decreased blinking, inability to close eyes, irritation to eyes

Outcome Criteria

✔ Patient will have absence of any injury to eyes.

NOC: *Risk Detection*

INTERVENTIONS	RATIONALES
Assess patient's visual acuity, sclera for clearness, cornea for damage, and irritation or dryness of eyes.	Hyperthyroidism or Graves' disease may result in exophthalmos, which has the potential for patient to receive corneal abrasions and other injuries to eye.
Provide eye pads and tape lids shut, if difficult to close.	Protects eyes from environmental particles.
Provide isotonic eye drops and/or cool compresses to eyes as needed.	Promotes comfort for dry, irritated eyes.
Raise head of bed during rest or sleep.	Promotes fluid drainage from periorbital area.
Instruct patient to wear sunglasses in bright light situations.	Helps to protect the eyes from light or particulate matter from the environment caused by inability to completely close lids.
Instruct patient in extraocular muscle exercises.	Helps to maintain strength of ocular muscles and ocular movement.

NIC: *Eye Care*

Discharge or Maintenance Evaluation

- Patient will be free of irritation of eyes, corneal damage, or other injury to eyes.
- Patient will be compliant in the use of eye drops and protective measures for eyes.

HYPOTHERMIA

Related to: decreased metabolic rate, hypothyroidism

Defining Characteristics: shivering, cool skin, perceived feeling of coldness

Outcome Criteria

✔ Patient will achieve increased comfort in environmental temperature.

NOC: *Thermoregulation*

INTERVENTIONS	RATIONALES
Assess patient for perception of cold, chilling, or shivering.	Impaired temperature adaptation may be caused by decreased secretion of thyroid hormones.

INTERVENTIONS	RATIONALES
Provide warmer clothing, additional blankets, and increase environmental temperature.	Promotes comfort and warmth.
Instruct patient that cold intolerance will decrease with treatment.	Information promotes understanding of condition.
Suggest warm liquids.	Provides warmth.

NIC: *Temperature Regulation*

Discharge or Maintenance Evaluation

- Patient will be able to verbalize feelings of increased comfort in normal environmental temperatures with treatment.
- Patient will exhibit an absence of chilling and shivering.
- Patient will suffer no complications from feelings of coldness.

Thyroid Dysfunction

(Aging, Radiation, Immune diseases)

↓

Atrophy of thyroid gland

↓

Decreased thyroid production
Hypothyroidism

↓

Slowing of body processes
Personality changes

↓

Bradycardia, decreased cardiac output
Decreased gastrointestinal motility
Decreased erythropoiesis
Mental sluggishness, lethargy
Dry, coarse skin and hair
Cold intolerance
Decreased metabolism
Decreased muscle tone, weakness
Sexual dysfunction, menorrhagia
Weight gain

Increased secretion of thyroid hormones
Diffuse thyroid hyperplasia

↓

Hyperthyroidism

Increase in oxygen
consumption
Increase in metabolism
Increase in sympathetic
activity

Edema of orbital
structure

↓

Graves' disease
Exophthalmos

↓

Weight loss
Tachycardia, increased cardiac output
Irritability, fatigue
Heat intolerance
Diarrhea
Thin, silky skin and hair
Increased muscle tone
Retraction of eyelids

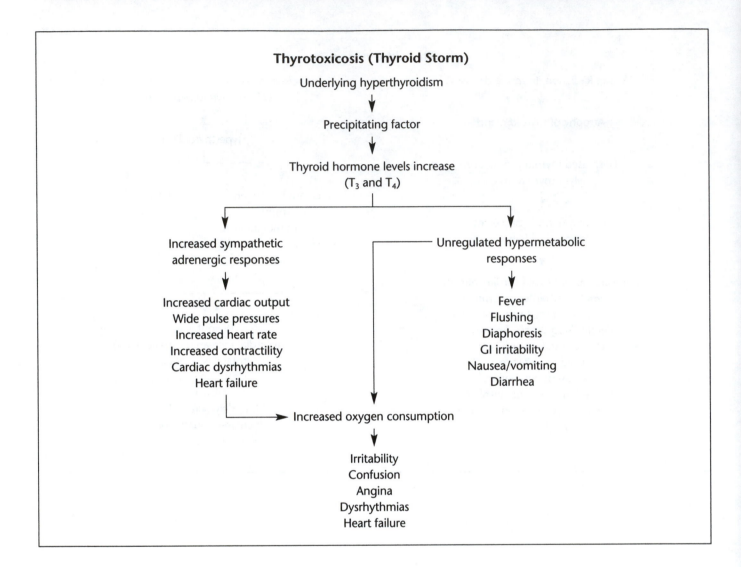

Thyrotoxicosis (Thyroid Storm)

Underlying hyperthyroidism

↓

Precipitating factor

↓

Thyroid hormone levels increase
(T_3 and T_4)

Increased sympathetic adrenergic responses	Unregulated hypermetabolic responses
↓	↓
Increased cardiac output Wide pulse pressures Increased heart rate Increased contractility Cardiac dysrhythmias Heart failure	Fever Flushing Diaphoresis GI irritability Nausea/vomiting Diarrhea

Increased oxygen consumption

↓

Irritability
Confusion
Angina
Dysrhythmias
Heart failure

UNIT 9

MUSCULOSKELETAL SYSTEM

CHAPTER 9.1

ARTHRITIS

Arthritis is a wide-ranging label for a number of different conditions that have to do with swollen, painful, or stiff joints. The joints connect bones together and each joint is supported by a layer of cartilage and sheathed by a fibrous capsule that contains synovial fluid. When disease, wear and tear, or infection cause this fluid or the tissues to swell or become inflamed, the joints can develop into scar tissue and result in deformity.

There are several types of arthritis, but osteoarthritis, or OA, is the most common cause of disability in the elderly population over 65 years of age. Aging, in itself, does not cause osteoarthritis, but age-related changes in the cellular matrix in cartilage predispose the elderly to this disease. Cartilage breaks down and the bones begin to grate against each other, resulting in pain and degeneration progression. Over a period of time, the bones may thicken and result in the appearance of additional growth of bone spurs. Osteoarthritis occurs in joints that are exposed to weight bearing and stress, especially the knees, hips, and spine.

Symptoms of OA include pain to the joints, degenerative changes with erosive osteophyte formation, especially to the hands. Pain is usually relieved by rest and worsened by movement and weight-bearing exercise. Crepitus, or a grating-type noise, may be heard when the joint is moved because of deterioration in the cartilage. Other diseases may occur in conjunction with osteoarthritis, such as bursitis, rheumatoid arthritis, gout, pseudogout, and polymyalgia rheumatica.

Treatment of OA involves supportive care, with NSAIDs or COX-2 inhibitors, braces or splints, therapy, or exercise, until the pain becomes unbearable, and then surgical intervention is the treatment of choice. Sometimes an intra-articular injection of corticosteroids is tried. Either surgical reconstruction of the joint, or complete joint replacement with an artificial appliance can frequently relieve pain and restore function for the patient.

Rheumatoid arthritis, or RA, is a systemic inflammatory disease of the joints that leads to deformity and progressive immobility and activity impairment. Because RA is systemic, it not only involves the swollen and painful joints, but also affects the organs of the body. RA may be caused by a virus or an autoimmune reaction, or a combination of the two factors, but the cause is unknown. When RA begins after the age of 60, the condition is known as elderly-onset rheumatoid arthritis and it comprises several conditions including RA and polymyalgia rheumatica. The incidence of RA increases up to age 80. The synovium of the diarthrodial joints become severely inflamed, causing the synovial tissue to become hyperplastic and permeated with lymphocytes and plasma cells. Inflammatory mediators are present in the synovial fluid.

The patient usually presents with pain to the joints of the hands and feet, elbows, shoulders, and knees, with stiffness and swelling, especially in the morning. Stiffness lasts at least an hour before mobility is improved. Late symptoms and signs include periarticular osteoporosis, joint space narrowing, and marginal erosions.

Treatment of RA is based on therapy, assistive devices, rest, heat or cold for pain relief, and regular use of NSAIDs or COX-2 inhibitors. Low-dose corticosteroids may help with reduction of disability and pain, and intra-articular injections of corticosteroid esters may be of some help temporarily. Slow-acting antirheumatoid drugs (SAARDS) may help to slow the disease process and reduce morbidity, but may take up to 6 months to act. Surgical interventions for RA include synovectomy or freeing the trapped median nerve in people with carpal tunnel syndrome in early stages of RA, up to total joint replacement or osteotomy in advanced cases.

MEDICAL CARE

Laboratory: RA factor testing used to identify patients with rheumatoid arthritis; CBC to identify anemia, thombocytosis, leukocytosis, presence of infection; synovial fluid analysis used to identify leukocytosis in OA and RA; fluid is usually cloudy, with increased WBCs, decreased complement components with RA; ESR used to identify the rate at which red blood cells settle to the bottom of a container, with increases in patient with RA; uric acid used to identify presence of gout; ANA used to rule out systemic lupus erythematosus; coagulation studies used to identify any coagulopathy; anti-Ro and anti-La tests used to identify the presence of Sjogren's disease; glucose levels used to identify dysfunction related to medications

Radiography: X-rays of the different parts of the body in which symptoms are present used to identify evidence of osteoarthritis bone destruction, as well as osteophyte formation, subchondral bony sclerosis and cyst formation, or joint space narrowing; X-rays not specifically diagnostic for RA, but may show articular cartilage destruction, erosion, and deformity, and be helpful in evaluating efficacy of treatment

Magnetic resonance imaging (MRI): MRI of the particular part of the body being investigated in order to visualize the joint and soft tissues with OA

Therapy: physical therapy, with applications of heat and/or cold for pain reduction, assistance with mobility, water exercise programs to reduce stress on joints while maintaining mobility

Nonsteroidal anti-inflammatories (NSAIDs): diclofenac potassium or sodium (Cataflam, Voltaren), etodolac (Lodine), fenoprofen calcium (Nalfon), flurbiprofen (Ansaid, Ocufen), ibuprofen (Advil, Motrin, Genpril, Nuprin, Trendar), indomethacin (Indocin, Indocid PDA), ketoprofen (Actron, Orudis, Oruvail), ketorolac tromethamine (Toradol), meloxicam (Mobic), nabumetone (Relafen), naproxen (Naprosyn, Aleve, Naprelan, Anaprox), oxaprozin (Daypro), piroxicam (Feldene), or sulindac (Clinoril) used to inhibit prostaglandin biosynthesis in the treatment of arthritis; may contribute to gastrointestinal bleeding

Cyclooxygenase-2 inhibitors (COX-2): celecoxib (Celebrex) or rofecoxib (Vioxx), used to inhibit COX-2, which is responsible for the conversion of arachidonic acid to prostaglandins, which in turn results in analgesic, antipyretic, and anti-inflammatory effects without the undesirable gastrointestinal bleeding side effects

Corticosteroids: betamethasone (Celestone), cortisone acetate (Cortone), dexamethasone acetate or sodium phosphate (Decadron, Dexone, Hexadrol, Solurex LA, Cortastat, Dalalone, Dexasone), hydrocortisone acetate, sodium phosphate, or sodium succinate (Cortef, Cortenema, Hydrocortone, Solu-Cortef), methylprednisolone acetate or sodium succinate (Medrol, Depo-Medrol, Duralone, Medralone, Solu-Medrol), prednisolone acetate, sodium phosphate, or terbutate (Delta-Cortef, Prelone, Cotolone, Predalone, Predate, Prenisol), prednisone (Deltasone, Meticorten, Orasone, Prednisone Intensol, Sterapred), or triamcinolone (Aristocort, Atolone, Kenacort, Azmacort, Trilog, Amcort, Trilone) used orally or by intra-articular injection to reduce pain and inflammation

Immunosuppressants: azathioprine (Imuran) and cyclosporin (Neoral, Sandimmune) used to treat rheumatoid arthritis unresponsive to conventional therapy to modify the disease process by inhibiting T-lymphocytes

Antirheumatics: methotrexate (Rheumatrex, Methotrexate), hydroxychloroquine (Plaquenil), sulfasalazine (Azulfidine, Sulfasalazine), used to suppress the inflammatory process in the joints by suppressing the immune response in the treatment of rheumatoid arthritis and connective tissue disease; biologic response modifiers (etanercept [Enbrel] and leflunomide [Arava] help to block the action of the inflammatory cytokine tumor necrosis factor or inhibit pyrimidine synthesis; gold compounds (auranofin [Ridaura], aurothioglucose [Solganal], or gold sodium thiomalate [Aurolate]) used to inhibit sulfhydryl systems that alter the cellular metabolism and have anti-inflammatory effects; these drugs, although older and not used as much anymore, are still viable options for patients who cannot tolerate the other antirheumatic drugs; D-penicillamine (Cuprimine, Depen) is a chelating agent that binds with lead, mercury, copper, iron and zinc ions and has been found to be helpful with rheumatoid arthritis treatment; cyclophosphamide (Cytoxan, Neosar) inhibits enzymes that allow synthesis of amino acids and is used to treat RA that is refractory to other treatment

Apheresis: new treatment used only for severely advanced RA cases; immunoadsorption therapy based on filtering the patient's plasma through a staphylococcus protein A (Prosorba) column to remove antibodies

Surgery: total joint replacement may be required if pain is unbearable and conservative methods have failed for both OA and RA; reconstruction of joints may be feasible for OA; synovectomy or release of the median nerve may help patients with RA

COMMON NURSING DIAGNOSES

IMPAIRED PHYSICAL MOBILITY (see ALZHEIMER'S DISEASE)

Related to: osteoarthritis, rheumatoid arthritis, pain and musculoskeletal impairment, inability to bear weight, impairment in range of motion from joint and cartilage dysfunction and/or destruction

Defining Characteristics: joint pain, swelling, stiffness, limited movement, limited function of joint, crepitus, inability to move at will, weakness, inability to bear weight, immobility, gait disturbances, balance and coordination deficits, difficulty turning, decreased range of motion, tremors, instability while standing, presence of joint space narrowing, osteophyte formation, subchondral cysts

RISK FOR IMPAIRED SKIN INTEGRITY (see PERIPHERAL VASCULAR DISEASE)

Related to: physiologic changes associated with the aging process, pressure on skin surfaces, external mechanical factor of pressure from splints and/or braces

Defining Characteristics: thin, dry skin on extremities, redness to pressure areas, edema, ulcerations or lesions to extremities, dermatitis, warmth to area, disruption of skin surface, excoriation of skin, decreased tactile sensation, pain, irritation to skin

CHRONIC PAIN (see PERIPHERAL VASCULAR DISEASE)

Related to: chronic physical disability, decreased joint movement, decreased joint stability, inflammatory process

Defining Characteristics: verbal report of pain for more than 6 months, altered ability to continue previous activities, physical withdrawal, social withdrawal, guarded behavior, protective behavior of affected joints, facial grimacing, crying, moaning, atrophy of muscle, irritability, restlessness, hypersensitivity, depression, fatigue, insomnia

INEFFECTIVE COPING (see DEPRESSION)

Related to: multiple life changes, limitations imposed by disease processes, depression, lack of coping skills

Defining Characteristics: verbalizations of inability to cope, inability to meet role expectations, inability to meet basic needs, social isolation and withdrawal, chronic fatigue, chronic worry, sleep disturbances, inappropriate coping strategies, inability to ask for help

DISTURBED BODY IMAGE (see PACEMAKERS)

Related to: changes in physical appearance, deformities of joints, biophysical factors

Defining Characteristics: verbal response to actual change in structure and/or function, fear of rejection, fear of reaction from others, negative feelings about body, refusal to participate in care, refusal to look at self, withdrawal from social contacts, withdrawal from family, presence of deformities to joints, biophysical changes

DRESSING/GROOMING SELF-CARE DEFICIT (see ALZHEIMER'S DISEASE)

Related to: arthritis, musculoskeletal impairment, cognitive impairment, pain, limited joint movement, loss of joint function

Defining Characteristics: inability to put on or take off clothing, inability to maintain appropriate appearance, inability to fasten clothing, inability to pick up clothing, inability to brush/comb hair, inability to shave, inability to brush teeth

BATHING/HYGIENE SELF-CARE DEFICIT (see ALZHEIMER'S DISEASE)

Related to: arthritis, impaired mobility status, pain, musculoskeletal impairment, limited joint movement, loss of function

Defining Characteristics: inability to wash body or body parts, inability to obtain bath supplies, inability to obtain water source, inability to get into and out of bathroom, inability to dry body, inability to take off necessary clothing, inability to maintain appearance at satisfactory level, inability to brush teeth, inability to comb/brush hair, inability to shave

ADDITIONAL NURSING DIAGNOSES

 DEFICIENT KNOWLEDGE

Related to: lack of knowledge and understanding of arthritis disease process and changes associated with the aging process, lack of cognitive skill, pain

Defining Characteristics: verbalized questions about disease, inability to follow instructions, lack of recall, inappropriate behavior, presence of preventable complications

Outcome Criteria

✔ Patient will be able to verbalize a basic understanding of his disease process and treatment modalities.

NOC: *Knowledge: Disease Process*

INTERVENTIONS	RATIONALES
Instruct patient/family regarding type of arthritis, the differences between types, and symptoms of each.	Facilitates knowledge of disease process and what to expect. Osteoarthritis is the most common joint disease in patients

INTERVENTIONS	RATIONALES
	over 65 and involves the hyaline cartilage and subchondral bone. Rheumatoid arthritis is a syndrome of inflammatory changes in the peripheral joints that progressively destroys articular and periarticular structures, and increases in prevalence up to age 80.
Evaluate patient's ability to understand information, and if necessary, instruct family members.	Patient may have other concurrent disease processes that impair cognitive ability.
Provide quite, calm environment for learning.	Helps patient to be able to process information without distracting stimuli.
Provide small increments of knowledge at a time; do not overwhelm patient/family with all information in one sitting.	Abundance of knowledge will overwhelm both patient and family member. Gradually increasing knowledge base will facilitate better recall and compliance with regimen.
Provide instruction in written form, with large print.	Elderly patients may require larger print in order to be able to see information. Written information will provide reference once patient is discharged from hospital.
Instruct patient/family regarding specific treatment modalities for his type of arthritis, with effects, side effects, and symptoms to report to physician or nurse.	NSAIDs are commonly used to decrease inflammation and pain, but have a high incidence of GI bleeding and toxicity in elderly patients over 65 years old. Corticosteroids help to reduce pain and disability effects, but must be tapered off, and are difficult to discontinue. They also have long-term side effects, such as osteoporosis, cataracts, poor wound healing, and hyperglycemia. Antirheumatic drugs used for treatment of RA may slow the disease process, improve function and reduce morbidity only if used early in the course to prevent joint destruction and disability. Elderly patients who receive

(continues)

(continued)

INTERVENTIONS	RATIONALES
	methotrexate should be monitored for liver toxicity, interstitial pneumonitis, bone marrow suppression, and GI bleeding. Gold compounds are older drugs sometimes used in patients who cannot tolerate other drugs, but may have side effects of pruritis, dermatitis, stomatitis, and pancytopenia. COX-2 inhibitors are used for their anti-inflammatory effects as well as having less GI irritation and antiplatelet action. Side effects can occur in the form of renal dysfunction, and sodium and water retention.
Instruct patient/family regarding surgery and prepare patient for surgery as warranted.	Surgery may be the patient's only option if all drug therapy and other conservative methods have failed. The treatment of choice for OA is total joint replacement, and for RA is synovectomy.

INTERVENTIONS	RATIONALES
Instruct patient/family regarding the need for continuing mobility exercises unless exacerbational flare-up occurs.	Therapy, exercises, and movement help to maintain mobility in joints and decrease pain.

NIC: *Teaching: Disease Process*

Discharge and Maintenance Evaluation

- Patient/family will be able to accurately verbalize understanding of the differences between OA and RA, and their treatments.

- Patient/family will be able to accurately verbalize understanding of patient's medication regimen and be compliant with dosages and timing.

- Patient/family will be able to accurately verbalize understanding regarding the need for surgery and can discuss post-op care.

- Patient/family will be able to ask questions and verbalize concerns and receive appropriate answers from caregivers.

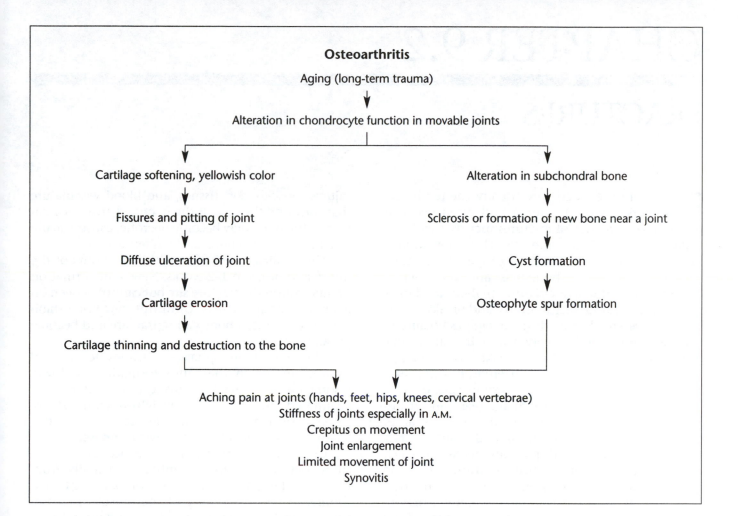

Osteoarthritis

Aging (long-term trauma)

↓

Alteration in chondrocyte function in movable joints

Cartilage softening, yellowish color

↓

Fissures and pitting of joint

↓

Diffuse ulceration of joint

↓

Cartilage erosion

↓

Cartilage thinning and destruction to the bone

Alteration in subchondral bone

↓

Sclerosis or formation of new bone near a joint

↓

Cyst formation

↓

Osteophyte spur formation

Aching pain at joints (hands, feet, hips, knees, cervical vertebrae)
Stiffness of joints especially in A.M.
Crepitus on movement
Joint enlargement
Limited movement of joint
Synovitis

CHAPTER 9.2

FRACTURES

Fractures in the elderly are usually the result of a low-energy type of trauma and often occur at home. The incidence of fractures increases with age beginning in one's 60s and 70s. This population is predisposed to fractures because of age-related osteoporosis, which reduces bone mass and causes deterioration of the microvasculature, making the bones more fragile and subject to injury and breaks.

Falls are greatly feared in the elderly because of the significant rise in incidence of fractures. They lose muscle tone, have muscle weakness and changes in gait and balance, encounter environmental hazards, have neurosensory and neuromuscular deficits, foot disorders, peripheral vascular disease, and arthritis, and are usually on multiple medications, all of which can contribute to falling and potential fractures. Types of falls include premonitory falling which occurs as a result of tripping or stumbling, drop attacks which occur as a result of loss of consciousness without warning for some unknown reason, and falling that is the result of multiple falls from either physical or mental impairment or disease. Pathologic fractures which result from the underlying disorder that undermines the bone structure are normally the result of osteoporosis, malignancy, metabolic disorders, infection, or benign bone tumors.

A long bone is divided into the shaft, or diaphysis, the articular area at each end of the bone (the epiphysis), and the flared areas joining the diaphysis and epiphysis (the metaphysis). The strength of the trabecular bone that comprises the epiphyses and metaphyses is directly proportional to its density, and density decreases with age. The bone density at which the risk of fracture becomes likely is approximately 0.77 g/cm^3 for the proximal femur and bone density less than this increases the risk of fracture (Dowd & Cavalieri, 1999).

Fractures tend to heal in three stages composed of inflammation, repair, and remodeling. Inflammatory phases begin as an immediate reaction to the injury. The trauma that makes the bone fracture also injures muscles, soft tissues, and blood vasculature that surround the area. If the fractured area devascularizes, the bone may become necrotic, causing acute inflammation, swelling, and tenderness.

The repair phase begins within 24 hours of the injury and peaks in 1–2 weeks. New bone formation occurs around the fracture site but cannot be seen on X-ray for about 6 weeks. Until this new bone stabilizes, the fractured bone can re-fracture and become misaligned.

The remodeling phase continues for several months in which the callus formation is slowly resorbed and replaced by stronger bone that is disseminated to withstand weight-bearing stress. Patients normally feel some degree of discomfort when performing activity during this phase.

Complications that may occur because of fractures include pulmonary embolism, usually from blood or fat particulate, and compartment syndrome, in which swelling of the muscle increases pressure and decreases normal tissue perfusion to the point of ischemia and potential necrosis.

MEDICAL CARE

Laboratory: CBC used to identify presence of infection, loss of blood, or platelet dysfunction; coagulation profiles used to identify presence of coagulopathy or to determine efficacy of anticoagulant therapy; alkaline phosphatase levels used to identify fracture healing; levels increase with remodeling phase or with malignancies or metabolic disorders; calcium levels may be used to identify imbalances, metastatic disease, or endocrine disorders; electrolyte profiles used to identify deficiencies or imbalances

Radiography: used to identify the presence, site, and type of fracture

CT scan: may be used as an adjunctive test to show occult fractures, and to determine extent of articular surface disruption with joint fractures; CT scans may also be used to identify bone destruction or soft tissue masses

Magnetic resonance imaging: MRIs show soft tissue damage and can identify occult fractures, pathological fractures, and osteonecrosis and osteomyelitis that mimic fractures

Bone scan: may be done to detect focal injury; occult fractures can be identified 3–5 days after injury; used to evaluate for metastatic and metabolic bone disease if pathologic fracture is diagnosed or suspected

Analgesics: buprenorphine hydrochloride (Buprenex), butophanol tartrate (Stadol), codeine phosphate, hydromorphone hydrochloride (Dilaudid), meperidine hydrochloride (Demerol), methadone hydrochloride (Dolophine), morphine hydrochloride or sulfate (Duramorph, Infumorph, Morphine, MS Contin, Roxanol, Statex), nalbuphine hydrochloride (Nubain), oxycodone hydrochloride (OxyContin), oxymorphone hydrochloride (Numorphan), pentazocine hydrochloride or lactate (Talwin), or tramadol hydrochloride (Ultram) used to relieve pain of inflammation and infection

Casting: used to maintain alignment of the bones while they heal; cast should extend one joint above and one joint below the fracture site

Traction: should be used when casting or surgery contraindicated for the elderly patient because fracture is too fragmented or the patient's medical conditions make them unstable and poor surgical risks; traction in the elderly extremely hazardous because of potential for complications, such as PE, DVT, pressure sores, and pulmonary infection

Surgery: may be required to realign the bones or stabilize the fracture in order to restore function; may be required if compartment syndrome occurs to release pressure to preserve tissue and muscle integrity; joint replacement may be required depending on the site of the fracture

COMMON NURSING DIAGNOSES

 IMPAIRED PHYSICAL MOBILITY (see PACEMAKERS, ALZHEIMER'S DISEASE)

Related to: pain, limb immobilization, fracture, falls, trauma

Defining Characteristics: inability to move as desired, imposed restrictions on activity, decreased muscle strength, decreased muscle coordination, pain, limited range of motion, impaired gait, foot problems, loss of physical function, swelling at fracture site

 RISK FOR TRAUMA (see DIABETES MELLITUS)

Related to: fracture, weakness, lack of safety precautions, cognitive or emotional difficulties, history of previous trauma, impairment of physical condition, impaired sensory perception, compartment syndrome

Defining Characteristics: joint dysfunction, foot drop, ulceration of leg or foot, slow healing, bruising of tissues, fractures of bones, unsafe environment, improper medication administration, impaired mobility, falls

 ACUTE PAIN (see CAD)

Related to: fracture, trauma, compartment syndrome, falls

Defining Characteristics: communication of pain, facial grimacing, restlessness, changes in pulse and blood pressure, diaphoresis, protective behavior of fracture site, hypoactive reflexes, decreased motor activity, decreased muscle strength, tissue bruising, swelling

CHRONIC PAIN (see PERIPHERAL VASCULAR DISEASE)

Related to: chronic pain during remodeling phase of fracture healing, inflammatory process

Defining Characteristics: verbal report of pain for more than 6 months, altered ability to continue previous activities, physical withdrawal, social withdrawal, guarded behavior, protective behavior of affected fracture site, facial grimacing, crying, moaning, atrophy of muscle, irritability, restlessness, hypersensitivity, depression, fatigue, insomnia

 DECREASED CARDIAC OUTPUT (see CAD)

Related to: bleeding into tissues from fracture, insufficient blood to the heart, complications from fracture

Defining Characteristics: decreased hemoglobin and hematocrit, dehydration, electrolyte imbalances, ECG changes, dysrhythmias, chest pain, coughing, dyspnea, adventitious breath sounds, wheezing, fatigue, syncope, restlessness, cold, clammy skin, decreased peripheral pulses, jugular vein distention, skin color changes, pallor, cyanosis, changes in blood pressure, edema, cardiac gallops, changes in mental status, disorientation

RISK FOR IMPAIRED SKIN INTEGRITY (see PERIPHERAL VASCULAR DISEASE)

Related to: fracture, fall, application of traction, surgical intervention, aging process, pressure on skin surfaces, bed rest, immobility, alteration in arterial and venous circulation, alterations in tissue perfusion, presence of shearing forces on skin

Defining Characteristics: thin, dry skin on extremities, redness to pressure areas, edema, ulcerations or lesions to extremities, dermatitis, mottling, cyanosis, pallor, decreased or absent pulses, warmth to area, disruption of skin surface, excoriation of skin, decreased tactile sensation, presence of traction apparatus

DEFICIENT FLUID VOLUME (see GI BLEEDING)

Related to: bleeding into soft tissues, bleeding from fracture

Defining Characteristics: hypotension, tachycardia, decreased skin turgor, weakness, decreased urinary output, pallor, diaphoresis, decreased capillary refill, mental changes, restlessness, decreased filling pressures, decreased hemoglobin and hematocrit, dry mucous membranes, increased hematocrit initially, concentrated urine, thirst, weakness

INEFFECTIVE TISSUE PERFUSION: CARDIOPULMONARY, CEREBRAL, PERIPHERAL (see CAD, CVA, AND PERIPHERAL VASCULAR DISEASE)

Related to: complications from fracture, pulmonary embolism, compartmental syndrome, reduced oxygen supply, hypovolemia, hypoxia, vasoconstrictive therapy, hypoperfusion, coexisting disease processes, age-related vascular structure changes, inactivity, surgery

Defining Characteristics: chest pain, conduction disturbances, dysrhythmias, vital sign changes, ECG changes, delayed capillary refill time, chest retractions, dyspnea, nasal flaring, use of accessory muscles, increased work of breathing, tachypnea, bradypnea, changes in mental status, weakness, paralysis, behavioral changes, abdominal distention, ileus, hypoactive or absent bowel sounds, nausea, vomiting, edema, weak or absent peripheral pulses, skin temperature changes, skin color changes, decreased peripheral tactile sensation

ADDITIONAL NURSING DIAGNOSES

RISK FOR INJURY

Related to: sensory dysfunction, integrative dysfunction, aging, decreased cardiac output, decreased cerebral flow, mobility impairment, medications, decreased tissue perfusion, pain

Defining Characteristics: verbalization of pain, changes in mentation, alterations in visual and tactile perception, decreased functional ability of body systems, decreased effects of interrelationships of systems, depression, bone loss, weak muscle, support system, decreased muscle tone, poor posture, drowsiness, impaired judgment, decreased pulses, changes in skin temperature, inability to move at will, polypharmacy

Outcome Criteria

✔ Patient will have no complications from trauma or fracture caused by falls.

NOC: *Risk Control*

INTERVENTIONS	RATIONALES
Assess type of medications, effect of medications, and number of medications being taken.	Several medications may be prescribed for more than one medical condition. Drug absorption, distribution, and excretion are altered in the aged, causing confusion, and forgetfulness leading to falls.
Assess patient's accident proneness, presence of agitation, ambulatory status, interference with thinking, balance, gait, hostility, depression or suicidal tendency, and need for attention.	Conditions may predispose falls in the elderly.

INTERVENTIONS	RATIONALES
Maintain vigilance and supervision when needed.	Accident prevention maintains safety of patient.
Reduce unsafe activities and behaviors, or modify, if appropriate.	Reduces risk of falls.
Evaluate patient for coexisting diseases and their effect on patient's current problem.	Additional medical conditions may cause increased symptoms for injury, and predispose patient to additional complications.
Assess patient's pulses distal for fracture, presence of edema, or color changes.	May indicate the presence of compartment syndrome, which requires emergency treatment to prevent necrosis and loss of tissue.
Monitor lab work, especially CBC and electrolytes.	Patient may have lost significant amounts of blood into the soft tissues and require transfusions for decreased circulating blood volume. Electrolytes may become imbalanced and result in cardiac and mental changes. Toxic levels of prescribed medications may occur as a result of dehydration, other medicines' potentiating action, or inhibition of medication action that may cause injury to patient.

INTERVENTIONS	RATIONALES
Instruct patient in safe operation of wheelchair or other assistive devices.	Promotes safety.
Instruct patient in responsible administration of all medications.	Prevents mistakes causing overdoses and untoward side effects, leading to accidents.

NIC: *Traction/Immobilization Care*

Discharge or Maintenance Evaluation

- Patient will have no accidental falls or injury.
- Patient will exhibit no other fractures or tissue trauma.
- Patient will be able to administer correct doses of medications at correct times.
- Patient will have stable mentation status, and have no complications from fracture injury.
- Patient will not exhibit any signs or symptoms of compartment syndrome, anemia, or electrolyte imbalance.
- Patient will not have any adverse reaction to medications being given.

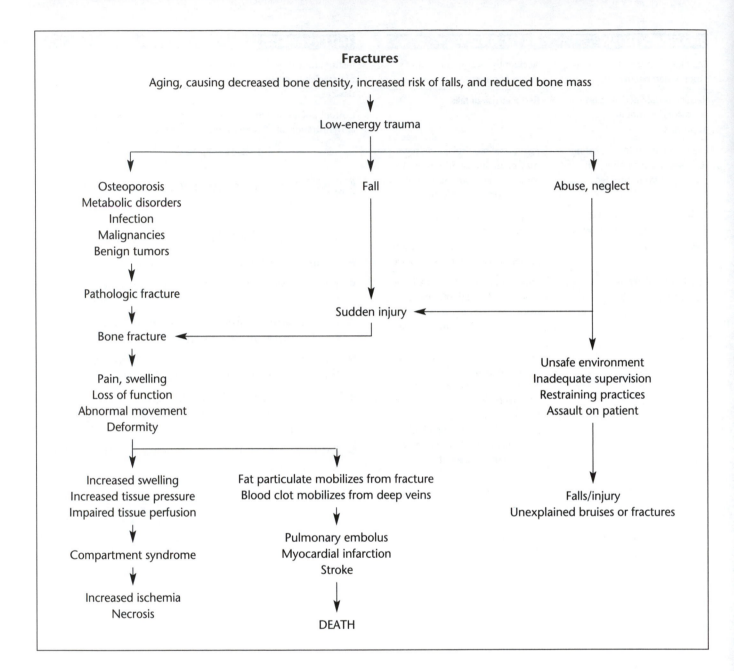

Fractures

Aging, causing decreased bone density, increased risk of falls, and reduced bone mass

Low-energy trauma

Osteoporosis
Metabolic disorders
Infection
Malignancies
Benign tumors

Fall

Abuse, neglect

Pathologic fracture

Sudden injury

Bone fracture

Unsafe environment
Inadequate supervision
Restraining practices
Assault on patient

Pain, swelling
Loss of function
Abnormal movement
Deformity

Increased swelling
Increased tissue pressure
Impaired tissue perfusion

Fat particulate mobilizes from fracture
Blood clot mobilizes from deep veins

Falls/injury
Unexplained bruises or fractures

Compartment syndrome

Pulmonary embolus
Myocardial infarction
Stroke

Increased ischemia
Necrosis

DEATH

CHAPTER 9.3

OSTEOPOROSIS

Osteoporosis is a disease that causes the bones to gradually lose mass by mineral resorption that exceeds bone formation, and results in brittle, porous, thinning bones and an increased potential for fractures. This deterioration of the bone is common to all elderly patients, but is increased by immobility, decreased estrogen secretion, altered intestinal absorption of calcium, short stature, lack of weight-bearing use, and decreased intake of calcium. When there is not enough calcium in the blood to maintain essential components of the body, such as the heart, nerves, and muscles, osteoclast cells liberate calcium from the bone, which results in gaps and decreased solidity.

Osteoporosis, which literally means "porous bones," develops over long periods of time and causes the eventual loss in height, kyphosis (dowager's hump), a shorter trunk, and decreased thorax movement that lead to respiratory problems and self-image disturbances. Smoking, alcohol abuse, and a calcium-deficient diet increase the potential for the disease. Lack of sun exposure also places patients at risk because the skin requires the absorption of some ultraviolet light in order to synthesize vitamin D, which is essential for strong bones.

Some medical disorders and medications that may lead to the increased development of secondary osteoporosis include diabetes, hyperthyroidism, Cushing's syndrome, kidney dysfunction, and the use of thyroid hormone replacement, corticosteroids, and phenytoin.

Osteoporosis in the elderly is classified as type I or II, with type I being menopausal osteoporosis that occurs in patients aged 51–75 and is connected with vertebral and Colles' fractures. Type II, or senescent osteoporosis, happens in patients over the age of 60, and results in vertebral or hip fractures (Dowd & Cavalieri, 1999).

The most universal symptom of osteoporosis is a fracture, usually of the vertebrae, wrists, or hips. Osteoporotic bones may collapse from the everyday pressure of standing or walking, or merely from stepping off a curb. These fractures often cause severe pain, and if surgery is required, as in the instance of hip fractures, morbidity is high from the complications of surgery, such as immobilization in the elderly.

Once osteoporosis is diagnosed, treatment is aimed at prevention of further deterioration in bone mass and treating the underlying disease process that may have contributed to osteoporosis in the first place. Analgesics, heat, massage, orthopedic support and therapy, and surgery are often required. Estrogen replacement therapy helps to slow bone loss and prevent fractures in women who already have osteoporosis because of its ability to improve calcium absorption. Calcitonin has been shown to inhibit osteoclast function so that bone tissue does not deteriorate.

MEDICAL CARE

Laboratory: calcium and phosphorus levels used to identify changes related to bone destruction, to evaluate treatment, and to identify potential for hyperparathyroidism, vitamin D abnormalities, liver disease, renal disease, thyroid disease, myeloma, or Cushing's disease; alkaline phosphatase used to identify presence of fracture or neoplasm with increased levels; thyroid profiles used to identify presence of thyroid dysfunction as cause of osteoporosis; renal and liver profiles used to identify dysfunction as a cause of disease, to identify sodium increases that can result in increased urinary calcium loss, and to monitor for complications from medication therapy; vitamin D levels used to identify malabsorption or toxicity; vitamin K levels used to identify deficiency that can increase fracture risk; glucose levels used to identify dysfunction from medication interaction

Radiography: X-rays used to identify fractures and other causes of bone disease

CT scan: used to identify true volumetric bone density

Dual energy X-ray absorptiometry (DEXA): bone density testing used to measure bone mineral density but does not measure true volumetric density

Bone densitometry: the only method for diagnosing or confirming osteoporosis without the presence of a fracture; measurement in the elderly frequently complicated by the presence of osteoarthritis, degenerative disk disease, or by aortic calcifications

Dual-proton absorptiometry: used to identify bone density in the hand, but not accurate at predicting fractures

Calcium: used to replace inadequate intake

Vitamin D: used to regulate serum calcium in the management of metabolic bone disease; vitamin D is necessary for calcium absorption in the intestines

Antiresorptive therapy: several different types of drugs used to prevent bone resorption and the progression of bone loss; vitamin D analogues (calcifediol [Calderol] or calcitriol [Calcijex, Rocaltrol]) stimulate calcium absorption from the GI tract and help to increase movement of calcium from the bone to the blood system; biphosphonates (calcitonin, human or salmon [Cibacalcin, Calcimar, Miacalcin, Osteocalcin, Salmonine], or etidronate disodium [Didronel]) directly inhibit osteoclast activity and reduce the incidence of fractures, but must be taken on an empty stomach and have been shown to have adverse GI effects; calcitonin inhibits osteoclast function and also relieves pain of vertebral fractures; estrogen replacement (17 beta-estradiol/norgestimate [Ortho-Prefest], estradiol cypionate or valerate [Alora, Climara, Estrace, Fempatch, Depo-Estradiol, Depogen, Clinagen, Menaval], estradiol/norethindrone acetate [Combipatch], conjugated estrogens [Premarin], estropipate [Ogen, Eortho-Est], ethinyl estradiol and desogestrel [Desogen, Ortho-Cept], ethinyl estradiol and norethindrone acetate [Loestrin], ethinyl estradiol and norgestimate [Ortho-Cyclen], medroxyprogesterone acetate [Amen, Curretab, Cycrin, Depo-Provera, Provera], and norethindrone [Micronor, Aygestin]); can help prevent menopausal bone loss in most women, and when given in conjunction with progestin, prevents endometrial hyperplasia and avoids the potential for malignancy; it improves calcium absorption and decreases excretion via the kidneys; selective estrogen receptor modulators (SERMs) (raloxifene hydrochloride [Evista]) used to prevent postmenopausal bone loss and decrease the incidence of vertebral fractures, as well as reducing the risk of

breast cancer; these drugs reduce the resorption of bone and increase bone mineral density, but are antiestrogenic in the breast and uterus

Fluoride: used as adjunctive treatment with calcium and vitamin D to help prevent bone loss

COMMON NURSING DIAGNOSES

 ### IMPAIRED PHYSICAL MOBILITY (see ALZHEIMER'S DISEASE)

Related to: pain, fractures, bone loss

Defining Characteristics: inability to move as desired, imposed restrictions on activity, decreased muscle strength, decreased muscle coordination, pain, limited range of motion, reluctance to attempt movement; presence of fracture restricting movement

 ### RISK FOR TRAUMA (see DIABETES MELLITUS)

Related to: fracture, bone loss, weakness from bone demineralization as a result of changes from aging and osteoporosis, falls

Defining Characteristics: spontaneous fracture, difficulty bending or climbing stairs, fracture resulting from minimal or no trauma, unsafe environment, past fractures from falls, bruising of tissues, impaired mobility

ACUTE PAIN (see CAD)

Related to: fracture, trauma, falls related to osteoporitic changes in bones associated with aging process

Defining Characteristics: communication of pain, facial grimacing, restlessness, changes in pulse and blood pressure, diaphoresis, protective behavior of fracture site, hypoactive reflexes, decreased motor activity, decreased muscle strength, tissue bruising, swelling

ADDITIONAL NURSING DIAGNOSES

 ### RISK FOR POISONING

Related to: drug toxicity, interactions with medications prescribed, polypharmacy, analgesic abuse, physiologic changes associated with the aging process, cognitive limitations

Defining Characteristics: use of numerous medications, adverse medicine effects, drug toxicity levels, inability to take medications correctly, pain, use of analgesic in doses sufficient to cause toxicity or interact with other medicines, inhibition of the action of medicines by use of another medication, use of alcohol, confusion, disorientation, impaired vision, multiple health care providers, multiple pharmacies, inability to understand drug interactions or usage

Outcome Criteria

✔ Patient will be able to take prescribed medications in correct quantities at correct times, and will not exhibit signs or symptoms of drug interactions or toxicity.

NOC: *Knowledge: Medication*

INTERVENTIONS	RATIONALES
Evaluate patient's entire collection of medications, including over-the-counter drugs, vitamin and mineral supplements, herbal remedies, and dietary regimen.	Provides information as to what drugs and substances are being utilized concurrently and what drug interactions may occur with concurrent use, as well as with dietary consumption. Incorrect administration of medications to be taken on an empty stomach may cause inhibition of the appropriate action of the drug. Concurrent use of other medications can result in potentiation of action and create drug toxicity.
Encourage patient/family to utilize one primary doctor to coordinate care.	Prevents utilization of several physicians who are unaware of each other's treatment regimens and may duplicate medication or prescribe medication that may affect other drugs.
Administer drugs as ordered, being cognizant of any interactions that might be possible.	Frequently elderly patients are on several medications, and the medicines used in the treatment of osteoporosis can interact with other drugs, causing either a decrease or potentiation of their action.
Provide instructions for use of medications, quantity, frequency, number of doses and times, and under what conditions they are to be taken.	Facilitates understanding of medication regimen and provides reference material once patient is discharged.

INTERVENTIONS	RATIONALES
Ensure medication labels are inscribed in large print with dosage instructions.	Prevents medication errors for patients with visual impairments.
Assist patient/family to establish a system for following medication regimen accurately, such as calendars, charts, medication boxes that are labeled for each day of the week, and so forth.	Assists in reduction of medication errors and assists family to be involved in patient's care.
Discuss medications with physician about potential for using alternative long-acting drugs that require only one daily dosage.	May help to decrease the number of medications per day and simplify the patient's regimen and facilitate compliance.
Monitor lab work for toxicity levels, imbalances of electrolytes and other factors pertinent to patient's medication profile.	Helps to reduce risk of toxicity. Age-related changes in the body, such as renal or liver impairment, decrease metabolism of drugs, so what may be considered a normal dosage may become toxic for patient with impaired function.
Instruct patient/family regarding all medications, their use, effect, side effects, and adverse reactions that should be reported to physician.	Helps to promote knowledge and facilitates compliance.
Instruct patient/family to store drugs in a secure area away from the bedside.	Elderly patients may have memory loss, forgetting that they have already taken medicine, and double the dose taken. Frequently, elderly patients keep their medications in their bedside table to prevent the need to get up at night.
Instruct patient/family regarding interactions that may occur with concurrent medication usage.	SERMs decreased the action of anticoagulants and ampicillin; biphosphanates can result in hypercalcemia; estrogens can decrease the action of anticoagulants and oral hypoglycemics, and other drugs, such as anticonvulsants, barbiturates, rifampin, and calcium can decrease the action of estrogens.

NIC: *Teaching: Prescribed Medication*

Discharge or Maintenance Evaluation

■ Patient will be able to accurately verbalize understanding of need for one medical provider to control care.

- Patient/family will be able to accurately verbalize understanding of all medications, their effects, side effects, and potential drug interactions.
- Patient/family will be compliant with providing safe environment for the patient by keeping medications in a secure location.
- Patient/family will be able to accurately verbalize understanding of appropriate medication administration and will devise a method that works for promoting this.
- Patient will exhibit no signs or symptoms of drug toxicity, or suffer problems with drug interactions.

DEFICIENT KNOWLEDGE

Related to: lack of exposure to information regarding medications, dietary modifications, or safe activity program

Defining Characteristics: verbalization of the problem, request for information, fear of further bone loss and fracture, presence of preventable complications

Outcome Criteria

✔ Patient will achieve increased knowledge and compliance with medical regimen to minimize bone demineralization and injury.

NOC: *Knowledge: Medication*

INTERVENTIONS	RATIONALES
Assess patient's knowledge of disease, diet, medication, and exercise program to arrest progression of bone deterioration.	Provides basis for teaching and techniques to promote compliance. Disease is not usually detected until 25–40% of calcium in bone is lost.
Provide support of body image and lifestyle changes.	Assists patient to cope with chronicity of disease and potential fractures causing pain and immobility.
Assist to plan exercise program according to capabilities; to avoid flexion of spine and wear corset if appropriate (walking is preferred to jogging).	Exercise will strengthen bone. Vertebral collapse is common and corset provides support.

INTERVENTIONS	RATIONALES
Instruct patient in methods to perform activities of daily living and to avoid lifting, bending, or carrying heavy objects.	Prevents injury that can occur in osteoporosis with minimal trauma.
Instruct patient/family in administration of calcium, vitamin D, estrogens, and other drug therapy for osteoporosis.	Provides replacement of calcium and helps to decrease bone loss.
Instruct patient/family regarding the need to include calcium in dietary management.	Provides calcium supplementation by dietary intake.
Instruct patient/family regarding potential referrals to therapy as warranted.	May help to provide exercise and the development of an activity program to maintain bone condition and encourage independence in ADLs.
Instruct patient/family regarding the use of assistive devices and safety precautions that are available to maintain mobility.	Prevents further trauma or fractures from falls resulting from lack of support.

NIC: *Teaching: Disease Process*

Discharge or Maintenance Evaluation

- Patient will be compliant with medication and dietary instructions.
- Patient will be able to perform daily exercises within identified limitations and to prevent further bone loss/deterioration.
- Patient will exhibit no injury, fall, or trauma that might predispose to a fracture.
- Patient will be independent in performing ADLs with modifications.
- Patient/family will be able to accurately verbalize understanding of medications and methods of administration.

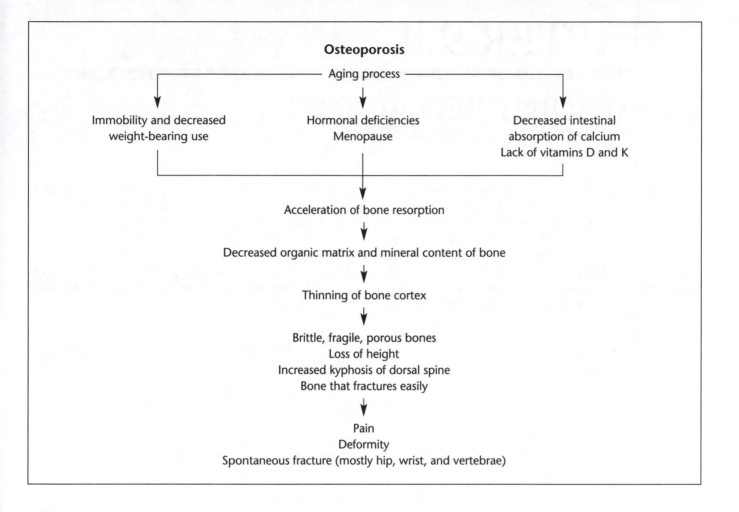

Osteoporosis

Aging process

Immobility and decreased
weight-bearing use

Hormonal deficiencies
Menopause

Decreased intestinal
absorption of calcium
Lack of vitamins D and K

Acceleration of bone resorption

Decreased organic matrix and mineral content of bone

Thinning of bone cortex

Brittle, fragile, porous bones
Loss of height
Increased kyphosis of dorsal spine
Bone that fractures easily

Pain
Deformity
Spontaneous fracture (mostly hip, wrist, and vertebrae)

CHAPTER 9.4

TOTAL JOINT REPLACEMENT

Total joint replacement, or total joint arthroplasty, is a procedure, usually of the knee or hip, in which an artificial joint is inserted in place of the patient's own joint which is usually fractured, diseased, or deteriorated. For a total hip replacement the femoral head and acetabulum of the hip joint are surgically removed and a prosthetic device is placed. Total knee replacement is the surgical removal of the surfaces where the tibia and femur articulate at the knee joint, and of the patella, if necessary, with a prosthetic replacement.

Joint replacement in the elderly requires less physiologic demands on their impaired musculoskeletal system, and usually provides for a more speedy recovery of return to normal function and weight-bearing use. In fact, hip replacement was originally introduced for patients over the age of 65 who had severe osteoarthritis. Total joint replacement is the treatment of choice when displaced fractures cannot be managed with an open reduction and internal fixation intervention due to postoperative osteonecrosis or nonunion of the bone, for patients with unrelenting pain and irreversibly damaged joints, for congenital hip disease, for pathologic fractures resulting from metastatic carcinoma, and for failure from previous reconstructive orthopedic surgery or complications, such as avascular necrosis.

The prosthetic devices are made of metal and polyethylene and replace the damaged bone fragments to restore skeletal strength. The hip prosthesis consists of a smooth metal ball attached to a stem that is lodged into the medullary canal of the femur and an internal metal-polyethylene prosthesis that is placed in the acetabulum, into which the ball then fits. Other prostheses are designed to be stabilized inside the femur and coated with an acrylic cement of porous metal to attach it directly to the bone. The selection of the prosthesis depends on the specific patient's needs, including bone structure, age, activity level, and joint stability.

Contraindications for these types of procedures include the presence of an active infection or neurotrophic joint disease. Any patient whose pain is severe enough to interfere with sleep or daily activities is considered a candidate for total joint replacement in the absence of any contraindications. Complications that can ensue following surgery include infection and the potential that the prosthetic device will require repair or replacement after 10–12 years.

MEDICAL CARE

Laboratory: CBC used to identify anemia and infection, and to evaluate for blood loss post-op; electrolyte profiles used to identify potential imbalances; renal profiles used to evaluate for renal insufficiency postoperatively; coagulation profiles may be drawn for potential coagulopathies

Radiography: used to identify fracture site, type of fracture, and presence of nonunion from previous surgeries; also used to identify any postoperative nonalignment of new joint and bones

Magnetic resonance imaging: to be done prior to insertion of joint replacement; used to identify complications such as avascular necrosis, soft tissue injury, or metastatic lesions

Analgesics: acetaminophen (Tylenol), ibuprofen (Motrin, Advil, Genpril, Ibuprofen, Nuprin, Trendar), and acetylsalicylic acid (ASA, aspirin) used to alleviate mild to moderate pain and to help reduce inflammation; buprenorphine hydrochloride (Buprenex), butophanol tartrate (Stadol), codeine phosphate, hydromorphone hydrochloride (Dilaudid), meperidine hydrochloride (Demerol), methadone hydrochloride (Dolophine), morphine hydrochloride or sulfate (Duramorph, Infumorph, Morphine, MS Contin, Roxanol, Statex), nalbuphine hydrochloride (Nubain), oxycodone hydrochloride (OxyContin), oxymorphone hydrochloride (Numorphan), pentazocine hydrochloride or lactate (Talwin), or tramadol hydrochloride (Ultram) used to relieve the pain immediately post-op and for severe pain

Surgery: joint reformation or total joint replacement done to restore function to the elderly patient

COMMON NURSING DIAGNOSES

DEFICIENT FLUID VOLUME (see GI BLEEDING)

Related to: surgical wound bleeding, hemorrhage, vasculature that has not been completely sealed during surgery

Defining Characteristics: hypotension, tachycardia, decreased skin turgor, weakness, decreased urinary output, pallor, diaphoresis, decreased capillary refill, mental changes, restlessness, decreased filling pressures, decreased hemoglobin and hematocrit, dry mucous membranes, increased drainage in suction container (more than 200–500 cc/24 hours), concentrated urine, thirst, weakness, pallor

IMPAIRED PHYSICAL MOBILITY (see PACEMAKER)

Related to: pain, immobilization, intolerance of activity, surgery

Defining Characteristics: inability to move as desired, imposed restrictions on activity, decreased muscle strength, decreased muscle coordination, pain, limited range of motion, decreased endurance, surgical procedures, presence of drainage tubes, reluctance to attempt movement, fear of falling or dislocating prosthesis, impaired weight-bearing ability, impaired movement of operative side, inability to move within bed easily, inability to transfer or ambulate without assistance

RISK FOR TRAUMA (see DIABETES MELLITUS)

Related to: fracture, surgery, weakness, lack of environmental safety

Defining Characteristics: joint dysfunction, foot drop, slow healing, bruising of tissues, fractures of bones, unsafe environment, improper medication administration, impaired mobility, falls, slippery floors, littered pathways, poor lighting, unsteady gait, incoordination, improper use of assistive aids for support when ambulating, poor-fitting shoes, impaired vision, confusion, medications

ACUTE PAIN (see INTERSTITIAL CYSTITIS)

Related to: surgery, inflammation, infection, muscle spasms

Defining Characteristics: communication of pain, fever, malaise, abdominal pain, abdominal distention, elevated white blood cell count, surgical wound, drains, guarding of surgical site, tachycardia, hypotension, hypertension, bradypnea, tachypnea, facial grimacing, crying, moaning, muscle spasms following surgery

ADDITIONAL NURSING DIAGNOSES

RISK FOR INFECTION

Related to: total joint replacement surgery, delayed wound healing related to the aging process, chronic comorbidities

Defining Characteristics: fever, tachycardia, tachypnea, elevated white blood cell count, shift to the left on differential, reddened wound, purulent drainage, drain tubes, edema, pain, sepsis, bleeding, allergic reaction to prosthetic device or to the orthopedic cement

Outcome Criteria

✔ Patient will exhibit no signs or symptoms of infection to surgical wound site, or systemic infection.

NOC: *Wound Healing: Primary Intention*

INTERVENTIONS	RATIONALES
Monitor vital signs every 1–2 hours postoperatively. Notify physician of significant changes.	Increased temperature, tachycardia, and/or tachypnea may indicate the presence of infection.
Observe surgical wound site for drainage, redness, swelling, dehiscence, and presence of drains.	Drains provide a method of removal of excessive drainage from the surgical site, but also provide a pathway for pathogenic entry and may result in infection. Purulent drainage from the wound indicates infection. Redness and swelling to the surgical area indicates that tissues are inflamed, and may progress to dehiscence of surgical wound.

(continues)

(continued)

INTERVENTIONS	RATIONALES
Change dressing as ordered using aseptic technique.	Provides for inspection of wound for signs of infection of dehiscence, cleaning of drainage from skin surfaces, and prevents infection.
Evaluate patient's complaints of pain, and medicate as ordered. If patient complains of sudden change in pain status, evaluate and notify physician.	Postoperative pain is to be expected, but sudden, severe pain may be indicative of further complications.
Administer IV fluids as ordered.	Provides hydration and venous access for administration of medications.
Administer antimicrobials as ordered.	Helps to prevent infection.
Encourage coughing and deep breathing every 2 hours. Use incentive spirometry prn and as ordered.	Helps to expand lungs and prevent atelectasis and pneumonia.
Turn patient every 2 hours, using special pillows to maintain alignment of body.	Helps to mobilize secretions, expand lungs, and decrease potential for respiratory complications. Maintenance of body alignment is crucial to avoid complications from dislocation of prosthesis.
Instruct patient regarding signs and symptoms of wound infection, increasing pain, or increased drainage, and to notify nurse or physician.	Provides for prompt notification and timely intervention.
Instruct patient in turning, coughing, and deep breathing, emphasizing the reasons behind this.	Helps promote understanding and facilitates compliance.
Instruct patient/family regarding the need to comply with diet.	Increased protein helps to facilitate cellular and wound healing and minimizes development of complications.
Instruct patient regarding methods of moving in bed while decreasing discomfort. Use of a trapeze bar, as well as ensuring sufficient help is present during turning procedure, will assist in maintaining good body alignment.	Assists in patient knowledge and facilitates compliance and assistance from patient with movement in bed. Decreases pain by use of smooth moves and gentle positioning. Having sufficient personnel during movement of patient also helps to prevent injury to the patient and to nursing staff.

NIC: *Wound Care*

Discharge or Maintenance Evaluation

■ Patient will be free of infection.

■ Patient's surgical wound will be clean, well-approximated, without redness, swelling, or drainage.

■ Patient will be able to accurately verbalize and demonstrate appropriate techniques for moving in bed, changing position, and coughing and deep breathing.

■ Patient will be compliant with dietary ingestion to facilitate prompt healing.

DEFICIENT KNOWLEDGE

Related to: lack of information regarding preservation of independence, mobility and exercises, and rehabilitation regimen

Defining Characteristics: request for information, fear of joint damage during rehabilitation regimen

Outcome Criteria

✔ Patient will achieve adequate knowledge to comply with follow-up care and progressive resumption of routine activities.

NOC: *Knowledge: Treatment Regimen*

INTERVENTIONS	RATIONALES
Assess patient's knowledge of exercise program according to capabilities and reason for rehabilitation regimen.	Provides basis for teaching and techniques to promote compliance.
Continue physical therapy and transfer techniques to chair or commode and use of aids for ambulation and personal care (raised toilet seat, walker, cane).	Provides for support and continued rehabilitative progress and promotes independence in self-care.
Continue muscle and joint exercises including ROM following rehabilitation regimen.	Maintains muscle strength and promotes endurance.
Instruct patient in use of walker or cane as appropriate. Instruct in gait training, weight bearing, and the use of proper footwear.	The elderly do not utilize crutches well. Use of assistive aids allows for mobility and allows the patient to be nonweight-bearing, partial- or full-weight–bearing. Proper shoes prevent slipping and danger of falls.

INTERVENTIONS	RATIONALES
Instruct patient to avoid leaning forward and reaching for articles on floor. Instruct to use pillow between knees, and avoid positions that cause internal rotation, flexion, or adduction of hip.	Prevents hip or knee flexion of more than 90° which may predispose the patient to prosthetic dislocation.
Instruct patient to avoid crossing legs, prolonged sitting, or sitting in low chairs with soft seats.	Prevents potential for injury and putting strain on affected side.
Instruct patient regarding keeping scheduled follow-up appointments with physician for X-rays, rehabilitation, therapy, and so forth.	Provides for further care postdischarge; The length of time for rehabilitation continues until the patient is able to ambulate and perform other activities independently.

NIC: *Teaching: Disease Process*

Discharge or Maintenance Evaluation

- Patient will be compliant with follow-up appointments with physician and participation in therapy and rehabilitation programs.
- Patient will be able to perform activities within limitations of chronic disease processes.
- Patient will be able to modify the environment to enhance independence in activity.
- Patient will be able to verbalize understanding of instructions and demonstrate compliance with limitations of mobility to avoid potential prosthetic dislocation.
- Patient will exhibit no signs or symptoms of complications from prosthetic device.

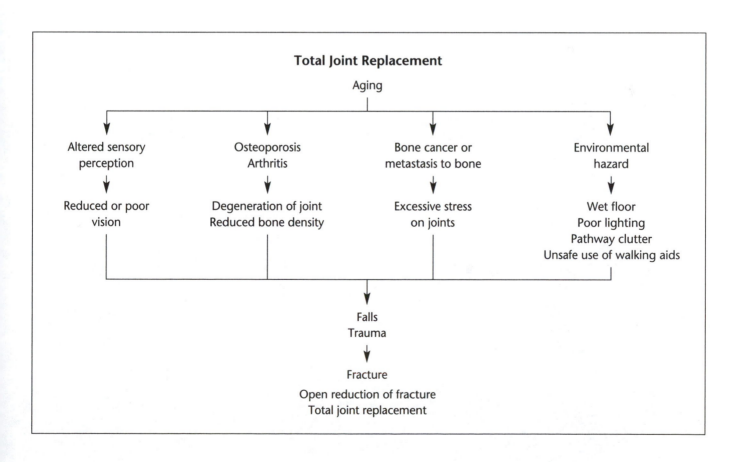

UNIT 10

INTEGUMENTARY SYSTEM

CHAPTER 10.1

HYPOTHERMIA

Systemic hypothermia results from exposure to prolonged or extreme cold with an unintended decrease in body temperature below 94° F or 34.4° C. It may occur even in cool temperatures if there are alterations in the patient's hemodynamics of homeostasis resulting from debility or chronic disease. Elderly patients who live in colder climates are particularly susceptible to cold injury, and of the recognized cases of hypothermia, morbidity is approximately 50%. The elderly who are 75 years of age and older are 5 times more likely to become a statistic of what is known as "winter deaths" (Beers & Berkow, 2000).

In patients who have concurrent cardiovascular or cerebrovascular disease, malnutrition, alcoholism, hypothyroidism, and hypopituitarism, there is an increased prevalence for accidental hypothermia. Other causes besides exposure to cold, either by air temperature or by water immersion, include postoperative hypothermia and with the administration of large volumes of stored blood which has not been rewarmed.

Reduction in core body temperature causes reduced oxygen consumption, decreased myocardial repolarization, decreased gastrointestinal motility, decreased peripheral nerve conduction, and decreased respiratory status. The body's defense system tries to compensate for the cold by constricting superficial blood vessels and increasing metabolic heat production by shivering. Blood is shunted to vital organs, such as the heart and brain, which need more oxygen than the periphery.

Initially, the first symptoms of hypothermia may be weakness, drowsiness, irritability, confusion, and incoordination as the cold decreases the body's temperature. When temperatures go below 35° C, the patient is usually delirious, drowsy, or comatose, and, frequently, breathing will cease. Pulse and blood pressure are difficult to obtain, if at all. Metabolic acidosis, ventricular fibrillation, glucose imbalances, and coagulopathies occur. Systemic hypothermic death results from cardiac asystole or ventricular fibrillation.

Prior to this cardiac standstill, the patient may manifest an Osborne wave, or J wave, following the QRS on an ECG, which is diagnostic for hypothermia.

Treatment consists of active rewarming with supportive care to maintain adequate cardiovascular and respiratory status. If resuscitation efforts have been started, they should not be stopped until the patient is rewarmed to at least 35° C. The prognosis depends on the severity of the metabolic acidosis and if aspiration pneumonia has occurred. If the pH is less than 6.6, the prognosis is very poor, and morbidity is high.

The patient should be monitored in an intensive care unit because in the elderly, mild hypothermia is an emergency, leading to numerous cardiac dysrhythmias and hemodynamic alterations.

MEDICAL CARE

Laboratory: CBC used to identify infection, anemia, platelet function; coagulation studies used to identify coagulopathy; renal profiles and liver function testing to identify dysfunction; electrolyte levels used to identify imbalances; glucose levels initially may be elevated, followed by hypoglycemia during the rewarming phase

Radiography: chest X-rays used to identify presence of pulmonary infiltrates and effusions; used to identify aspiration pneumonia which is common with hypothermia

Arterial blood gases: used to identify acid–base disturbances, hypoxia, hypoxemia

Rewarming therapies: different methods used depending on severity of hypothermia; warming blankets, warm air flow blankets, warmed IV solutions, warmed peritoneal lavage solutions, warmed solutions for bladder instillation, warm baths, extracorporeal rewarming in extreme cases, peritoneal dialysis, heated, humidified air through a face mask or endotracheal tube, and warm colonic or nasogastric irrigations

IV fluids: used to restore circulating volume and prevent dehydration, and may be used to assist with rewarming

Antimicrobials: may be used to treat infection if patient has open wounds or systemic infection and are based on the patient's specific condition, other disease processes, and the suspected site of infection, or based on actual culture sensitivity reports

Analgesics: acetaminophen (Tylenol), ibuprofen (Motrin, Advil, Genpril, Ibuprofen, Nuprin, Trendar), and acetylsalicylic acid (ASA, aspirin) used to alleviate mild to moderate pain and to help reduce inflammation; aspirin may be used to decrease platelet aggregation and sludging; buprenorphine hydrochloride (Buprenex), butophanol tartrate (Stadol), codeine phosphate, hydromorphone hydrochloride (Dilaudid), meperidine hydrochloride (Demerol), methadone hydrochloride (Dolophine), morphine hydrochloride or sulfate (Duramorph, Infumorph, Morphine, MS Contin, Roxanol, Statex), nalbuphine hydrochloride (Nubain), oxycodone hydrochloride (OxyContin), oxymorphone hydrochloride (Numorphan), pentazocine hydrochloride or lactate (Talwin), or tramadol hydrochloride (Ultram) used to relieve severe pain from cold injuries

Surgery: may be required; fasciotomy may be needed to reduce tissue pressure caused from edema; debridement may be required for necrotic tissues

COMMON NURSING DIAGNOSES

 ### ACUTE PAIN (see CAD)

Related to: tissue damage, rewarming, hypothermia, surgery, altered hemodynamics related to aging process

Defining Characteristics: communication of pain, facial grimacing, restlessness, changes in pulse and blood pressure, diaphoresis, protective behavior of extremities, hypoactive reflexes, decreased motor activity, decreased muscle strength, anxiety

 ### RISK FOR INFECTION (see TOTAL JOINT REPLACEMENT)

Related to: frozen tissue, open wounds, decreased tissue perfusion, edema, changes in thermoregulatory

center and hemodynamic status related to the aging process, chronic comorbidities

Defining Characteristics: fever, tachycardia, tachypnea, elevated white blood cell count, shift to the left on differential, reddened wound, drainage, edema, pain, sepsis

ADDITIONAL NURSING DIAGNOSES

 ### INEFFECTIVE THERMOREGULATION

Related to: exposure to cold, suppressed shivering response, physiologic changes with thermoregulation related to aging

Defining Characteristics: temperature below 95° F, cold skin, mottling, cyanosis, pallor, poor judgment, apathy, decreased mental ability, level of consciousness changes, coma, lack of shivering, cardiopulmonary arrest, anuria, oliguria, decreased peripheral perfusion

Outcome Criteria

✔ Patient will achieve and maintain an acceptable temperature with no complications.

NOC: *Thermoregulation*

INTERVENTIONS	RATIONALES
Obtain baseline temperature, and monitor every 15 minutes until stable.	Temperatures below 90° F result in suppression of normal body mechanisms to self-warming. Rewarming that is done too rapidly may cause peripheral vasodilation and may actually impede rewarming efforts.
Rewarm patient per hospital protocol, preferably in an intensive care unit.	Early rewarming decreases tissue damage from potential ice crystal formation as seen in frostbite, and helps to decrease cardiac instability and predisposition to ventricular fibrillation.
Observe for mental changes and return of shivering response, or rigidity.	Shivering is suppressed at temperatures below 90° F and is the body's normal response to facilitate self-warming. This response is somewhat different in the elderly patient, and may be seen

(continues)

(continued)

INTERVENTIONS	RATIONALES
	as rigidity. Patients have decreased mental abilities and levels of consciousness dependent on severity of hypothermia, with hypoxia and hypoxemia occurring from decreased perfusion.
Instruct patient/family on appropriate procedures for rewarming.	Provides knowledge and reduces anxiety. Patient may be unconscious and family will require information.
Instruct patient/family in notifying nurse for subtle changes in mentation, speech, and orientation.	May indicate complications after rewarming has been accomplished.
Instruct patient/family in methods of avoiding hypothermia exposure, such as sufficient housing, heating, and so forth. Refer to community agencies or social workers as warranted.	Because the elderly usually live on fixed incomes, the patient may try to economize by decreasing ambient temperature to lower fuel bill, or may not have access to adequate housing. Social workers and other agencies may be required to assist in obtaining adequate and safe housing for patient after discharge.

NIC: *Hypothermia Treatment*

Discharge or Maintenance Evaluation

- Patient will be normothermic, with stable vital signs.
- Patient will be awake, alert, and oriented, with no alterations in cognitive abilities.
- Patient will be able to maintain thermoregulation.
- Patient will exhibit no complications from hypothermia.
- Patient/family will be able to avoid patient becoming hypothermic from inadequate facilities, heating, and living circumstances.
- Patient/family will be able to access community resources for financial, housing, and other assistance as needed.

INEFFECTIVE TISSUE PERFUSION: CARDIOPULMONARY, CEREBRAL, GASTROINTESTINAL, PERIPHERAL, RENAL

Related to: exposure to cold temperatures, hypothermia, tissue necrosis, sludging of red blood cells, tissue ischemia, alterations in hemodynamics associated with the aging process

Defining Characteristics: skin mottling, grayish skin color, purplish-blue color, cold skin, burning, tingling, numbness, pain, skin blisters, gangrene, diminished or absent pulses, decreased capillary refill, cardiac dysrhythmias, cardiac standstill, apnea, dyspnea, mental changes, unconsciousness, change in consciousness level, coma, oliguria, anuria, absent bowel sounds, ileus, hypotension, dysrhythmias

Outcome Criteria

✔ Patient will achieve and maintain normal body temperature with no lasting complications of decreased perfusion.

NOC: *Tissue Perfusion*

INTERVENTIONS	RATIONALES
Monitor vital signs every 15 minutes until stable, then every 1–2 hours, and prn.	During initial period after exposure, pulses and blood pressure may be too weak to be detectable. Rewarming too rapidly may result in heart irregularities.
Monitor ECG for rhythm changes, dysrhythmias, and treat per protocol.	Patient should be in ICU or telemetry unit where cardiac rhythm can be monitored constantly. Hypothermia affects the heart rate and rhythm, and may cause heart irregularities from hypoxemia and conduction problems. Heart rhythm may be difficult to restore to sinus when the body temperature is too low because of the increased ventricular fibrillation threshold. A 12-lead ECG may show an early J wave in the left ventricular leads.
Administer oxygen as ordered, with warmed humidification.	PaO_2 should be maintained above normal levels to treat hypoxia and hypoxemia that occurs with acidosis as a result of the injury and exposure.
Monitor oximetry levels and notify physician if <90%. Monitor ABGs for trends and changes.	Facilitates prompt identification of acid–base imbalances and changes in ventilation/oxygenation.

INTERVENTIONS	RATIONALES
Monitor peripheral pulses for presence, character, quality, and changes.	Decreased or absent pulses may indicate impairment in circulation to extremities and may predispose patient to tissue ischemia and necrosis.
Move and handle patient gently when required.	Excessive movement may trigger lethal dysrhythmias or may cause tissue damage.
Administer warmed IV solutions as ordered.	Restores circulating volume, helps to maintain hydration and output, assists with rewarming efforts, and assists with treatment of hypotension.
Monitor I&O hourly and notify physician for significant changes, such as urinary output <30 cc/hr.	Anuria or oliguria may indicate decreased perfusion to renal vessels or dehydration.
Evaluate patient's level of consciousness and mental status, and notify physician for significant changes.	Patients may have weakness, incoordination, apathy, drowsiness, and confusion with hypothermia. When the body temperature is less than 90° F, stupor and coma are common.
Observe for muscle tremors, rigidity, decreased reflexes, seizures, and Parkinson-like muscle tone.	Neurologic symptoms may occur from hypothermic influences.
Remove constricting jewelry and clothing from patient.	Constriction, especially in the presence of edema, may impair circulation and perfusion.
Rewarm patient per protocol.	Prompt rewarming reverses ice crystal formation in tissues. Warm water should not be more than tepid temperature because of the potential for burns. The appearance of skin flushing indicates that circulatory flow has been established.
Avoid rubbing the extremities, and handle the patient's body carefully and gently.	Helps to prevent further tissue damage.

INTERVENTIONS	RATIONALES
Encourage patient to take warm liquids if possible.	Helps with rewarming.
Monitor for pulses to extremities after rewarming procedure, and notify physician if pulse is absent.	When extremities have rewarmed, pulses should be palpable. An absence of pulse may indicate decreased or absent circulation that requires emergency treatment.
Instruct patient/family regarding long-term effects of hypothermia: increased sensitivity to cold, tingling, burning, increased sweating, and so forth.	Provides knowledge and identifies symptoms that patient may be faced with during lifetime.
Instruct patient to avoid smoking.	Smoking causes vasoconstriction and may inhibit healing process.
Prepare patient for fasciotomy as warranted.	Edema may impair circulation requiring a fasciotomy to relieve the pressure.

NIC: *Cardiac Care*

NIC: *Circulatory Precautions*

Discharge or Maintenance Evaluation

- Patient will achieve optimal circulation and peripheral perfusion with equal palpable pulses.
- Patient will be able to recall and adhere to instructions and avoid preventable complications.
- Patient will be able to verbalize understanding of instructions accurately.
- Patient will have no impediment to circulation and will not require treatment for circulatory constriction.
- Patient will have healed wounds, if fasciotomy is required.

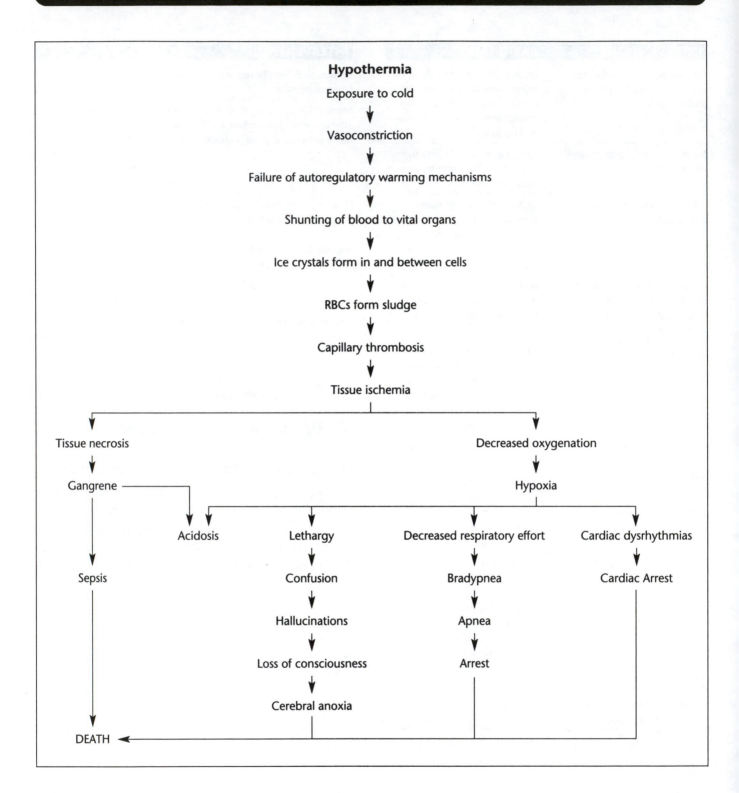

Hypothermia

Exposure to cold
↓
Vasoconstriction
↓
Failure of autoregulatory warming mechanisms
↓
Shunting of blood to vital organs
↓
Ice crystals form in and between cells
↓
RBCs form sludge
↓
Capillary thrombosis
↓
Tissue ischemia

Tissue necrosis
↓
Gangrene
↓
Sepsis
↓
DEATH

Acidosis

Lethargy
↓
Confusion
↓
Hallucinations
↓
Loss of consciousness
↓
Cerebral anoxia

Decreased oxygenation
↓
Hypoxia

Decreased respiratory effort
↓
Bradypnea
↓
Apnea
↓
Arrest

Cardiac dysrhythmias
↓
Cardiac Arrest

CHAPTER 10.2

HYPERTHERMIA

Hyperthermia is the presence of an uncharacteristically high body temperature that is the result of inadequate responses of the body's heat-regulatory mechanisms. Age-related factors reduce the efficacy of the mechanism of sweating in order to cool the body. In the elderly, the exocrine glands become fibrotic or do not function appropriately, and adjacent connective tissue has less vascularity, so the elderly patient only begins to sweat at higher core body temperatures.

With normal physiologic functioning, the hypothalamus regulates any heat loss through neuroendocrine and autonomic nervous system mechanisms. Heat causes the vasculature in the skin to dilate, and sweating occurs as a result of cholinergic discharge. Concurrent conditions that may occur in the elderly also impair the normal heat regulatory system because heat makes chronic illnesses worse, and heatstroke can result in pathophysiologic changes within the body. At least 80% of persons who die from heatstroke are over the age of 50 (Beers & Berkow, 2000).

There are three major types of disorders that are caused by excessive heat: heat cramps, heat exhaustion, and heatstroke. Heat cramps occur during extreme physical activity that is performed in hot, humid weather. Profuse sweating and polydipsia precede the muscle cramps because fluids and electrolytes are lost through sweating and may only be replaced with water. Treatment with electrolyte-containing beverages will help to prevent this disorder.

Heat exhaustion may be caused by water depletion that results in hypertonic dehydration, or salt depletion, when fluids and salt are lost through sweating and water is all that is replaced. This disorder usually presents with anorexia, nausea, vomiting, disorientation, and postural hypotension. Body temperature may or may not be elevated. Patients are thirsty and weak, with dizziness, light-headedness, or a loss of consciousness. Elderly patients with this dis-

order usually present with late symptomatology, and are treated with IV fluids and electrolyte replacement.

Heatstroke is a dangerous condition, especially in the elderly, in which the heat loss mechanisms are inadequate or fail to reduce elevated body temperatures, and the patient has a noticeable absence of sweating and the presence of severe CNS disturbances. The elderly, who usually have coexisting disease processes, also have risk factors, such as fixed incomes, impairment of the ability to take care of oneself, alcoholism, mental illness, and nonavailability of air-conditioning. Drugs can also affect the patient and cause heatstroke to occur, as well as decreasing the ability of the person to be aware of the heat and to respond appropriately.

A high temperature of at least 105–106° F, an absence of sweating, light-headedness, headache, weakness, dyspnea, and nausea, and loss of consciousness usually distinguish heatstroke. The elderly usually have a hypodynamic response to the elevated temperature, and have a slow, thready pulse, extreme hypotension or imperceptible blood pressure, and hypovolemia.

Treatment of heatstroke is aimed at fluid and volume replacement with electrolyte solutions, reduction of the temperature, and preservation of metabolic and cardiovascular dynamics. It is a medical emergency and patients should be treated in the intensive care unit because of the potential for lethal dysrhythmias, renal and hepatic damage, and coagulation defects.

MEDICAL CARE

Laboratory: CBC used to evaluate hydration, bleeding, anemia, and presence of infection; renal profiles used to identify renal failure and acute tubular necrosis; lactate levels usually elevated; urinalysis used to show proteinuria, elevated RBCs, and potential for rhabdomyolysis; electrolyte profiles used to identify imbalances, with hypokalemia being common secondary to aldosterone production; liver profiles used to identify transient increases in transaminases and jaundice; coagulation profiles used to identify coagulopathy, with usual increases in prothrombin and PTT, and decreased fibrinogen; CSF used to rule out possible neurologic causes for loss of consciousness

Electrocardiogram: used to show cardiac rate and rhythm, conduction disturbances, dysrhythmias; tachycardias seen in younger patients, bradycardias seen in elderly patients; ECG usually shows changes in ST segments and T waves; may have dysrhythmias as a result of electrolyte imbalances

Cooling techniques: cool IV solutions, cooling blankets, sponge baths, ice packs to groin and axilla used to reduce temperature

IV fluids: used to maintain hydration and provide circulating fluid volume with electrolyte solutions; also provide access for emergency drugs

Antipyretics: acetaminophen (Tylenol), ibuprofen (Motrin, Advil, Genpril, Ibuprofen, Nuprin, Trendar), and acetylsalicylic acid (ASA, aspirin) used to reduce temperature by the action on the hypothalamus control center

COMMON NURSING DIAGNOSES

 ### DEFICIENT FLUID VOLUME (see GI BLEEDING)

Related to: hyperthermia, heatstroke, heat exhaustion

Defining Characteristics: hypotension, tachycardia, decreased skin turgor, weakness, decreased urinary output, pallor, diaphoresis, decreased capillary refill, mental changes, restlessness, decreased filling pressures, decreased hemoglobin and hematocrit, dry mucous membranes, increased hematocrit initially, concentrated urine, thirst, weakness

 ### INEFFECTIVE TISSUE PERFUSION: CARDIOPULMONARY, CEREBRAL, PERIPHERAL, GASTRO-INTESTINAL, RENAL (see CAD)

Related to: hyperthermia, heatstroke, heat exhaustion, reduced oxygen supply, hypoperfusion, hypovolemia, dysrhythmias, coexisting disease processes, age-related vascular structure changes, inactivity

Defining Characteristics: chest pain, conduction disturbances, dysrhythmias, vital sign changes, ECG changes, delayed capillary refill time, chest retractions, dyspnea, nasal flaring, use of accessory muscles, increased work of breathing, tachypnea, bradypnea, changes in mental status, weakness, paralysis, behavioral changes, abdominal distention, ileus, hypoactive or absent bowel sounds, nausea, vomiting, edema, weak or absent peripheral pulses, skin temperature changes, skin color changes, decreased peripheral tactile sensation, hematuria, oliguria, anuria, increased BUN and creatinine, fever, rhabdomyolysis, dehydration

ADDITIONAL NURSING DIAGNOSES

 ### HYPERTHERMIA

Related to: dehydration, heatstroke, decreased ability in the aged to maintain body temperature or recognize signs of heatstroke

Defining Characteristics: increased core body temperature, usually above 105° F, hot skin, flushed, increased respiratory rate, tachycardia, cardiac conduction problems, dysrhythmias, electrolyte imbalances, coagulation problems, rhabdomyolysis, seizures

Outcome Criteria

✔ Patient will have temperature within normal range and fluid status will be stable.

NOC: *Thermoregulation*

INTERVENTIONS	RATIONALES
Monitor vital signs, especially body temperature every 15 minutes, until stable, then every 1–2 hours, and prn.	Identifies problem and monitors efficacy of treatment. Hypotension and tachycardia may indicate hypovolemia that requires emergency treatment.
Administer IV fluids as ordered.	Maintains hydration status, replaces electrolytes, and provides access for administration of emergency medications.
Administer antipyretics as ordered.	Reduces fever.
Utilize techniques and methods of reducing temperature, such as applying ice packs to axilla and	These methods promote patient comfort and lower body temperature. If cooling blanket is

INTERVENTIONS	RATIONALES
groin, using cooling blanket, and so forth.	utilized, it should be closely monitored and turned off when temperature decreases to 102° F to prevent rebound hypothermia.
Monitor heart rhythm and hemodynamics if possible.	Tachycardia, decreased CVP, and hypotension may indicate hypovolemia, which may cause reduced tissue perfusion. Cool, blanched skin may also indicate reduced perfusion.
Monitor patient's mentation status and notify physician for changes.	Changes in level of consciousness may occur as a result of hypoxia or hypoxemia.
Instruct patient/family regarding the need for avoiding situations that predisposed patient to this hyperthermic episode.	Provides knowledge and helps to prevent recurrences.
Instruct patient/family to ingest sufficient fluids of patient's preference.	Provision of preferred liquids will help facilitate intake for adequate hydration.

INTERVENTIONS	RATIONALES
Instruct patient/family regarding community resources, supportive organizations, and so forth that can provide fans, or air-conditioning.	Patient may be on a limited income and not able to afford air-conditioning; access to community resources that can assist in obtaining help will be invaluable.

NIC: *Heat Exposure Treatment*

Discharge or Maintenance Evaluation

- Patient will have stable vital signs with no signs or symptoms of impaired perfusion.
- Patient will have adequate fluid hydration as shown by equivalent intake and output.
- Patient/family will be able to access community resources to obtain needed assistance.
- Patient will be able to prevent recurrence of hyperthermia.
- Patient will suffer no organ system dysfunction as a complication from hyperthermia

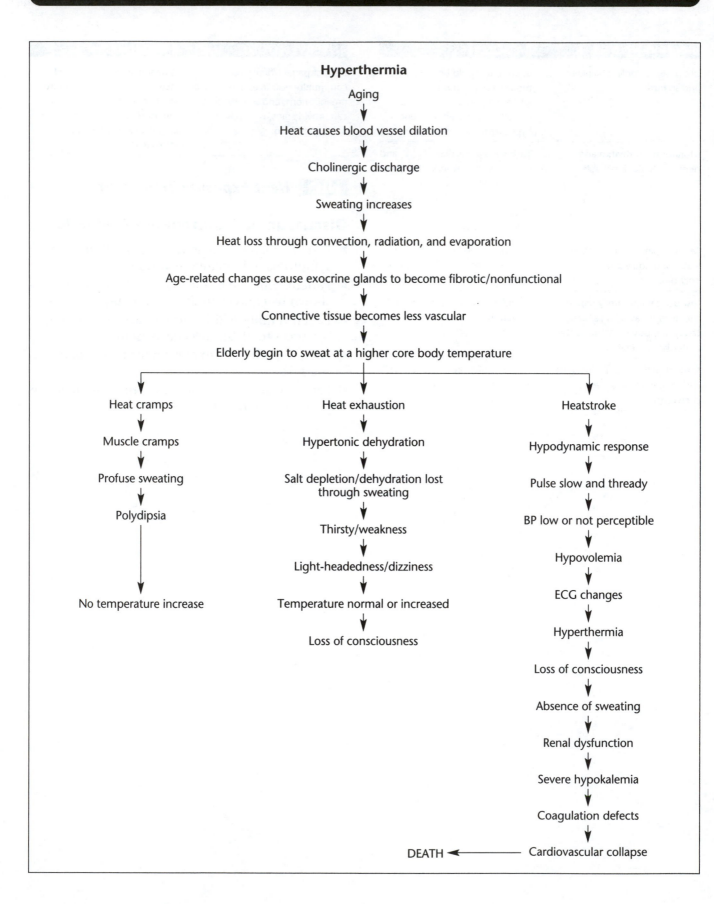

Hyperthermia

Aging

Heat causes blood vessel dilation

Cholinergic discharge

Sweating increases

Heat loss through convection, radiation, and evaporation

Age-related changes cause exocrine glands to become fibrotic/nonfunctional

Connective tissue becomes less vascular

Elderly begin to sweat at a higher core body temperature

Heat cramps	Heat exhaustion	Heatstroke
Muscle cramps	Hypertonic dehydration	Hypodynamic response
Profuse sweating	Salt depletion/dehydration lost through sweating	Pulse slow and thready
Polydipsia	Thirsty/weakness	BP low or not perceptible
	Light-headedness/dizziness	Hypovolemia
No temperature increase	Temperature normal or increased	ECG changes
	Loss of consciousness	Hyperthermia
		Loss of consciousness
		Absence of sweating
		Renal dysfunction
		Severe hypokalemia
		Coagulation defects
	DEATH ◄────	Cardiovascular collapse

CHAPTER 10.3

DECUBITUS ULCER

Pressure sores, or decubitus ulcers, are one of the most frequently seen complications in the elderly population with mobility impairment. Whenever extended pressure is exerted on skin surfaces, perfusion is impaired, resulting in ischemia and the ensuing necrosis of the area. Vasculature is more fragile in the aged patient, and shearing forces cause pressure, irritation, erythema, and, eventually, open wounds. Wound healing is affected by age also, so once a wound develops, the repair rate also decreases.

Patients who have concurrent diagnoses of diabetes and peripheral vascular disease are more predisposed to acquire a decubitus ulceration because of the disease process neuropathy.

Decubitus ulcers are created by the application of pressure, friction, shearing, or maceration. Pressure, especially over bony prominences, compromises blood supply and lymphatic drainage at the affected site. Friction when the skin rubs against another surface results in epidermal cell destruction and loss. Shearing forces when two layers of skin slide on each other, moving in opposite directions, damage the underlying tissue or the tissues become stretched. Maceration is triggered by moisture or drainage that remains on the skin and causes deterioration of the skin surface.

Pressure sores are classified by four stages according to the depth of the wound and degree of damage. In stage I, the skin has nonblanchable erythema, and sometimes warmth, hardness, and indurations to intact skin; this stage can be reversed if treated promptly. Stage II ulcers have a partial thickness skin loss that comprises the dermis and/or the epidermis, and appears as a blister, abraded area, or shallow crater on the skin's surface. This stage, also, is reversible with prompt treatment. Stage III ulcers involve a full thickness of skin loss and the damage to subcutaneous tissues may extend down to the underlying fascia. It appears as a deep crater with or without injury to adjacent tissues. Signs of infection may be present, and if so, cultures should be taken and wound and skin precautions followed. Necrotic

tissues may have to be removed to achieve a clean wound base in order to provide the potential for healing. This stage can be life-threatening, and may require surgical intervention. Stage IV ulcers have full-thickness skin loss with destruction, necrosis, or damage to muscle, bone, or supporting structures. There may also be fistulas and tunneling tracts. These types of wounds in the elderly may be fatal because of the susceptibility of the aged to infection and sepsis.

Prevention of decubitus ulcers is the most essential issue in management of these sores. Appropriate wound care should be performed, and patients evaluated frequently to ensure that pressure areas are not deteriorating. The Norton Scale or Braden Scale has been designed to assess risk for ulceration based on six categories: sensory perception, activity, mobility, moisture, nutrition, and friction/shear.

MEDICAL CARE

Laboratory: CBC used to identify presence of infection and anemia; albumin levels used to identify nutritional status; vitamin and mineral levels used to identify deficiencies; cultures of drainage in wound sites to identify causative organism of infection; specific antimicrobials levels to identify efficacy and/or toxicity, albumin, prealbumin and protein levels to determine nutritional status that may affect healing

Debridement: can be done surgically mechanically, autolytically, or enzymatically; the method selected is specific to the patient's condition, illnesses, and goals; surgical debridement used when sepsis or worsening cellulitis is a factor and the need urgent; other methods used when removal of necrotic tissue not as urgent or when patient unable to tolerate surgical intervention; mechanical debridement occurs when a wet-to-dry dressing is applied into the wound after cleansing wound of purulent material and left to dry so any loosened necrotic tissue adheres onto the dressing and is removed with each dressing change; autolytic debridement involves using occlusive or semi-occlusive dressings to allow the body's enzymes to soften and digest the devitalized tissue, but cannot be used if infection is present in the wound; enzymatic debridement consists of topical substances applied to clean wounds to debride any damaged tissues

Hydrogels: polymers that are used to absorb exudates and form a gelatinous substance to provide a moist atmosphere for wound healing

Calcium alginate dressings: made of substances found in seaweed, these dressings able to absorb up to 20 times own weight in exudates, forming a soft gel and moist environment to promote wound healing

Debriding enzymes: fibrinolytics and proteolytic substances help to act against injured tissues, and usually more effective with superficial wound layers because enzymes must be in actual contact with wound; may be used adjunctively with surgical or mechanical debridement

Absorption dressings: hydrophilic agents that help absorb the excessive wound exudates and necrotic debris that restrict new tissue generation; beads or grains most often used, gently packed into the wound and then covered with a dry dressing that is changed 1–2 times per day

Hydrocolloid dressings: semipermeable occlusive dressings made of hydrophobic olymers with hydrocolloid particles that swell upon contact with wound exudates to form a moist gel; help to increase cell migration, debridement, cleansing of the wound, and granulation of new tissues; can usually be left on up to 1 week unless the exudates leak from the dressing

Liquid barrier dressings: substances that contain alcohol and plasticizing agents to provide a protective waterproof covering over an affected area of tissue; can be dissolved using soapy solutions but allow healing to occur while preventing fluids from further injuring skin surfaces

Film dressings: clear, nonabsorbent dressings that are gas permeable but not fluid permeable and are left on the wound for up to 1 week; help to keep the exudative material against the wound to increase epithelial cell migration across the wound; exudates can be aspirated through the dressing using a small-gauge needle and, if the dressing does not reseal itself, can be patched

Enzyme debriding agents: fibrinolysin and desoxyribonuclease (Elase), sutilains (Travase) used to reduce necrotic material and most effective when used with mechanical or surgical debridement

Wound cleansers: dextranomer (Debrisan) used to absorb tissue exudates and remove bacteria and protein degradation products; reduce healing time by preventing scab formation and decreasing inflammation and edema

Antimicrobials: used to treat infection; specific agent dependent on culture results to eradicate the causative organism

Vacuum assisted closure (VAC) system: used in treatment of deep wounds; a special sponge-like dressing applied into the cleaned wound, a hose then applied over or into the sponge dressing, and entire system covered with occlusive dressing; tubing connected to a low-pressure suction system that draws fluid and exudates into dressing to quickly clean and heal the wound

Specialized beds: kinetic air beds that use a Gore-Tex sheet over pillows of air to reduce pressure on the patient's skin helps to heal wounds, and to prevent wounds in high-risk patients

COMMON NURSING DIAGNOSES

INEFFECTIVE TISSUE PERFUSION: PERIPHERAL (see PERIPHERAL VASCULAR DISEASE)

Related to: interruption of arterial and venous flow from pressure, friction, or shearing forces to skin, decubitus ulcer, decreased vascularity caused by changes associated with aging

Defining Characteristics: reddish-brown color to skin, pressure changes, slow healing, tissue edema, impaired tissue nutrition, impaired tissue oxygenation, ulcer formation, erythema, indurations, hardened areas, necrosis, drainage from wounds

DISTURBED SENSORY PERCEPTION: TACTILE (see ALZHEIMER'S DISEASE)

Related to: alteration in sensory reception, transmission, and or integration of neurologic deficit from neuropathy; altered status of sense organ, diabetes, medications, aging

Defining Characteristics: reported loss of sensation when pressure applied, posture alteration, inability to change position, inability to feel pain, paresthesias, loss of sensitivity to touch, temperature changes to skin, numbness

FUNCTIONAL URINARY INCONTINENCE (see INTERSTITIAL CYSTITIS)

Related to: sensory, cognitive, or mobility deficits, increased tissue injury due to constant wetness

Defining Characteristics: urge to void or bladder contractions strong enough to result in loss of urine before reaching commode or bathroom, lack of caretaker availability or interest, decreased bladder size and capacity, urgency, frequency, incontinent episodes, inability to find and reach commode or bathroom in time, lack of awareness, memory, poor bladder control, unpredictable passage of urine, intermittent loss of urine, urine remaining on skin for lengthy periods of time resulting in excoriation, lesions, or open wounds, increased susceptibility to pressure wounds because of consistent fluid environment

ADDITIONAL NURSING DIAGNOSES

IMPAIRED SKIN INTEGRITY

Related to: external mechanical factors, shearing, pressure, friction, physical immobilization, altered nutritional state, circulation, sensation, skeletal prominence

Defining Characteristics: disruption of skin surface, skin discoloration, destruction of skin layers, open wound, exudate, drainage

Outcome Criteria

✔ Patient will have skin intact with absence of factors that predispose patient to skin impairment.

NOC: *Tissue Integrity: Skin*

INTERVENTIONS	RATIONALES
Assess patient's risk for pressure sore formation with the Norton scale chart or Braden scale.	A Norton score of 12–15 indicates a high risk for decubitus formation. Severely limited status level in 6 areas indicates a pre-

INTERVENTIONS	RATIONALES
	diction of risk for decubitus on the Braden scale.
Assess skin over bony prominences, soft tissue for reddish-brown color, warmth, firmness, induration, drainage, and foul odor.	Signs of impending or existence of decubitus ulcer with most common sites at sacrum, heels, elbows, trochanters, and scapulae.
Assess patient's mobility status, presence of urinary/fecal incontinence, ability to move in bed, sensitivity to pain, and edema.	May be the most common causes of decubitus in elderly.
Provide position change q 2 hours, maintain body alignment and support with pillows, trochanter rolls, or pads.	Unrelieved pressure will cause beginning of skin breakdown. Proper position and support prevents contractures.
Administer debriding or wound cleansing agents as appropriate.	Absorbs tissue exudate and assists in healing in stages III and IV decubitus.
Wash, rinse and dry skin with mild soap, warm water, soft towel after each incontinent episode. Apply skin barrier if appropriate or external devices.	Removes body excretions that macerate skin and predispose patient to breakdown of skin.
Maintain bed that is wrinkle and crumb free. Change if wet or soiled.	Prevents discomfort and ulcer formation.
Protect all bony prominences. Avoid positioning on any reddish or pink area.	Prevents compromised circulation that reduces oxygen and nutrients to tissues.
Apply treatments as appropriate (heat lamp, irrigations, wet-to-dry compresses, whirlpool).	Promotes healing of decubitus.
Raise head of bed no higher than semi-Fowler's, if tolerated.	Elevated head of bed promotes pressure on lower torso from sliding, causing friction.
Instruct patient of need for fluid intake of at least 2 L/day, high protein dietary intake, and suggest nutritionist, if appropriate.	Promotes tissue integrity and wound healing which is slower in the elderly.
Maintain mobility and avoid sitting or lying for prolonged periods.	Maintains circulation and prevents pressure on tissues.
Instruct patient/family how to care for skin and complications of immobility.	Promotes knowledge of skin protection.

NIC: *Pressure Management*

NIC: *Pressure Ulcer Care*

Discharge or Maintenance Evaluation

- Patient will exhibit no presence of decubitus ulceration.

- Patient will have restoration of skin integrity with appropriate treatment modalities.

- Patient will be able to avoid infection and necrosis to skin.

- Patient will be able to demonstrate progressive wound healing of open decubitus.

- Patient will be compliant with fluid intake and dietary inclusions of protein and increased carbohydrates.

- Patient/family will be able to perform wound care as needed, with no exacerbation or worsening of wounds exhibited.

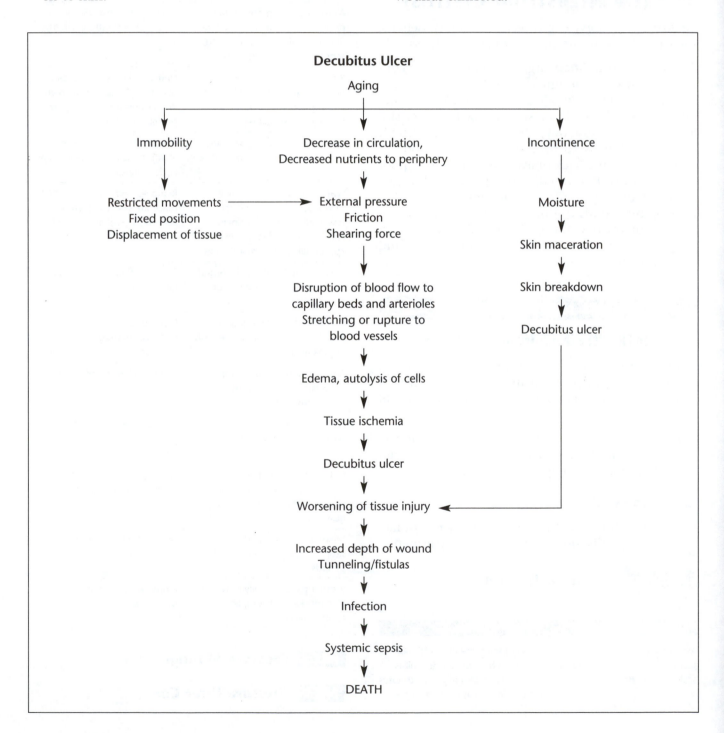

UNIT 11

OTHER CONSIDERATIONS

CHAPTER 11.1

CANCER (MALIGNANCIES)

Cancer, also known as carcinoma or malignancy, is a tumor that invades the surrounding tissue with the capability of spreading to other tissues at distant site(s) in the body, which is then termed, metastasis. This unregulated cell destruction is the result of uncontrolled and abnormal cell growth. Any body system can be affected by a tumor—either solid organ sites, or blood-forming organ sites. Physical changes result from the disease process, and the treatments as well as the psychological responses of the patient to the disease have a great impact on the patient's quality and quantity of life. This section deals with all malignancies, and is not specific to any one particular type.

Cancer is a leading cause of death in the elderly; the most common malignancies in the older adult include neoplasms of the lung, breast, and prostate, leukemia, lymphoma, and colorectal carcinoma. Although each diagnosis presents in its own unique way, this chapter deals with generic nursing care planning for all malignancies, regardless of which organs or body systems they affect.

Chemotherapy is one treatment for malignancy that utilizes chemical agents to cure, prevent, or relieve the disease or the symptoms presented by the disease. These drugs use different methods of action to eradicate the cancer cells that have invaded the body and possibly spread, as a way of preventing the spread from a tumor in its early stages, or as a palliative way to help prolong life by alleviating pain or discomfort in terminal cancer.

Cancer chemotherapy drugs are numerous, and are used singly or in combination, to inhibit and interfere with the cancer cell's ability to reproduce and grow. Usually there are side effects from the medication, such as nausea, vomiting, bone marrow suppression, loss of hair, and anemia, and the consequences of benefit versus risk should be weighed in each specific case. The elderly may not tolerate some of the chemotherapy agents because of the changes that occur with age, such as poorer wound healing, comorbidities, and less organ reserve, but usually

nausea and vomiting have a tendency to be less intense in the elderly patient. Neurotoxicity is especially problematic because of the occurrence of several neuropathies that may occur from the drugs. Frail elderly patients may not be able to tolerate the episodes of diarrhea or stomatitis from some drugs. Renal dysfunction can decrease tolerance to other drugs, and require adjustments in choice of drug utilized and dosage.

Radiation therapy is utilized for the treatment of cancer with high-energy X-rays or other types of radiation, in which rapidly dividing cells are killed by damage to the DNA cell structure. Irradiation therapy may be used alone as the primary tool in the treatment of some cancers, or in combination with chemotherapy to help shrink tumors prior to surgery or to kill any wayward cells. Radiation therapy is usually performed 5 times a week for several weeks, and may have some side effects, such as blistering of the skin, swallowing dysfunction, loss of appetite, fatigue, hair loss, and excessive sleepiness. Radiation therapy can weaken bones and make them more susceptible to fracture, which is already a high risk for the elderly. The elderly patient also has an increased risk of lung damage, coronary artery injury, esophagitis, and enteritis from the radiation, which can lead to rapid dehydration or severe disease exacerbation.

MEDICAL CARE

Laboratory: too numerous to mention all the lab tests that can be done; CBC used to identify infection, anemia, and decreasing platelet counts that may cause deletion or changes in treatment; prostate specific antigen used as a diagnostic tool and evaluation means for therapy; sputum or bronchial washings used to identify cytology and malignancy from pulmonary-related cancers; occult blood screening used to identify risk for colorectal cancer, bone marrow aspiration used to identify abnormalities that may indicate leukemia; biopsies of a particular site to identify the stage of a malignancy, or to identify metastasis; electrolytes used to identify imbalances that may result from dehydration or medications; carcinogenic embryonic antigen (CEA) used to identify invasion of cancer cells and to monitor efficacy of treatment

Analgesics: buprenorphine hydrochloride (Buprenex), butophanol tartrate (Stadol), codeine phosphate, fentanyl (Sublimaze, Duragesic, Actiq), hydromorphone hydrochloride (Dilaudid), meperidine hydrochloride (Demerol), methadone hydrochloride (Dolophine), morphine hydrochloride or sulfate (Duramorph, Infumorph, Morphine, MS Contin, Roxanol, Statex), nalbuphine hydrochloride (Nubain), oxycodone hydrochloride (OxyContin), oxymorphone hydrochloride (Numorphan), pentazocine hydrochloride or lactate (Talwin), or tramadol hydrochloride (Ultram); combinations of other drugs may be used to potentiate these analgesics or to interact with them; pain management specialists should always be consulted for cancer patients

Antineoplastic drugs: alkylating agents (busulfan [Myleran], carboplatin [Paraplatin], carmustine [BCNU, BiCNU, Gliadel Wafer], chlorambucil [Leukeran], cisplatin [Platinol, CDDP, Cisplatin], cyclophosphamide [Cytoxan, Neosar], ifosfamide [Ifex], lomustine [CeeNu, CCNU], mechlorethamine hydrochloride [Mustargen, Nitrogen Mustard], melphalan [Alkeran], streptozocin [Zanosar], temozolomide [Temodar], or thiotepa [Thioplex, TESPA, TSPA]) probably interfere with cross-linking DNA strands and RNA transcription and result in cellular death by alkylation; antimetabolites (capecitabine [Xeloda], cladribine [Leustatin], cytarabine [Cytosar-U], floxuridine [FUDR], fludarabine phosphate [Fludara], fluorouracil [5-FU, Adrucil, Efudex, Fluoroplex], hydroxyurea [Droxia, Hydrea], mercaptopurine [Purinethol, 6-MP], methotrexate [Folex, Rheumatrex, MTX], or thioguarine [6-TG]) use a variety of actions but probably impair the synthesis of new DNA and cell division; antibiotic antineoplastics (bleomycin sulfate [Blenoxane], dactinomycin [Actinomycin D, Cosmegen], daunorubicin citrate [DaunoXome], daunorubicin hydrochloride [Cerubidine], doxorubicin hydrochloride [Adriamycin, Rubex, Doxil], epirubicin hydrochloride [Ellence], idarubicin hydrochloride [Idamycin], mitomycin [Mutamycin, Mitomycin-C], pentostatin [Nipent, 2-Deoxycoformycin], plicamycin [Mithracin, Mithramycin], or valrubicin [Valstar]) used to inhibit

enzymes or increase deoxyadenosine triphosphate and result in cellular damage and death; antineoplastics with hormone alteration actions (anastrozole [Arimidex], bicalutamide [Casodex], exemestane [Aromasin], flutamide [Eulexin], goserelin acetate [Zoladex], letrozole [Femara], leuprolide acetate [Lupron], megestrol acetate [Megace], nilutamide [Nilandron], tamoxifin citrate [Nolvadex, Tamoxifen], or testolactone [Teslac]) with actions varying dependent on drug; other miscellaneous antineoplastics (asparaginase [Elspar], bacille Calmette-Guerin [BCG, TICE BCG, TheraCys], bexarotene [Targretin], dacarbazine [DTIC, DTIC-Dome], docetaxel [Taxotere], etoposide [VP-16, VePesid, Etopophos], gemcitabine hydrochloride [Gemzar], gemtuzumab ozogamicin [Mylotarg], irinotecan hydrochloride [Camptosar], mitotane [Lysodren], mitoxantrone hydrochloride [Novantrone], paclitaxel [Taxol], pegaspargase [PEG-$_L$-asparaginase, Oncaspar], porfimer sodium [Photofrin], procarbazine hydrochloride [Matulane], rituximab [Rituxan], teniposide [VM-26, Vumon], topotecan hydrochloride [Hycamtin], trastuzumab [Herceptin], tretinoin [Vesanoid], vinblastine sulfate [VLB, Velban], vincristine sulfate [VCR, Oncovin, Vincasar PFS], and vinorelbine tartrate [Navelbine]) which have varying methods of action to kill carcinogenic cells

Antiemetics: chlorpromazine hydrochloride (Thorazine), dimenhydrinate (Dramamine, Dimetabs, Tinate, Triptone), dolesetron mesylate (Anzemet), dronabinol (Marinol), granisetron hydrochloride (Kytril), meclizine hydrochloride (Antivert, Bonine, Vergon), metoclopramide hydrochloride (Clopra, Reclomide, Reglan), ondansetron hydrochloride (Zofran), prochlorperazine (Compazine, PMS), thiethylperazine maleate (Torecan), trimethobenzamide hydrochloride (Arresting, Tebamide, Ticon, Tigan, Triban), used to reduce nausea and vomiting by depressing the chemoreceptor trigger zone or by inhibiting serotonin receptors to block nausea response

Antianxiety drugs: alprazolam (Xanax), buspirone hydrochloride (BuSpar), chlordiazepoxide hydrochloride (Libritabs, Librium), clorazepate dipotassium (Tranxene, Gen-XENE), diazepam (Valium, Diazepam), hydroxyzine embonate or hydrochloride (Atarax, Anx, Vistaril, Hydroxacen), lorazepam (Ativan, Lorazepam, Intensol), meprobamate (Equanil, Miltown, Probate, Trancot), midazolam hydrochloride (Versed), or oxazepam (Serax) may be used to inhibit the action of serotonin or to depress subcortical levels of the central nervous system to help relieve anxiety

Laxatives, stool softeners, enemas: bisacodyl (Bisacolax, Dulcolax, Fleet Laxative, Fleet Enema), calcium polycarbophil (Equalactin, Fiberall, FiberCon, Mitrolan), cascara sagrada, castor oil (Emulsoil, Purge), docusate calcium or sodium (DC Softgels, Sulfolax, Surfak, Colace, Coloxyl, Diocto, DOS, DUOsol, Modane, Pro-Sof), glycerin (Fleet Babylax, Sani-Supp), lactulose (Cephulac, Cholac, Chronulac, Constilac, Duphalac, Enulose), magnesium citrate, hydroxide or sulfate (Citroma, Citro-Mag, Milk of Magnesia, Epsom salts), methylcellulose (Citrucel), psyllium (Fiberall, Genfiber, Hydrocil, Konsyl, Metamucil, Perdiem, Prodiem, Serutan, Unilax, V-Lax), senna (Black-Draught, Fletcher's Castoria, Senexon, Senokot), or sodium phosphate (Fleet Phospho-Soda); bulk laxatives used to provide sufficient bulk to stool to promote peristalsis and bowel elimination; osmotic laxatives used to promote bowel elimination on a daily or every other day basis; laxatives that contain magnesium should be utilized on a short-term basis only and cautiously in patients with renal impairment; stimulant laxatives used for acute constipation but can result in abdominal cramping and fluid and electrolyte imbalances, and are frequently abused by laxative-dependent patients; stool softeners help soften stools to allow for easier elimination; suppositories may be required for acute constipation or as part of a bowel program; enemas used when impaction of stool exists; soapsuds enemas may result in mucosal damage and cramping and should be avoided; oil enemas are used to soften impacted stool for easier removal

Antidiarrheal drugs: attapulgite (Diasorb, Donnagel, Kaopectate, Parepectolin, Rheaban), bismuth subsalicylate (Bismatrol, Pepto-Bismol, Pink Bismuth), diphenoxylate hydrochloride and atropine sulfate (Logen, Lomotil, Lonox), loperamide (Imodium), octreotide acetate (Sandostatin) or opium tincture (Paregoric) to relieve diarrhea resulting from chemotherapy or radiation therapy by decreasing bowel motility and fecal water content

Astringents: chlorhexidine gluconate or Domboro solutions used as cleansing agents to treat desquamation caused by radiation therapy

Chest and bone X-rays: reveal lung involvement and aid in staging process; bone metastasis if present with osteoblastic changes

Mammography: reveals lesion prior to surgery or in remaining breast

Bronchoscopy: views area for diagnosis, tumor excision, or biopsy

Colonoscopy/proctosigmoidoscopy: reveals polyp/tumor location and allows for removal or biopsy

Barium enema: used to reveal colonic tumor site

Radionuclide scans: computerized scanning following an IV injection of a radionuclide specific to organ uptake for presence of tumor

External radiation: may be done as primary treatment to destroy tumor, adjunct therapy to surgery or chemotherapy to prevent recurrence or shrink tumor to size that is operable, or palliation of symptom of pain depending on tumor staging

Surgery: prostatectomy with or without radical resection, bilateral orchiectomy in advanced stage; pneumonectomy, lobectomy to remove tumor; removal of tumor with right or left colectomy with anastomosis, abdominoperineal resection with permanent colostomy; lumpectomy, simple, modified-radical, or radical mastectomy, depending on need for biopsy, tumor removal, or staging of disease

COMMON NURSING DIAGNOSES

 ### INEFFECTIVE BREATHING PATTERN (see TB)

Related to: pain of tumor invasion, pneumonia, inflammatory process of disease, decreased lung expansion, decreased energy and fatigue from treatments, tracheobronchial obstruction by tumor

Defining Characteristics: cough, tachypnea, hemoptysis, cyanosis, dyspnea, use of accessory muscles, adventitious breath sounds, excessive mucus production, stasis of secretions, bronchial obstruction by tumor mass, pulmonary edema, fever, weakness, diaphoresis, fatigue, leukopenia, sputum, warm, flushed skin, effects of analgesia, inability to cough up secretions, abnormal chest X-rays

 ### RISK FOR DEFICIENT FLUID VOLUME (see HTN)

Related to: bleeding, anemia, lack of adequate blood volume, excessive losses through normal routes associated with chemotherapy and/or radiation therapy, diarrhea, nausea/vomiting

Defining Characteristics: nausea, vomiting, thirst, diarrhea, dry skin, dry mucous membranes, concentrated urine, hypotension, tachycardia, decreased skin turgor, weakness, decreased urinary output, pallor, diaphoresis, decreased capillary refill, mental changes, restlessness, decreased filling pressures, hemorrhage, confusion, dysrhythmias

EXCESS FLUID VOLUME (see HEART FAILURE)

Related to: compromised regulatory mechanism resulting from radical surgery, removal of or irradiation of lymph nodes, inability of elderly regulatory mechanisms to compensate for excessive fluid imbalances

Defining Characteristics: interstitial edema, lymphedema in arm on affected side, heaviness, pain, impaired motor function, numbness and paresthesias of fingers

DIARRHEA (see BOWEL DISORDERS)

Related to: medications and/or radiation to treat the tumor, inflammation of the bowel mucosa, infection, inflammation, irritation, or malabsorption of bowel from gastrointestinal disorders

Defining Characteristics: frequent passage of stools, loose, liquid, or watery stools, abdominal pain, cramping, increased bowel sounds, changes in color of stool, fever, malaise, bloody stools, mucoid stools, fatty substances in stool, fecal urgency, increased bowel sounds

SEXUAL DYSFUNCTION (see SEXUAL DISORDERS)

Related to: changes in body structure and function from radical surgery, biopsychosocial alteration of sexuality from altered body structures, prostatectomy, medications, alteration in function resulting from radiation therapy

Defining Characteristics: verbalization of problems with sexual function, avoidance of engaging in sexual intercourse, need for confirmation of desirability, actual or perceived limitation imposed by BPH, anxiety, erectile dysfunction, impotence, inability to achieve sexual satisfaction, limitations imposed

by hormonal therapy or surgery (colostomy, prostatectomy, orchiectomy)

ANXIETY (see CAD)

Related to: threat to body image, threat to role functioning, pain, change in health status, fear of death, presence of cancer, uncertain prognosis, effect of therapy and disease on lifestyle

Defining Characteristics: communication of fear and apprehension, uncertainty of treatment regimen and outcome, communication of increased helplessness, dependence on others, restlessness, insomnia, anorexia, increased respirations, increased heart rate, increased blood pressure, difficulty concentrating, dry mouth, poor eye contact, decreased energy, irritability, crying

DISTURBED SLEEP PATTERN (see HEART FAILURE)

Related to: impaired medication clearance, emotional and psychological concerns related to cancer diagnosis, pain interfering with sleep, fear of going to sleep, depression, anxiety, lack of activity, metabolic disturbances related to internal factors of carcinogenic evolution

Defining Characteristics: interrupted sleep, difficulty falling asleep, awakening early, fatigue, lethargy, irritability, disorientation, complaints of not feeling rested, insomnia, sleeplessness, naps during the day, sleepiness during the day, yawning, morning headache, pain, dyspnea, feelings of anxiety, depression, and fear

ACUTE PAIN (see CAD)

Related to: biologic injuring agents, tumor invasion, compression of body structures, radiation

Defining Characteristics: communication of pain, facial grimacing, restlessness, changes in pulse and blood pressure, guarding behavior, protective behavior of radiation site

FATIGUE (see HEART FAILURE)

Related to: decreased metabolic energy production, overwhelming psychological or emotional demands, cancer and treatment regimen, pain, dyspnea

Defining Characteristics: verbalization of fatigue, lack of energy, inability to maintain usual routine activity, lethargy, emotionally labile, inability to achieve rest even with sleep, decreased performance, irritability, increased physical complaints, dyspnea, pain

 INEFFECTIVE PROTECTION (see ANEMIA)

Related to: abnormal blood profiles, leukopenia, thrombocytopenia, anemia, drug therapy, antineoplastics, corticosteroids, radiation therapy

Defining Characteristics: deficient immunity, altered clotting, tissue hypoxia, weakness, anemia, low blood counts, decreased hemoglobin and hematocrit, altered coagulability

 IMPAIRED SKIN INTEGRITY (see LIVER FAILURE)

Related to: poor nutrition, radiation therapy, medications, altered metabolic state, renal involvement causing uremia resulting in pruritis, ascites, bile deposits on skin, liver failure, immobility

Defining Characteristics: edema, ascites, jaundice, pruritis, deposits of bile salts on skin, increased ammonia levels, decreased mental sensorium, dry, scaly skin, destruction of skin layers, skin discoloration, diarrhea, uremia, uremic frost on skin

 DISTURBED BODY IMAGE (see PACEMAKERS)

Related to: changes in physical appearance, ascites, biophysical factors, alopecia, presence of colostomy, disfigurement of mastectomy

Defining Characteristics: fear of rejection, fear of reaction from others, negative feelings about body, refusal to participate in care, refusal to look at self, withdrawal from social contacts, withdrawal from family, presence of ascites, biophysical changes, fear of death, fear of the unknown, verbal response to actual change in structure or function, alopecia, preoccupation with loss, persistent lymphedema of arm on affected side postmastectomy, inability to adjust to alterations in sexual patterns

ADDITIONAL NURSING DIAGNOSES

 ANTICIPATORY GRIEVING

Related to: perceived potential loss of physiopsychosocial well-being, potential death from fatal illness

Defining Characteristics: expression of distress at potential loss, guilt, anger, sorrow

Outcome Criteria

✔ Patient will progressively move through the stages of grieving.

NOC: *Psychosocial Adjustment: Life Change*

INTERVENTIONS	RATIONALES
Assess stage of grieving process experienced. Discuss patient's feelings about cancer, prognosis, treatment, and alterations in body.	Stages are normal responses leading to acceptance of loss and include shock and disbelief, anger, and depression.
Provide opportunity for patient to express emotions related to anticipated loss.	Allows for venting of feelings.
Be honest in communications and acknowledge reality of fears expressed.	Promotes trusting relationship.
Identify support system of family, significant other, or clergy and assist to mobilize.	Positive support system and feelings for relationships enhance movement through grieving process.
Encourage maintenance of rest, nutrition, and activity needs.	Promotes continuous self-care.
Provide quiet and privacy when requested.	Allows for thoughtful relaxation.
Recognize and respect religious, economic, educational, and cultural aspects of patient.	Promotes sense of identity and positive self-worth.
Assist patient/family to identify coping mechanisms, verbalization of feelings, and concerns over diagnosis and prognosis.	Assists patient to utilize current strategies for coping with new diagnosis, and potential for fatal illness, and allows for new strategies to be explored. Expression of feelings and concerns allows both the patient and family time to grieve and come to terms with diagnosis and eventual outcome, and enables them to make hard decisions to avoid difficulty in patient's latter stages of the disease process.
Instruct patient/family regarding the stages of the grieving process.	Provides understanding of behaviors associated with grieving and anticipated loss.

INTERVENTIONS	RATIONALES
	Grieving is a natural reaction and progression of feelings starting with denial, fear of losing control, parting from family members, facing the uncertainty of the future, and potential for suffering. The family will also need emotional support during this time in dealing with their own grief.
Instruct patient of importance of communication with family and other support systems.	Promotes needed support at the most critical times. Allows for communication between the patient and others who want to achieve closure of issues.
Instruct patient/family regarding referral sources for counseling, ministerial, financial, and other professional services that are available within the community.	Financial care of the patient who is dying as well as the patient's concern for the family's financial welfare if he or she dies may be diminished with factual knowledge of what options are available. Counseling and other resources will be of help for the patient once discharged.

NIC: *Dying Care*

Discharge or Maintenance Evaluation

- Patient will be able to discuss feelings regarding anticipated loss.
- Patient will be able to maintain significant relationships and support systems.
- Patient/family will be able to effectively understand the stages of grief and grieving.
- Patient will be able to maintain self-care and basic needs, or to have family/support systems assist with needs.
- Patient will be able to identify plans for changes in lifestyle and potential premature death.

 IMBALANCED NUTRITION: LESS THAN BODY REQUIREMENTS

Related to: inability to take in enough food, increased metabolism caused by disease process, decreased level of consciousness, inability to absorb nutrients because of biologic or psychologic factors, chemotherapy, radiation therapy

Defining Characteristics: actual inadequate food intake, altered taste, altered smell sensation, weight loss, body weight 20% or more under ideal for height and frame, anorexia, absent bowel sounds, decreased peristalsis, muscle mass loss, decreased muscle tone, changes in bowel habits, nausea, vomiting, abdominal distention, lack of interest in food, satiety immediately after ingesting food, abdominal pain or discomfort, sore, inflamed buccal cavity, depression, anxiety, social isolation, difficulty in feeding self, changes in mental status, fatigue from work of breathing

Outcome Criteria

✔ Patient will exhibit no evidence of weight loss and will be able to have sufficient intake of caloric nutrients by oral route, enteral route, or parenteral route.

NOC: *Nutritional Status: Nutrient Intake*

INTERVENTIONS	RATIONALES
Assess patient's dietary status, ability to eat, presence of nausea and vomiting, anorexia, and actual intake. Obtain calorie count.	Provides information regarding identification of specific problem of lack of sufficient nutrition, and helps establish plan of care for meeting needs. Caloric counts give fairly accurate estimates of ingested calories, and can be used to identify specific caloric needs based on patient's condition and metabolism.
Weigh patient every day, on same scale, at same time.	Provides accurate measurement of efficacy of dietary regimen. If patient continues to lose weight, oral intake may not be sufficient and patient may require alternate source of nutrition. Weight loss is the single best identifying factor for prediction of malnutrition.
Identify whether patient is terminal, whether patient wishes to have life prolonged by supplemental feedings, or if patient is suffering from effects of chemotherapy or radiation therapy.	Anorexia is common among patients who are receiving chemotherapy as well as among dying patients, so the nurse must identify if increased nutritional efforts are desired by the dying patient.
Identify food preferences and encourage family members to bring foods from home.	Familiar foods may entice the patient to eat. Specific food preferences may be given but supplemented in such a way as to increase their caloric value.

(continues)

(continued)

INTERVENTIONS	RATIONALES
Administer antiemetics as ordered.	Prevention of nausea and vomiting will enhance appetite. Nausea and vomiting may be caused by reduced gastric emptying, obstruction, opioids effects, gastritis, ulcers, or toxic drug effects. Metoclopramide can be helpful if nausea is caused by decreased gastric motility by its action of increasing peristalsis and relaxation of the pyloric sphincter. Ondansetron (Zofran) helps to control the nausea caused by chemotherapy.
Provide small, frequent meals, with dense caloric intake.	Helps to encourage patient to eat. A large meal tray may be overwhelming to the elderly cancer patient. Sometimes a small portion of the patient's favorite alcoholic beverage half an hour prior to mealtime may help stimulate appetite.
If patient/family desires, and patient is unable to ingest sufficient calories to meet metabolic needs, provide for and administer enteral or parenteral nutrition.	Enteral feedings are less costly and more efficient if the patient's gut is functional. If not, obstruction and increased gastric residuals may occur. Parenteral nutrition can be utilized and prescribed specifically for patient's metabolic needs to prevent further weight loss, but provides potential for infection.
Instruct patient/family regarding need for nutritional intake.	Promotes healing of cells and tissues, maintains body strength, reduces fatigue, and maintains weight.
Instruct patient/family regarding tube feedings/TPN administration as warranted.	Provides information and knowledge regarding the need for additional calories for metabolic demands while patient is receiving therapy for cancer.
Instruct patient/family in use of medications to help control symptoms related to therapy for cancer.	Antiemetics and corticosteroids can help decrease nausea and stimulate appetite.

NIC: *Nutrition Management*

Discharge or Maintenance Evaluation

- Patient will achieve a stable weight, and be able to orally ingest sufficient nutrition.
- Patient will avoid any further weight loss, and will be able to verbalize understanding of the need for daily weights to ensure proper nutrition.
- Patient/family will be compliant with encouraging familiar foods.
- If patient and family so desire, nursing staff will adhere to patient's wishes regarding withholding of nutritional alternatives if advanced directives are in place.
- Patient will exhibit no further nausea, vomiting, or anorexia.

SPIRITUAL DISTRESS

Related to: diagnosis of cancer, current health crisis, age, treatment regimen

Defining Characteristics: questioning about meaning of one's life, questions of why cancer has affected them, questions of what will happen after death, anger toward God, displaced anger toward ministerial and religious authorities, questions about belief systems, verbalization of inner conflicts, questioning one's moral and ethical mores regarding therapy and suffering, feelings of guilt that one's spirituality or lack of it has caused the illness, suicidal ideations, expressed desire to die

Outcome Criteria

✔ Patient will be able to express his feelings about his current religious beliefs and will work through grieving process and be able to utilize coping mechanisms successfully.

NOC: *Spiritual Well-Being*

INTERVENTIONS	RATIONALES
Assess patient for desire to discuss religious concerns, and if patient wants to talk about this, be accepting and nonjudgmental.	Allows patient to have unconditional regard, which fosters self-esteem and feelings of worth.

INTERVENTIONS	RATIONALES
Identify patient's religious affiliation, if patient has one, and offer to seek clergy from that denomination should patient so desire.	Provides for opportunity for patient to discuss certain religious beliefs with clergy to dispel any misperceptions, and to help alleviate fears and concerns regarding relationship with God.
Allow sufficient time for patient to continue with religious practices and provide for specific religious restrictions, such as dietary restrictions.	Helps to support patient by accepting beliefs and religious practices, and conveys a caring attitude that fosters further discussion.
Allow patient to verbalize feelings and concerns, and correct any misinformation that patient may believe regarding medical care.	Patients who are dying frequently evaluate their lives and may have both positive and negative emotions that are related to past injustices, family squabbles, relationships, and deeds. Patients need to find meaning and a purpose in their life, and may need assistance in reconciliation with themselves, with others, and with God. A belief in the afterlife and reunion with loved ones who have previously died may be comforting to the patient and family.
Provide opportunity and assist with devotional readings, prayers, religious rituals, meditation, guided imagery, music, and/or biofeedback.	Allows for patient to reconcile self with others and improve coping skills.
Instruct patient/family that patient wishes will be honored. If patient has a living will, or desires a Do Not Resuscitate order, ensure that all staff are aware of this.	Helps patient to know last requests will be completed.
Instruct patient/family that patient will be kept as comfortable as possible, discuss exactly what will happen, and address any concerns they may have.	Dying patients frequently fear the process of dying in pain more than death itself. Reassurance that pain medication will be available and given as often as needed, that the patient will be respected even if not conscious, and that the family may remain with the patient will benefit and enhance the patient's feelings and comfort.

INTERVENTIONS	RATIONALES
Discuss with the family members the options for the patient who is dying.	Hospice allows patients to die at home in the care of their family and helps reconcile differences and enhance bonding, but some families are hesitant to participate in this program and should not be made to feel cruel if their own distress will not permit them to utilize this avenue. Discussion with the family regarding decisions about religious rituals, burial, autopsy, organ donation, or legal matters will help to allay anxiety and worry about these issues.
Instruct family regarding financial resources, community resources, counselors, and so forth for patient's imminent death and burial.	Provides information to allow family time to prepare for emotional crisis and to seek resources that may be able to help with financial burdens.

NIC: *Spiritual Support*

Discharge or Maintenance Evaluation

- Patient will be able to discuss feelings about religious beliefs openly without fear of reprisal.
- Patient will achieve a sense of spiritual acceptance and be able to use coping skills to face medical crises.
- Patient/family will be able to resolve conflicts prior to death.
- Patient will be able to resolve any conflicts with religious beliefs prior to death.
- Family will be able to access community resources for care needed after discharge and/or patient's death.
- Patient/family will have any erroneous information regarding patient's medical condition corrected to allay fears and concerns.

IMPAIRED ORAL MUCOUS MEMBRANE

Related to: infection, inflammation resulting from chemotherapy or radiation therapy, stomatitis

Defining Characteristics: oral pain, discomfort, mucositis, stomatitis, bleeding, dysphagia, coated tongue, dysphasia, difficulty eating, anorexia, altered taste, fissures, dry mouth, gingival hyperplasia, halitosis, oral ulcers or lesions, purulent oral drainage, smooth, atrophic, sensitive tongue, white patches on tongue, curd-like exudates, vesicles, nodules, papules, plaque

Outcome Criteria

✔ Patient will have minimal to no complications from cancer therapies.

✔ Patient will have improvement or healed oral lesions and be able to perform oral care hygiene.

NOC: *Tissue Integrity: Mucous Membrane*

INTERVENTIONS	RATIONALES
Evaluate patient's mouth, teeth, and gums every shift, noting changes, and reporting significant changes to physician.	Assessment helps to identify problems, exacerbations, and prevent recurrence of oral injury caused by chemotherapy or radiation therapy.
Provide good oral hygiene at least every 4 hours and prn.	Refreshes mouth and provides comfort.
Administer antifungal solutions as ordered.	Nystatin is typically ordered to alleviate the pain and discomfort of thrush, and to eradicate the fungal pathogens that cause this condition.
Provide lubrication ointment to lips every 2–4 hours and prn.	Prevents cracking and drying to lips.
Administer artificial saliva drops as ordered.	Replenishes moisture to mouth when patient's therapy results in dry mouth.
Suction oral cavity if patient is not able to clear secretions on his own.	Removes excess saliva and prevents drooling and potential for aspiration of accumulated secretions that could lead to aspiration pneumonia, coughing, choking, or further trauma.
Provide diet that is soft or pureed as tolerated.	Reduces pain by refraining from irritating tissues with harsh, spicy foods. Thicker foods are easier to swallow.
Encourage patient to express feelings and concerns about	Assists patient to accept body changes, and allows for informa-

INTERVENTIONS	RATIONALES
disease process, and changes that affect his body image. Instruct on misperceptions.	tion to be exchanged. Permits corrections of misinformation.
Instruct patient regarding the use of soft-bristled toothbrush or other oral hygiene applicators.	Helps to minimize trauma to already-compromised oral cavity.
Instruct patient/family to avoid temperature extremes with foods, spicy foods, citrus foods, or fried foods.	Avoidance will prevent irritation to damaged tissues.
Instruct patient/family in oral hygiene regimen.	Provides knowledge regarding importance of oral hygiene, proper methods to use, and how to reduce pain, which ultimately will increase nutritional status by increasing intake.

NIC: *Oral Health Maintenance*

Discharge or Maintenance Evaluation

■ Patient will exhibit no lesions or oral wounds, or pain from these lesions will be reduced.

■ Patient will not achieve any further oral trauma or complication to oral mucosa.

■ Patient will be able to discuss concerns and have questions answered, with misinformation corrected.

■ Patient/family will be able to verbalize understanding of oral hygiene care and be able to give return demonstration.

■ Patient will be able to tolerate diet and be able to chew and swallow without difficulty.

DEFICIENT KNOWLEDGE

Related to: lack of information about care of colostomy, prevention or treatment of lymphedema, and care of remaining breast

Defining Characteristics: request for information on ability to care for colostomy, perform exercises to reduce edema on affected side and maintain shoulder mobility

Outcome Criteria

✔ Patient will be able to perform appropriate care of colostomy and achieve restoration of size and function of arm and shoulder on affected side.

NOC: *Knowledge: Treatment Regimen*

INTERVENTIONS	RATIONALES
Assess patient for knowledge of colostomy care and ability and desire to provide self-care of stoma and bowel elimination.	Provides basis for instruction and demonstration of procedures necessary for self-care.
Use written instructions and visual aids in all instructions.	Assists in effective teaching.
Demonstrate setting up and administration of colostomy irrigation.	Assists to establish regular pattern of elimination if colostomy is in descending colon.
Instruct patient in cleansing of stoma and application of skin barrier or skin sealant and adhesive for appliance.	Maintains cleanliness and prevents skin irritation from excreta.
Instruct patient in complete removal of appliance and materials with solvent, warm water, and soap.	Maintains skin integrity.
Instruct patient in measurement and appropriate application of appliance.	Proper fit prevents leakage.
Demonstrate and instruct patient in emptying pouch including cleansing and reclosing with use of deodorant.	Two-piece appliance allows for bag to be removed for emptying and only needs changing q 5 days.
Instruct patient to avoid foods that are constipating, gas-forming, odor-producing, or irritating to the colostomy stoma or mucosa.	Promotes proper elimination via colostomy without discomfort or excessive odor.
Instruct patient to report any change in color of stoma, presence of irritation or drainage, diarrhea, or constipation to nurse or physician.	May be indicative of disturbance in circulation to stoma or mucosa.
Assess patient for edema, pain, and reduced movement in arm on affected side after mastectomy.	Removal of lymph nodes impair lymph removal of fluid which results in edema.
Assess patient for knowledge and compliance in breast self-examination and mammography.	Promotes early detection of abnormality in remaining breast.
Instruct patient to elevate affected arm on pillows, and to avoid any dependent position of arm. Bed should be in semi-Fowler's position.	Promotes drainage of fluid.
Encourage to flex and extend fingers early after surgery and	Prevents contractures and muscle shortening and maintains muscle

INTERVENTIONS	RATIONALES
increase arm and shoulder exercises daily.	tone and circulation.
Refrain from using affected arm for BP monitoring.	Constricts circulation and promotes swelling.
Instruct patient regarding performing hourly ROM exercises, progressing from fingers to hand and wrist movements, and onward to elbow flexion and extension.	Prevents contractures and promotes mobility.
Instruct patient regarding post-mastectomy exercises, use of arm to brush hair, putting on makeup, pulling rope attached to a door knob, using a pulley over a shower rail, using fingers to climb up the wall, and flexion and extension of shoulder.	Promotes lymph and blood circulation to prevent or control lymphedema and maintain use of arm and shoulder.
Instruct patient regarding protecting arm from trauma or sunburn, and to report any injury to physician.	Infection is common in arm that has circulation problems.
Instruct patient regarding the use of an elastic arm sleeve or intermittent pneumatic compression sleeve and device.	Promotes circulation in arm in acute lymphedema by massage.
Instruct in breast self-examination in remaining breast.	Permits early detection of mass in breast by self-examination. Recurrence of breast cancer to the other noninvolved breast is likely.
Instruct patient regarding community resources, support groups for cancer, colostomy, and/or mastectomy patients, and so forth.	Provides for assistance from peers once patient is discharged from hospital.

NIC: *Teaching: Disease Process*

Discharge or Maintenance Evaluation

- Patient will be able to perform care of colostomy stoma and peristomal skin, irrigation, and appliance removal and reapplication accurately.

- Patient will be able to comply with dietary restrictions to avoid colostomy dysfunction.

- Patient will be able to accurately perform breast self-examination monthly.

- Patient will be able to perform postmastectomy exercises.
- Patient will have chronic lymphedema maintained at minimal levels by use of exercise and/or compression devices.
- Patient will maintain mobility of affected arm postmastectomy.

- Patient will be able to request information and ask questions when needed.
- Patient will be able to adequately access community resources and support groups for assistance postdischarge.

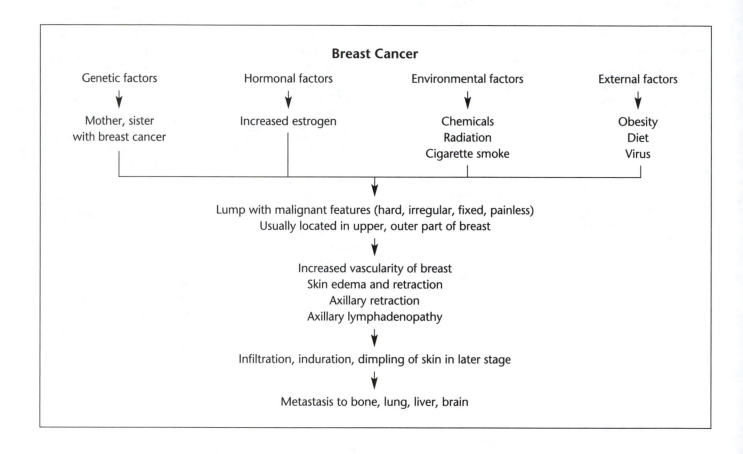

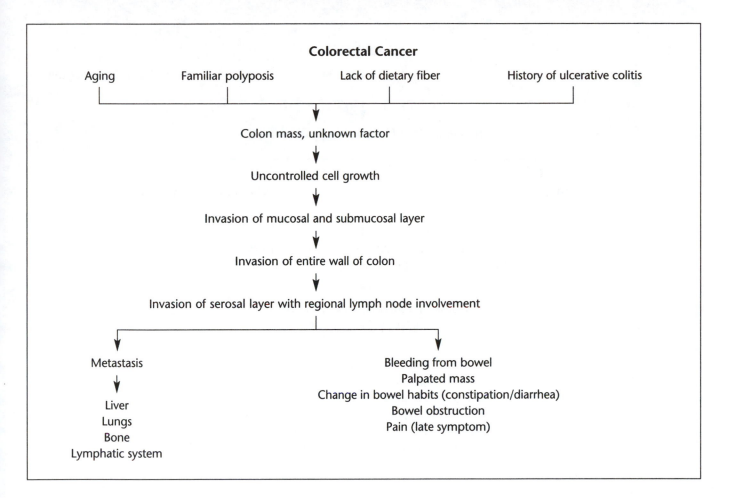

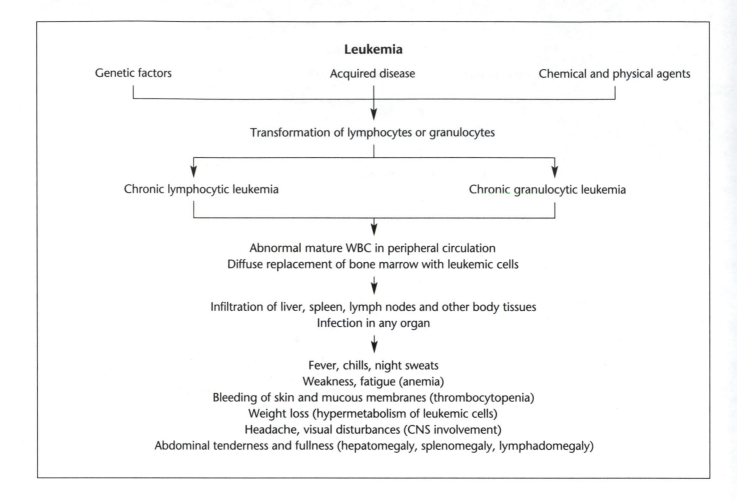

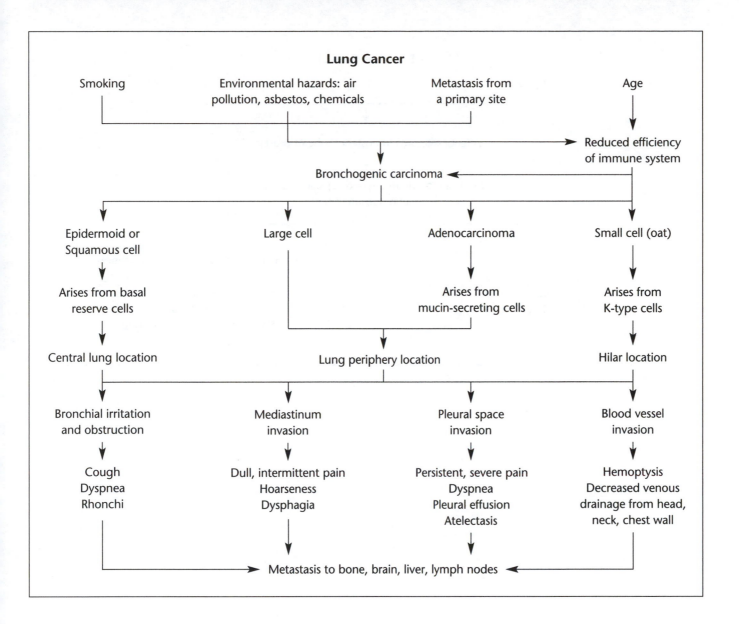

Lung Cancer

Smoking   Environmental hazards: air   Metastasis from   Age
                 pollution, asbestos, chemicals   a primary site

Reduced efficiency
of immune system

Bronchogenic carcinoma

Epidermoid or   Large cell   Adenocarcinoma   Small cell (oat)
Squamous cell

Arises from basal   Arises from   Arises from
reserve cells   mucin-secreting cells   K-type cells

Central lung location   Lung periphery location   Hilar location

Bronchial irritation   Mediastinum   Pleural space   Blood vessel
and obstruction   invasion   invasion   invasion

Cough   Dull, intermittent pain   Persistent, severe pain   Hemoptysis
Dyspnea   Hoarseness   Dyspnea   Decreased venous
Rhonchi   Dysphagia   Pleural effusion   drainage from head,
                                                         Atelectasis   neck, chest wall

Metastasis to bone, brain, liver, lymph nodes

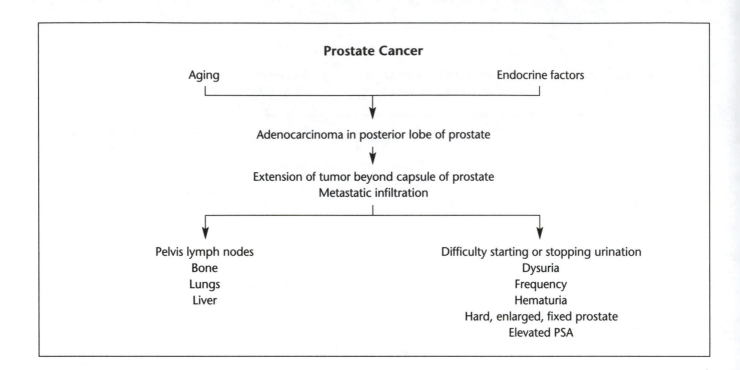

Prostate Cancer

Aging   Endocrine factors

Adenocarcinoma in posterior lobe of prostate

Extension of tumor beyond capsule of prostate
Metastatic infiltration

Pelvis lymph nodes   Difficulty starting or stopping urination
Bone   Dysuria
Lungs   Frequency
Liver   Hematuria
                                                          Hard, enlarged, fixed prostate
                                                                 Elevated PSA

CHAPTER 11.2

DRUG POISONING/OVERDOSE

The use of excessive amounts of medication may happen for many reasons. Active self-destructive behavior usually results from the patient's perception of an overwhelming catastrophic event in life, in conjunction with the lack of appropriate coping strategies, and is visualized as a means of escape from the sensed threat to self. Drug ingestion is the most frequent method utilized with suicidal attempts, partially because of the availability of medications, and partially to avoid more violent means of death, such as with weapons or by hanging.

Although the elderly may consider suicide, drug poisoning is usually an accident that is caused by memory impairment and taking medications twice, or an effect of physiologic impairment in which a "normal" dosage is not metabolized effectively, leading to toxicity of the particular drug. Age-related significant decreases in liver and renal mass and blood flow affect the elimination of drugs. Sometimes drug-receptor interaction among frail elderly patients results in toxicity and organ dysfunction. Dehydration, which the elderly are prone to, also affects how drugs are handled within the body.

Another factor that may predispose the elderly to overdosage/toxicity is polypharmacy. It is rare that an elderly patient takes only one or two medications, and a combination of numerous medications can potentiate or inhibit the action of a specific drug. Central nervous system sedation is increased in the elderly.

The elderly are more prone to have several physicians who are not aware of each other's treatment, and this can lead to repetitious care or prescription of drugs that interact or counteract with each other. Facilitation of one provider directing care helps to coordinate care and avoid duplication of types of drugs that may lead to toxicity.

Approximately one-third of drug-related hospitalizations and half the drug-related deaths that occur are seen in the elderly population (Beers & Berkow, 2000). Patients over age 60 are at great risk for toxicity from specific drugs, especially the long-acting benzodiazepines, NSAIDs, coumadin, aminoglycosides, thiazides, chemotherapy drugs, and anti-dysrhythmics. Toxicity can also be attributed to drug-related organic changes that may create potentiation of a drug reaction.

Dosages in the elderly must be decreased, depending on the patient, metabolism, and the presence of other disease processes. Usually starting doses are begun anywhere from one-third to one-half of the normal dosage and increased as tolerated.

MEDICAL CARE

Laboratory: CBC to identify infection, anemia, and platelet dysfunction; electrolyte profiles used to identify imbalances which can result in toxicity; renal and liver profiles to evaluate dysfunction and decreases in metabolism of drugs; drug screens may be used to identify the specific agent that may have been used in a suicidal attempt; alcohol level used to assess concurrent use or toxicity; specific drug levels used to identify therapeutic versus toxic reactions; coagulation profiles used to identify coagulopathy; urinalysis may show low specific gravity, increased protein, hematuria, oxalate crystals, or metabolic byproducts from a drug overdose

Radiography: chest X-rays may show aspiration pneumonia, pulmonary effusions, infiltrates, cardiac silhouette and hypertrophy

Electrocardiogram: used to identify conduction problems of dysrhythmias that may occur from drug toxicity, electrolyte disturbances, or with heart failure

Dialysis: hemodialysis or hemoperfusion may be performed to remove some drugs when levels are severely elevated

Diuretics: chlorthalidone (Hygroton, Thalitone), hydrochlorothiazide (Esidrix, Ezide, HydroDiuril, Microzide, Oretic), Indapamide (Lozol), and metolazone (Mykrox, Zaroxolyn) are thiazide-acting diuretics that increase sodium and water excretion by inhibiting reabsorption of sodium in the cortical diluting site of the ascending loop of Henle, or inhibit sodium and chloride reabsorption in the distal segment of the nephron; amiloride hydrochloride (Amiloride, Midamor), spironolactone (Aldactone), and triamterene (Dyrenium) are potassium-sparing diuretics that inhibit sodium reabsorption and potassium and hydrogen excretion by their action on the distal tubules; both promote diuresis and elimination of acebutolol hydrochloride sodium; diuretics may be required to manage certain forms of overdose

NURSING DIAGNOSES

RISK FOR INJURY
(see LIVER FAILURE)

Related to: drug overdose, drug toxicity

Defining Characteristics: respiratory depression, pulmonary edema, shock, dysrhythmias, encephalopathy, mental status changes, edema, visual changes, bronchoconstriction, blindness, hypotension, hypothermia, seizures, hypertension, rhabdomyolysis, oliguria, anuria, heart failure, liver failure, renal failure, coagulopathy

RISK FOR SUICIDE
(see DEPRESSION)

Related to: purposeful ingestion of toxic substances, purposeful overdosage, undiagnosed or untreated depression, significant losses, loneliness, decreased abilities, decreased ability to cope, hopelessness, terminal illness, chronic disease, chronic pain

Defining Characteristics: threats of killing oneself, previous history of suicide attempt, significant abrupt changes in behavior, loss of independence, terminal illness, debilitating disease, chronic pain, changing items in one's will, making plans, stockpiling medications, impulsively purchasing a gun, sudden euphoric mood swings after suffering from major depression

INEFFECTIVE COPING
(see DEPRESSION)

Related to: depression, lack of coping skills, physical or emotional impairment, loss of significant other, lack of support systems, change in lifestyle

Defining Characteristics: verbalizations of inability to cope, sleep disturbances, inappropriate coping strategies, social withdrawal, destructive behavior, irritability, aggressiveness, hostility, changes in communication pattern, inability to ask for help, fatigue, increased illness, poor concentration, decreased problem-solving ability, risk-taking behaviors, substance abuse, suicidal ideations and/or attempts

RISK FOR POISONING
(see OSTEOPOROSIS)

Related to: drug toxicity, interactions with medications prescribed, polypharmacy, analgesic abuse, memory changes and physiologic changes associated with the aging process, cognitive limitations

Defining Characteristics: use of numerous medications, adverse medicine effects, drug toxicity levels, inability to take medications correctly, pain, use of analgesic in doses sufficient to cause toxicity or interact with other medicines, inhibition of the action of medicines by use of another medication, use of alcohol, confusion, disorientation, impaired vision, multiple health care providers, multiple pharmacies, inability to understand drug interactions or usage

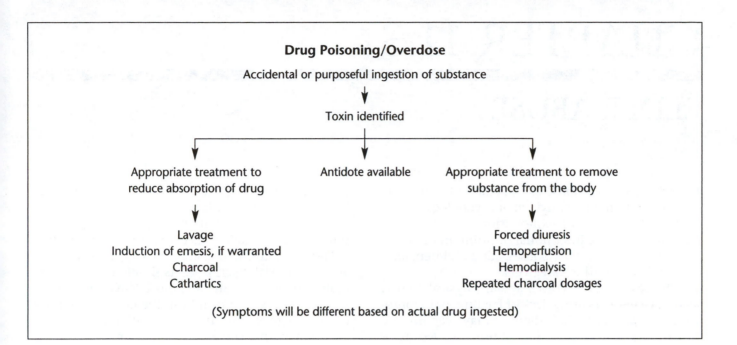

Drug Poisoning/Overdose

Accidental or purposeful ingestion of substance

↓

Toxin identified

Appropriate treatment to reduce absorption of drug	Antidote available	Appropriate treatment to remove substance from the body

Appropriate treatment to reduce absorption of drug

↓

Lavage
Induction of emesis, if warranted
Charcoal
Cathartics

Appropriate treatment to remove substance from the body

↓

Forced diuresis
Hemoperfusion
Hemodialysis
Repeated charcoal dosages

(Symptoms will be different based on actual drug ingested)

CHAPTER 11.3

ELDER ABUSE

In today's society, abuse of the elderly has become common. It involves physical or psychological maltreatment, neglect, or exploitation of the elderly. This abuse may be intentional or unintentional and is usually committed by spouses, adult children, family members, or other caregivers.

Physical abuse involves actual physical injury, such as shaking, beating, lack of feeding, or inappropriate restraining of the patient. It may even involve sexual assault. Psychological abuse uses words or actions to cause emotional distress and suffering, by either verbalizing threats, insults, or harsh comments, or by ignoring and refusing to speak to the patient. Patronizing the patient is a form of abuse that encourages the elderly victim to become reliant on the abuser.

Neglect involves a failure to provide the essentials of life to the elderly patient, such as food, clothing, care, or shelter.

Financial abuse involves taking advantage of the elderly by pressuring a person to buy something, dispensing his or her possessions or money to others, swindling the person of his or her money, or purposely managing the elderly patient's money in an irresponsible manner.

Risk factors for abuse include the presence of physical or cognitive impairment, social isolation, psychiatric disorders, and functional impairment. Frequently, abuse is difficult to identify because the signs may be understated. The patient may be unwilling or unable to discuss the abuse for fear of retribution and retaliation, as well as shame, and a desire to protect the abuser, who may be a family member.

Signs and symptoms of abuse may be ascribed to the patient's illness, but there are certain signs that are predominantly indicative of abuse, such as when the stories of the injury from the patient and the caregiver do not match, when the acuteness of the injury does not fit with the explanation being given by the caregiver, when the patient is seen in the emergency room frequently for chronic disease,

and when the caregiver is reluctant to accept home health care for the patient.

Patients may present with bruises, welts, pressure sores, rectal or vaginal bleeding, lesions to wrists or ankles, fractures, depression, anxiety, poor hygiene, and withdrawal. Such patients should be thoroughly evaluated for abuse, and if found, referred to adult protective services. Removal from the home, or removal of the caregiver from the home with an appropriate replacement, may be the desired treatment.

MEDICAL CARE

Laboratory: CBC used to identify infection, anemia, and platelet dysfunction, albumin level, prealbumin, and protein levels used to determine nutritional status; electrolytes used to identify imbalances and hydration status; many other profile tests to determine potential for abuse

Radiography: used to evaluate patient for fractures and other damage, aspiration, presence of foreign bodies

Reporting of incident: mandatory reporting is required for all suspected elder abuse from institutions in all states, and in most states, when the abuse occurs in the home; Adult Protective Services can assist with interventions tailored to each particular situation

NURSING DIAGNOSES

POST-TRAUMA SYNDROME

Related to: assault, physical abuse or neglect of the elderly

Defining Characteristics: excessive fear, dependent behavior, avoidance of abuser's touch, blames self, unexplained bruises or fractures, lack of supervision, unsafe environment, mismatching stories of event/injury from caregiver and patient

Outcome Criteria

✔ Patient will have an absence of injury and behavior associated with abuse.

✔ Patient will be able to identify and expose abuse, and have resolution of abuse.

NOC: *Abuse Recovery*

INTERVENTIONS	RATIONALES
Evaluate patient's history of injuries, crises, and evidence of abuse or neglect, ability to express abuse, anger, guilt, or fear when caregiver is present.	May be indicative of presence of abuse and identifies the pattern of abuse.
Evaluate patient's activities and perceptions regarding injury. Assess cognitive and emotional status.	Identifies whether patient is capable of separating the real from imagined causes of injury.
Provide protection from abuser.	Prevents continuing abuse.
Refer to community legal support and protective services, and report abuse if suspected.	Protects patient from further abusive behavior or neglect.
Provide privacy during assessments and care.	Patient may be more willing to discuss abuse, promotes trusting relationship, and reduces fear of the abuser.

INTERVENTIONS	RATIONALES
Instruct patient regarding reporting of abuse and advise patient to seek counseling.	Reporting of abuse is mandatory and patient will require counseling to deal with feelings and concerns relating to the abuse, especially if it involves sexual assault or a family member.
Inform family members of situation and patient's physical status, once abuser has been identified.	Helps patient to deal with feelings and to provide alternatives for patient.
Instruct patient/family regarding provision of safe environment and need for supervision.	Prevents injury as a result of neglect in removing hazards from environment.

NIC: *Abuse Protection: Elder*

Discharge or Maintenance Evaluation

■ Patient will be able to halt the physical and emotional abuse and neglect.

■ Patient will be able to reduce behaviors associated with past abuse.

■ Patient will have an absence of injury or trauma.

■ Patient will be able to access community support services for assistance.

CHAPTER 11.4

LONG-TERM CARE

Under normal conditions, the older adult lives in a home or apartment-type dwelling that allows for autonomy and privacy. Leaving this environment with all familiar belongings and memories to live with family members or in a long-term facility creates a sense of loss for the individual. Adjustment to relocation depends on minimal trauma during the transition, accomplished by proper emotional preparation, participation in the admission planning, decision-making, and family acceptance.

The elderly adult has several choices these days for long-term care, depending on the patient's medical, social, and financial needs and resources. If the patient is active, he or she may choose an independent senior-citizen housing development with his or her own apartment and on-site social services. There are facilities that cater to the individual who may be active, but possibly harmful regarding medication administration or food preparation for self; these facilities provide such services, and also personal care. Assisted living housing varies widely from area to area, but provides some or all of the patient's meals, personal care, oversight, housekeeping, and transportation. The majority of elderly patients are not able to afford these alternatives, and ultimately either live with a relative or are placed in a nursing home (Cleverly, 1997).

Skilled nursing facilities, or SNFs, are facilities that provide services to those who are disabled or over the age of 65 years who need daily skilled nursing care or rehabilitation and medical services. Medicare will reimburse a facility for skilled care if it is certified and has a licensed charge nurse on duty 24-hours/day, as well as certified nursing assistants, a social worker, and other licensed administrative personnel. To qualify for coverage for SNF care, a patient must be admitted to the SNF within 30 days after a hospital stay of at least 3 days.

Nursing homes are also expensive. Medicaid pays approximately half the bill, with approximately 37% paid by the patient. Although these facilities must be licensed, there are many instances of abuse and neglect of patients because of their vulnerability and inability to leave the facility. Medicare has a toll-free hotline and a public advocacy system also exists for reporting abuse and fraudulent care.

COMMON NURSING DIAGNOSES

DISTURBED THOUGHT PROCESSES (see DEPRESSION)

Related to: psychological conflicts, physiologic changes

Defining Characteristics: impaired ability for self-care, altered sleep pattern, anxiety, feeling of abandonment, presence of family conflict, involuntary placement or relocation

ADDITIONAL NURSING DIAGNOSES

RELOCATION STRESS SYNDROME

Related to: decreased physical health status, lack of support system, feeling of powerlessness, past, concurrent, and recent losses, moderate to high degree of environmental change

Defining Characteristics: change in environment/location, increased confusion, anxiety and apprehension, insecurity, sad affect, withdrawal, vigilance, verbalization of unwillingness to relocate or transfer

Outcome Criteria

✔ Patient will achieve relocation adjustment with adaptation to new environment.

NOC: *Psychosocial Adjustment: Life Change*

INTERVENTIONS	RATIONALES
Assess patient's need for new living quarters, feelings about loss of personal possessions, loneliness, meaning of independence, and feelings about sudden dependence.	Provides information useful in assisting adaptation to the new environment.
Assess patient for anxiety, anger, depression, and other negative emotions.	Responses to trauma or relocation.
Familiarize patient/family with admission process and planning. Allow patient to participate in decisions regarding daily needs.	Promotes smooth transition and some control over the environment.
Discuss feelings of family during relocations and presence of guilt, conflict, and/or supporting behaviors.	Family attitude can interfere with and create problems with adjustment.
Provide privacy, personal space, and personal objects. Allow patient to arrange items and furniture in own room.	Promotes satisfaction with new environment.
Encourage familiar coping skills and anxiety reduction techniques.	Increases autonomy and improves self-esteem.

INTERVENTIONS	RATIONALES
Instruct patient of choices to make regarding daily care and leisure activities within physical and mental limitations.	Promotes independence and empowers patient to meet obligations and responsibilities.
Review discharge plan and discuss implementation with patient and family.	Provides continuity of care if discharged from a hospital.

NIC: *Health System Guidance*

Discharge or Maintenance Evaluation

- Patient will progressively move through phases of adjustment to new environment.
- Patient will be able to maintain sense of autonomy, privacy, and personal space.
- Patient will be able to manage self-care and choice of activities within identified limitations.
- Patient will be able to participate in decision-making regarding planning of daily routines.
- Patient will be able to participate in decision-making regarding choice of long-term care facility.

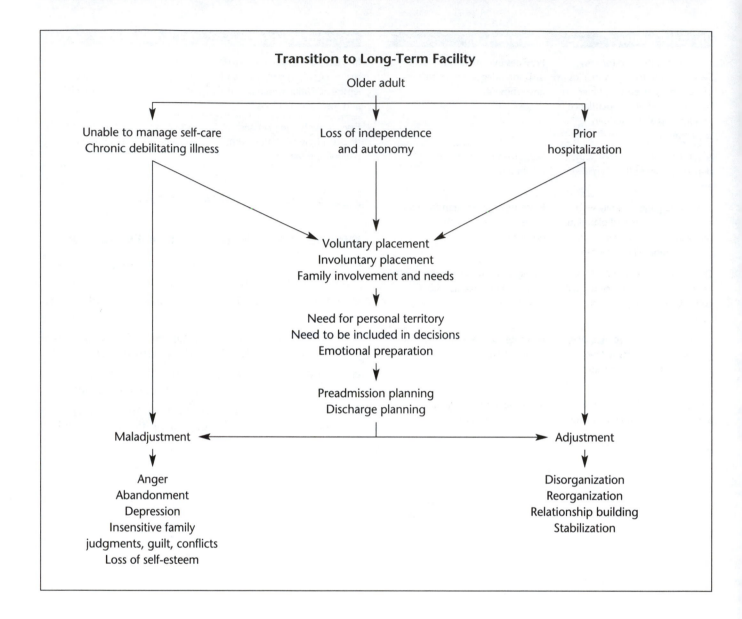

Transition to Long-Term Facility

Older adult

Unable to manage self-care
Chronic debilitating illness

Loss of independence
and autonomy

Prior
hospitalization

Voluntary placement
Involuntary placement
Family involvement and needs

Need for personal territory
Need to be included in decisions
Emotional preparation

Preadmission planning
Discharge planning

Maladjustment

Adjustment

Anger
Abandonment
Depression
Insensitive family
judgments, guilt, conflicts
Loss of self-esteem

Disorganization
Reorganization
Relationship building
Stabilization

BIBLIOGRAPHY

BOOKS

Alfaro-LaFevre, R. (2004). *Critical thinking in nursing: A practical approach* (3rd ed.). Philadelphia: W.B. Saunders Co.

Barnum, B.S. (1999). Teaching nursing in the era of managed care. New York: Springer Publishing.

Baron, R.B. (Ed.). (2001). *Current medical diagnosis and treatment 2001* (40th ed.). New York: McGraw-Hill Publishers.

Beers, M. & Berkow, R. (Eds.). (2000). *The Merck manual of geriatrics* (3rd ed.). Rahway, NJ: Merck, Sharp, & Dohme, Inc.

Beers, M. & Berkow, R. (Eds.). (1999). *The Merck manual* (17th ed.). Rahway, NJ: Merck, Sharp, & Dohme, Inc.

Black, J., Hokanson, J., & Keene, A. (2002). *Medical-Surgical nursing: Clinical management for positive outcomes* (7th ed.). St. Louis, MO: Mosby-Year Book Inc.

Blanchard, R. & Loeb, S. (2001). *Nurse's drug looseleaf.* Blue Bell, PA: Blanchard & Loeb Publishers, Inc.

Butler, R.N., Lewis, M., & Sunderland, T. (1998). *Aging and mental health* (5th ed.). New York: Macmillan and Co.

Carlson, K., Eisenstat, S., & Ziporyn, T. (1996). *The Harvard guide to women's health* (2nd ed.). Cambridge, MA: Harvard University Press.

Carpenito, L.J. (2002). *Nursing diagnosis: Application to clinical practice* (9th ed.). Philadelphia: Lippincott Williams & Wilkins.

Carpenito, L.J. (2004). *Nursing care plans and documentation: Nursing diagnosis and collaborative problems* (4th ed.). Philadelphia: Lippincott Williams & Wilkins.

Carpenito, L.J. (2004). *Handbook of nursing diagnosis* (10th ed.). Philadelphia: Lippincott Williams & Wilkins.

Carpenito, L. J. (2004). *Nursing diagnosis: Application to clinical practice* (10th ed.). Philadelphia: Lippincott Williams & Wilkins.

Chenitz, W.C., Stone, J.T., Wyman, J.F., & Salisbury, S.A. (Eds.). (1998). *Clinical gerontological nursing: A guide to advanced nursing practice.* Philadelphia: W.B. Saunders Co.

Christiansen, J.L. & Grzybowski, J.M. (1999). *Biology of aging: 2000 version.* St. Louis, MO: Mosby-Year Book.

Cleverly, W. 1997. *Essentials of health care finance* (4th ed.). Pacific Grove, CA: Aspen Publishing.

Comer, S. (2004). *Delmar's Critical care nursing care plans* (2nd ed.). Clifton Park, NY: Thomson Delmar Learning.

Cress, C. (2001). *Handbook of geriatric care management.* Pacific Grove, CA: Aspen Publishing.

DeLaune, S.C. & Ladner, P.K. (2002). *Fundamentals of nursing: Standards and practice* (2nd ed.). Clifton Park, NY: Thomson Delmar Learning.

Dochterman, J.M., & Bulechek, G.M. (2004). *Nursing Interventions Classificaton (NIC)* (4th ed.). St. Louis: Mosby, Inc.

Doenges, M.E., Geissler, A.C., & Moorhouse, M.F. (2002). *Nursing care plans: Guidelines for individualizing patient care* (5th ed.). Philadelphia: F.A. Davis Co.

Duthie, E.H., Kersey, R., & Katz, P.R. (Eds.). (1998). *Practice of geriatrics* (3rd ed.). Philadelphia: W.B. Saunders Co.

Ebersole, P. & Hess, P. (2001). *Geriatric nursing and healthy aging.* St. Louis, MO: Mosby-Year Book, Inc.

Eliopoulos, C. (1999). *Manual of Gerontologic Nursing* (2nd ed.). St. Louis, MO: Mosby-Year Book.

Fowles, D. (Ed.). (1993). *A profile of older Americans.* Washington, DC: American Association of Retired Persons.

Gardner, P. (2003). *Nursing process in action.* Clifton Park, NY: Thomson Delmar Learning.

Gomella, L. & Haist, S. (Eds.). (1997). *Clinician's pocket reference* (8th ed.). Philadelphia: McGraw-Hill Publishing.

Grif Alspach, J. (Ed.). (1998). *Core curriculum for critical care nursing* (5th ed.). Philadelphia: W.B. Saunders Co.

Gulanick, M. & Myers, J. (2003). *Nursing care plans: Nursing diagnosis and intervention* (5th ed.). St. Louis, MO: Mosby-Year Book.

Hamdy, R.C., Edwards, J., & Turnball, J.M. (1997). *Alzheimer's disease: A handbook for caregivers* (3rd ed.). St. Louis, MO: Mosby-Year Book.

Harkreader, H. (2004). *Fundamentals of nursing: Caring and clinical judgment* (2nd ed.). Philadelphia: W.B. Saunders Co.

Harvey, M. (2000). *Study guide to core curriculum for critical care nursing* (3rd ed.). Philadelphia: W.B. Saunders Co.

Hogstel, M., Zembrzuski, C., & Wallace, M. (2001). *Gerontology: Nursing care of the older adult.* Clifton Park, NY: Thomson Delmar Learning.

Katz, B.R. & Bressler, R. (2003). *Geriatric pharmacology.* New York: McGraw-Hill.

Kelly-Heidenthal, P. (2003). *Nursing leadership and management*. Clifton Park, NY: Thomson Delmar Learning.

Kozier, B., Erb, G., Blais, K., & Wilkinson, J. (2004). *Fundamentals of nursing: Concepts, process, and practice*. Upper Saddle River, NJ: Pearson Education.

Lewis, S.M., Collier, I., Heitkemper, M.M. & Dirksen, S.R. (2000). *Medical-Surgical nursing: Assessment and management of clinical problems* (5th ed.). St. Louis, MO: Mosby-Year Book.

Lueckenotte, A.G. (1998). *Pocket guide to gerontologic assessment* (3rd ed.). St. Louis, MO: Mosby-Year Book.

Lueckenote, A. (2000). *Gerontologic nursing* (2nd ed.). St. Louis: Mosby, Inc.

Maas, M., Buckwalter, K., Tripp-Reimer, T., Titler, M., & Hardy, M. (2000). *Nursing care of older adults: Diagnoses, outcomes, and interventions*. St. Louis, MO: Mosby-Year Book.

Maas, M., Johnson, M., & Moorhead (Eds.). (2000). *Nursing outcomes classification (NOC)* (2nd ed.). St. Louis, MO: Mosby-Year Book.

Matteson, M.A., McConnell, E.S., & Linton, A. (Eds.). (1997). *Gerontological nursing: Concepts and practice* (2nd ed.). Philadelphia: W.B. Saunders Co.

McCloskey, J.C. & Bulechek, G.M. (2000). *Nursing interventions classification (NIC)* (3rd ed.). St. Louis, MO: Mosby-Year Book.

Medical-Surgical nursing (10th ed.). Philadelphia: Lippincott Williams & Wilkins.

Mezey, M., Berkman, B., & Callahan, C. (2001). *The encyclopedia of elder care: The comprehensive resource on geriatrics and social care*. New York: Springer Publishing Co.

Mitly, E. (2000). *Handbook for directors of nursing in long-term care*. Clifton Park, NY: Thomson Delmar Learning.

Moorhead, S., Johnson, M., & Maas, M. (2004). *Nursing Outcomes Classification (NOC)* (3rd ed.). St. Louis: Mosby, Inc.

Nettina, S. (Ed.). (2000). *Lippincott's manual of nursing practice* (7th ed.). Philadelphia: Lippincott Williams & Wilkins.

Nettina, S. (2001). *The Lippincott manual of nursing practice* (7th ed.). Philadelphia: Lippincott Williams & Wilkins.

North American Nursing Diagnosis Association (NANDA) (2003). *Nursing diagnoses: Definitions & classification 2003–2004*. Philadelphia: North American Nursing Diagnosis Association.

Salzman, C. (Ed.). (1997). *Clinical geriatric psychopharmacology* (3rd ed.). Baltimore: Lippincott Williams & Wilkins.

Smeltzer, S. & Bare, B. (Eds.). (2004). *Brunner and Suddarth's textbook of medical-surgical nursing* (10th ed.). Philadelphia: Lippincott Williams & Wilkins.

Sodeman, W.A. & Kersey, R. (Eds.). (1999). *Instructions for geriatric patients*. Philadelphia: W.B. Saunders Co.

Sparks, S. & Taylor, C. (2001). *Nursing diagnosis reference manual* (5th ed.). Springhouse, PA: Springhouse Corporation.

Spratto, G., & Woods, A. (2004). *2004 PDR nurse's drug handbook*. Clifton Park, NY: Thomson Delmar Learning.

Stanley, M. & Beare, P.G. (Eds.). (1999). *Gerontological nursing* (2nd ed.). Philadelphia: F.A. Davis.

Stone, J., Wyman, J., & Salisbury, S. (1999). *Clinical gerontological nursing: A guide to advanced practice* (2nd ed.). Philadelphia: W.B. Saunders Co.

Ulrich, S., & Canale, W. (2001). *Nursing care planning guides: For adults in acute, extended and home care settings* (5th ed.). Philadelphia: W.B. Saunders Co.

Urden, L., Diann, S., Lough, M., and Urden, M. (2002). *Thelan's critical care nursing: Diagnosis and management*. St. Louis: Mosby, Inc.

Watson, J. & Cavanaugh, B. (1999). *Nurse's manual and laboratory and diagnostic tests* (2nd ed.). Philadelphia: F.A. Davis.

White, L. (2003). *Documentation and the nursing process*. Clifton Park, NY: Thomson Delmar Learning.

Wold, G. (1999). *Basic geriatric nursing* (2nd ed.). St. Louis, MO: Mosby-Year Book, Inc.

PERIODICALS

Alcoser, P. & Burchett, S. (1999). Bone marrow transplantation. *American Journal of Nursing, 99* (6), 26–31.

Barker, E. (1999). Brain attack! A call to action. *RN, 62* (5), 54–62.

Bockhold, K. (2000). Who's afraid of hepatitis C? *American Journal of Nursing, 100* (5), 26–31.

Calandra, J. & Petterson, R. (2001, October 1). Midlife sexuality—Understanding the social, biological, and emotional factors for women. *Nurseweek*.

Chua Patel, C., Kinsey, G., Koperski-Moen, K., & Bungum, L. (2000). Vacuum-Assisted wound closure. *American Journal of Nursing, 100* (12), 45–48.

Dilanchian, P. (2001, October 15). Hypertension—Staying informed about drug therapy. *Nurseweek*.

Dowd, R. & Cavalieri, R.J. (1999). Help your patient live with osteoporosis. *American Journal of Nursing, 99* (4), 55–60.

Fischer, C. & Hegge, M. (2000). The elderly woman at risk. *American Journal of Nursing, 100* (6), 54–58.

Goldsmith, C. (1999). Hypothyroidism. *American Journal of Nursing, 99* (6), 42–43.

Goldstein, L.E. & Henderson, D.C. (2000). Atypical antipsychotic agents and diabetes mellitus. *Primary Psychiatry* (7) 5, 65–68.

Gray, M. (2000). Urinary retention: Management in the acute care setting. *American Journal of Nursing, 100* (8), 36–42.

Habel, M. (2001, March 19). Brain attack—New stroke treatments, education can limit disabilities. *Nurseweek*.

Habel, M. (2001, May 14). Joint replacement—Coming soon to a person near you. *Nurseweek.*

Hailey, D. & Topfer, L.A. (2002). Extracorporeal immuno-adsorption therapy for rheumatoid arthritis. *Issues in Emergency Health Technology, 28* (1), 1–4.

Halm, M. & Penque, S. (1999). Heart disease in women. *American Journal of Nursing, 99* (4), 26–31.

Hoban, S. (2000). Elder abuse and neglect. *American Journal of Nursing, 100* (11), 49–50.

Kearney, K. (2000). Digitalis toxicity. *American Journal of Nursing, 100* (6), 51–52.

King, M. & Tomasic, D. (1999). Treating TB today. *RN, 62* (6), 26–30.

Kozuh, J. (2000). NSAIDs & antihypertensives: An unhappy union. *American Journal of Nursing, 100* (6), 40–42.

Mitchell, R. (1999). Sickle Cell Anemia. *American Journal of Nursing, 99* (5), 38–39.

Nestel, P.J., Shige, H., & Pomeroy, S. (2001). High-fat meals impair arterial elasticity and increase heart attack risk. *Journal of the American College of Cardiology, 37* (7), 1929–1935.

O'Hanlon-Nichols, T. (1999). Neurologic assessment: The basics of a comprehensive examination. *American Journal of Nursing, 99* (6), 44–50.

Orhon Jeck, A. (2001, April 2). Of human bondage—Alternatives to restraints help reduce risks to patients. *Healthweek*

Poznanski Hutchison, C. (1999). Healing touch: An energetic approach. *American Journal of Nursing, 99* (4), 43–48.

Ramsburg, K. (2000). Rheumatoid arthritis. *American Journal of Nursing, 100* (11), 40–43.

Schneidewind-Muller, J.M., Winkler, R.E., & Tiess, M. (2002). Changes in lymphocytic cluster distribution during extracorporeal immunoadsorption. *Artificial Organs, 26* (2), 140–144.

Schoofs, N. (1999). Sjogren's syndrome? *RN, 62* (4), 45–47.

Shovein, J., Damazo, R., & Hyams, I. (2000). Hepatitis A: How benign is it? *American Journal of Nursing, 100* (5), 43–47.

Valsa, M. & Lawrence, M. (2001, September 3). Post-acute care—Where does the money come from? *Nurseweek.*

Warner, P., Rowe, T., & Whipple, B. (1999). Shedding light on the sexual history. *American Journal of Nursing, 99* (6), 34–40.

Warzynski, D. (2001, June 25). Chronic care—How to achieve continuity across the continuum. *Nurseweek.*

Wilson, D. & Tracy, M. (2000). CABG and the elderly. *American Journal of Nursing, 100* (5), 24AA–24UU.

Zaccagnini, M. (1999). Prostate cancer. *American Journal of Nursing, 99* (4), 34–35.

APPENDIX A

NANDA NURSING DIAGNOSES

Activity Intolerance
Acute Confusion
Acute Pain
Adult Failure To Thrive
Anticipatory Grieving
Anxiety
Autonomic Dysreflexia

Bathing/Hygiene Self-Care Deficit
Bowel Incontinence

Caregiver Role Strain
Chronic Confusion
Chronic Low Self-Esteem
Chronic Pain
Chronic Sorrow
Compromised Family Coping
Constipation

Death Anxiety
Decisional Conflict (specify)
Decreased Cardiac Output
Decreased Intracranial Adaptive Capacity
Defensive Coping
Deficient Diversional Activity
Deficient Fluid Volume
Deficient Knowledge (specify)
Delayed Growth And Development
Delayed Surgical Recovery
Diarrhea
Disabled Family Coping
Disorganized Infant Behavior
Disturbed Body Image
Disturbed Energy Field
Disturbed Personal Identity
Disturbed Sensory Perception (specify: visual, auditory,
   kinesthetic, gustatory, tactile, olfactory)
Disturbed Sleep Pattern
Disturbed Thought Processes
Dressing/Grooming Self-Care Deficit
Dysfunctional Family Processes: Alcoholism
Dysfunctional Grieving
Dysfunctional Ventilatory Weaning Response

Effective Breast-Feeding
Effective Therapeutic Regimen Management
Excess Fluid Volume

Fatigue
Fear
Feeding Self-Care Deficit
Functional Urinary Incontinence

Health-Seeking Behaviors (specify)
Hopelessness
Hyperthermia
Hypothermia

Imbalanced Nutrition: Less Than Body Requirements
Imbalanced Nutrition: More Than Body Requirements
Impaired Adjustment
Impaired Bed Mobility
Impaired Dentition
Impaired Environmental Interpretation Syndrome
Impaired Gas Exchange
Impaired Home Maintenance
Impaired Memory
Impaired Oral Mucous Membrane
Impaired Parenting
Impaired Physical Mobility
Impaired Skin Integrity
Impaired Social Interaction
Impaired Spontaneous Ventilation
Impaired Swallowing
Impaired Tissue Integrity
Impaired Transfer Ability
Impaired Urinary Elimination
Impaired Verbal Communication
Impaired Walking
Impaired Wheelchair Mobility
Ineffective Airway Clearance
Ineffective Breast-Feeding
Ineffective Breathing Pattern
Ineffective Community Coping
Ineffective Community Therapeutic Regimen
   Management
Ineffective Coping

Ineffective Denial
Ineffective Family Therapeutic Regimen Management
Ineffective Health Maintenance
Ineffective Infant Feeding Pattern
Ineffective Protection
Ineffective Role Performance
Ineffective Sexuality Patterns
Ineffective Therapeutic Regimen Management
Ineffective Thermoregulation
Ineffective Tissue Perfusion (specify type: renal, cerebral, cardiopulmonary, gastrointestinal, peripheral)
Interrupted Breast-Feeding
Interrupted Family Processes

Latex Allergy Response

Nausea
Noncompliance (specify)

Parental Role Conflict
Perceived Constipation
Post-Trauma Syndrome
Powerlessness

Rape-Trauma Syndrome
Rape-Trauma Syndrome: Compound Reaction
Rape-Trauma Syndrome: Silent Reaction
Readiness for Enhanced Communicaton
Readiness for Enhanced Community Coping
Readiness for Enhanced Coping
Readiness for Enhanced Family Coping
Readiness for Enhanced Family Processes
Readiness for Enhanced Fluid Balance
Readiness for Enhanced Knowledge (specify)
Readiness for Enhanced Nutrition
Readiness for Enhanced Organized Infant Behavior
Readiness for Enhanced Parenting
Readiness for Enhanced Self-Concept
Readiness for Enhanced Sleep
Readiness for Enhanced Spiritual Well-Being
Readiness for Enhanced Therapeutic Regimen Management
Readiness for Enhanced Urinary Elimination
Reflex Urinary Incontinence
Relocation Stress Syndrome
Risk for Activity Intolerance
Risk for Aspiration
Risk for Autonomic Dysreflexia
Risk for Caregiver Role Strain
Risk for Constipation
Risk for Deficient Fluid Volume

Risk for Delayed Development
Risk for Disorganized Infant Behavior
Risk for Disproportionate Growth
Risk for Disuse Syndrome
Risk for Falls
Risk for Imbalanced Body Temperature
Risk for Imbalanced Fluid Volume
Risk for Imbalanced Nutrition: More Than Body Requirements
Risk for Impaired Parent/Infant/Child Attachment
Risk for Impaired Parenting
Risk for Impaired Skin Integrity
Risk for Infection
Risk for Injury
Risk for Latex Allergy Response
Risk for Loneliness
Risk for Other-Directed Violence
Risk for Perioperative-Positioning Injury
Risk for Peripheral Neurovascular Dysfunction
Risk for Poisoning
Risk for Post-Trauma Syndrome
Risk for Powerlessness
Risk for Relocation Stress Syndrome
Risk for Self-Directed Violence
Risk for Self-Mutilation
Risk for Situational Low Self-Esteem
Risk for Spiritual Distress
Risk for Sudden Infant Death Syndrome
Risk for Suffocation
Risk for Suicide
Risk for Trauma
Risk for Urge Urinary Incontinence

Self-Mutilation
Sexual Dysfunction
Situational Low Self-Esteem
Sleep Deprivation
Social Isolation
Spiritual Distress
Stress Urinary Incontinence

Toileting Self-Care Deficit
Total Urinary Incontinence

Unilateral Neglect
Urinary Retention
Urge Urinary Incontenance

Wandering

APPENDIX B

NURSING OUTCOMES CLASSIFICATIONS (NOC)

Abuse Cessation
Abuse Protection
Abuse Recovery Status
Abuse Recovery: Emotional
Abuse Recovery: Financial
Abuse Recovery: Physical
Abuse Recovery: Sexual
Abusive Behavior Self-Restraint
Acceptance: Health Status
Activity Tolerance
Adaptation to Physical Disability
Adherence Behavior
Aggression Self-Control
Allergic Response: Localized
Allergic Response: Systemic
Ambulation
Ambulation: Wheelchair
Anxiety Level
Anxiety Self-Control
Appetite
Aspiration Prevention
Asthma Self-Management

Balance
Blood Coagulation
Blood-Glucose Level
Blood Loss Severity
Blood Transfusion Reaction
Body Image
Body Mechanics Performance
Body Positioning: Self-Initiated
Bone Healing
Bowel Continence
Bowel Elimination
Breastfeeding Establishment: Infant
Breastfeeding Establishment: Maternal
Breastfeeding: Maintenance
Breastfeeding: Weaning

Cardiac Disease Self-Management
Cardiac Pump Effectiveness
Caregiver Adaptation to Patient Institutionalization
Caregiver Emotional Health

Caregiver Home Care Readiness
Caregiver Lifestyle Disruption
Caregiver-Patient Relationship
Caregiver Performance: Direct Care
Caregiver Performance: Indirect Care
Caregiver Physical Health
Caregiver Stressors
Caregiver Well-Being
Caregiving Endurance Potential
Child Adaptation to Hospitalization
Child Development: 1 Month
Child Development: 2 Months
Child Development: 4 Months
Child Development: 6 Months
Child Development: 12 Months
Child Development: 2 Years
Child Development: 3 Years
Child Development: 4 Years
Child Development: Middle Childhood
Child Development: Adolescence
Circulation Status
Client Satisfaction: Access to Care Resources
Client Satisfaction: Caring
Client Satisfaction: Communication
Client Satisfaction: Continuity of Care
Client Satisfaction: Cultural Needs Fulfillment
Client Satisfaction: Functional Assistance
Client Satisfaction: Physical Care
Client Satisfaction: Physical Environment
Client Satisfaction: Protection of Rights
Client Satisfaction: Psychological Care
Client Satisfaction: Safety
Client Satisfaction: Symptom Control
Client Satisfaction: Teaching
Client Satisfaction: Technical Aspects of Care
Cognition
Cognitive Orientation
Comfort Level
Comfortable Death
Communication
Communication: Expressive
Communication: Receptive
Community Competence

Community Disaster Readiness
Community Health Status
Community Health Status: Immunity
Community Risk Control: Chronic Disease
Community Risk Control: Communicable Disease
Community Risk Control: Lead Exposure
Community Risk Control: Violence
Community Violence Level
Compliance Behavior
Concentration
Coordinated Movement
Coping

Decision Making
Depression Level
Depression Self-Control
Diabetes Self-Management
Dignified Life Closure
Discharge Readiness: Independent Living
Discharge Readiness: Supported Living
Distorted Thought Self-Control

Electrolyte and Acid/Base Balance
Endurance
Energy Conservation

Fall Prevention Behavior
Falls Occurrence
Family Coping
Family Functioning
Family Health Status
Family Integrity
Family Normalization
Family Participation in Professional Care
Family Physical Environment
Family Resiliency
Family Social Climate
Family Support During Treatment
Fear Level
Fear Level: Child
Fear Self-Control
Fetal Status: Antepartum
Fetal Status: Intrapartum
Fluid Balance
Fluid Overload Severity

Grief Resolution
Growth

Health Beliefs
Health Beliefs: Perceived Ability to Perform
Health Beliefs: Perceived Control
Health Beliefs: Perceived Resources
Health Beliefs: Perceived Threat
Health Orientation
Health-Promoting Behavior

Health-Seeking Behavior
Hearing Compensation Behavior
Hemodialysis Access
Hope
Hydration
Hyperactivity Level

Identity
Immobility Consequences: Physiological
Immobility Consequences: Psycho-Cognitive
Immune Hypersensitivity Response
Immune Status
Immunization Behavior
Impulse Self-Control
Infection Severity
Infection Severity: Newborn
Information Processing

Joint Movement: Ankle
Joint Movement: Elbow
Joint Movement: Fingers
Joint Movement: Hip
Joint Movement: Knee
Joint Movement: Neck
Joint Movement: Passive
Joint Movement: Shoulder
Joint Movement: Spine
Joint Movement: Wrist

Kidney Function
Knowledge: Body Mechanics
Knowledge: Breastfeeding
Knowledge: Cardiac Disease Management
Knowledge: Child Physical Safety
Knowledge: Conception Prevention
Knowledge: Diabetes Management
Knowledge: Diet
Knowledge: Disease Process
Knowledge: Energy Conservation
Knowledge: Fall Prevention
Knowledge: Fertility Promotion
Knowledge: Health Behavior
Knowledge: Health Promotion
Knowledge: Health Resources
Knowledge: Illness Care
Knowledge: Infant Care
Knowledge: Infection Control
Knowledge: Labor and Delivery
Knowledge: Medication
Knowledge: Ostomy Care
Knowledge: Parenting
Knowledge: Personal Safety
Knowledge: Postpartum Maternal Health
Knowledge: Preconception Maternal Health
Knowledge: Pregnancy
Knowledge: Prescribed Activity

Knowledge: Sexual Functioning
Knowledge: Substance Abuse Control
Knowledge: Treatment Procedure(s)
Knowledge: Treatment Regimen

Leisure Participation
Loneliness Severity

Maternal Status: Antepartum
Maternal Status: Intrapartum
Maternal Status: Postpartum
Mechanical Ventilation Response: Adult
Mechanical Ventilation Weaning Response: Adult
Medication Response
Memory
Mobility
Mood Equilibrium
Motivation

Nausea & Vomiting Control
Nausea & Vomiting: Disruptive Effects
Nausea & Vomiting Severity
Neglect Cessation
Neglect Recovery
Neurological Status
Neurological Status: Autonomic
Neurological Status: Central Motor Control
Neurological Status: Consciousness
Neurological Status: Cranial Sensory/Motor Function
Neurological Status: Spinal Sensory/Motor Function
Newborn Adaptation
Nutritional Status
Nutritional Status: Biochemical Measures
Nutritional Status: Energy
Nutritional Status: Food and Fluid Intake
Nutritional Status: Nutrient Intake

Oral Health
Ostomy Self-Care

Pain: Adverse Psychological Response
Pain Control
Pain: Disruptive Effects
Pain Level
Parent-Infant Attachment
Parenting: Adolescent Physical Safety
Parenting: Early/Middle Childhood Physical Safety
Parenting: Infant/Toddler Physical Safety
Parenting Performance
Parenting: Psychosocial Safety
Participation in Health Care Decisions
Personal Autonomy
Personal Health Status
Personal Safety Behavior
Personal Well-Being
Physical Aging

Physical Fitness
Physical Injury Severity
Physical Maturation: Female
Physical Maturation: Male
Play Participation
Post Procedure Recovery Status
Prenatal Health Behavior
Preterm Infant Organization
Psychomotor Energy
Psychosocial Adjustment: Life Change

Quality of Life

Respiratory Status: Airway Patency
Respiratory Status: Gas Exchange
Respiratory Status: Ventilation
Rest
Risk Control
Risk Control: Alcohol Use
Risk Control: Cancer
Risk Control: Cardiovascular Health
Risk Control: Drug Use
Risk Control: Hearing Impairment
Risk Control: Sexually Transmitted Diseases (STDs)
Risk Control: Tobacco Use
Risk Control: Unintended Pregnancy
Risk Control: Visual Impairment
Risk Detection
Role Performance

Safe Home Environment
Seizure Control
Self-Care Status
Self-Care: Activities of Daily Living (ADL)
Self-Care: Bathing
Self-Care: Dressing
Self-Care: Eating
Self-Care: Hygiene
Self-Care: Instrumental Activities of Daily Living (IADL)
Self-Care: Nonparenteral Medication
Self-Care: Oral Hygiene
Self-Care: Parenteral Medication
Self-Care: Toileting
Self-Direction of Care
Self-Esteem
Self-Mutilation Restraint
Sensory Function Status
Sensory Function: Cutaneous
Sensory Function: Hearing
Sensory Function: Proprioception
Sensory Function: Taste and Smell
Sensory Function: Vision
Sexual Functioning
Sexual Identity
Skeletal Function
Sleep

Social Interaction Skills
Social Involvement
Social Support
Spiritual Health
Stress Level
Student Health Status
Substance Addiction Consequences
Suffering Severity
Suicide Self-Restraint
Swallowing Status
Swallowing Status: Esophageal Phase
Swallowing Status: Oral Phrase
Swallowing Status: Pharyngeal Phase
Symptom Control
Symptom Severity
Symptom Severity: Perimenopause
Symptom Severity: Premenstrual Syndrome (PMS)
Systemic Toxin Clearance: Dialysis

Thermoregulation
Thermoregulation: Neonate

Tissue Integrity: Skin and Mucous Membranes
Tissue Perfusion: Abdominal Organs
Tissue Perfusion: Cardiac
Tissue Perfusion: Cerebral
Tissue Perfusion: Peripheral
Tissue Perfusion: Pulmonary
Transfer Performance
Treatment Behavior: Illness or Injury

Urinary Continence
Urinary Elimination

Vision Compensation Behavior
Vital Signs

Weight: Body Mass
Weight Control
Will to Live
Wound Healing: Primary Intention
Wound Healing: Primary Intention

APPENDIX C

NURSING INTERVENTIONS CLASSIFICATIONS (NIC)

Abuse Protection Support
Abuse Protection Support: Child
Abuse Protection Support: Domestic Partner
Abuse Protection Support: Elder
Abuse Protection Support: Religious
Acid-Base Management
Acid-Base Management: Metabolic Acidosis
Acid-Base Management: Metabolic Alkalosis
Acid-Base Management: Respiratory Acidosis
Acid-Base Management: Respiratory Alkalosis
Acid-Base Monitoring
Active Listening
Activity Therapy
Acupressure
Admission Care
Airway Insertion And Stabilization
Airway Management
Airway Suctioning
Allergy Management
Amnioinfusion
Amputation Care
Analgesic Administration
Analgesic Administration: Intraspinal
Anaphylaxis Management
Anesthesia Administration
Anger Control Assistance
Animal-Assisted Therapy
Anticipatory Guidance
Anxiety Reduction
Area Restriction
Aromatherapy
Art Therapy
Artificial Airway Management
Aspiration Precautions
Assertiveness Training
Asthma Management
Attachment Promotion
Autogenic Training
Autotransfusion

Bathing
Bed Rest Care
Bedside Laboratory Testing
Behavior Management

Behavior Management: Overactivity/Inattention
Behavior Management: Self-Harm
Behavior Management: Sexual
Behavior Modification
Behavior Modification: Social Skills
Bibliotherapy
Biofeedback
Bioterrorism Preparedness
Birthing
Bladder Irrigation
Bleeding Precautions
Bleeding Reduction
Bleeding Reduction: Antepartum Uterus
Bleeding Reduction: Gastrointestinal
Bleeding Reduction: Nasal
Bleeding Reduction: Postpartum Uterus
Bleeding Reduction: Wound
Blood Products Administration
Body Image Enhancement
Body Mechanics Promotion
Bottle Feeding
Bowel Incontinence Care
Bowel Incontinence Care: Encopresis
Bowel Irrigation
Bowel Management
Bowel Training
Breast Examination
Breastfeeding Assistance

Calming Technique
Capillary Blood Sample
Cardiac Care
Cardiac Care: Acute
Cardiac Care: Rehabilitative
Cardiac Precautions
Caregiver Support
Care Management
Cast Care: Maintenance
Cast Care, Wet
Cerebral Edema Management
Cerebral Perfusion Promotion
Cesarean Section Care
Chemical Restraint
Chemotherapy Management

Chest Physiotherapy
Childbirth Preparation
Circulatory Care: Arterial Insufficiency
Circulatory Care: Mechanical Assist Device
Circulatory Care: Venous Insufficiency
Circulatory Precautions
Circumcision Care
Code Management
Cognitive Restructuring
Cognitive Stimulation
Communicable Disease Management
Communication Enhancement: Hearing Deficit
Communication Enhancement: Speech Deficit
Communication Enhancement: Visual Deficit
Community Disaster Preparedness
Community Health Development
Complex Relationship Building
Conflict Mediation
Constipation/Impaction Management
Consultation
Contact Lens Care
Controlled Substance Checking
Coping Enhancement
Cost Containment
Cough Enhancement
Counseling
Crisis Intervention
Critical Path Development
Culture Brokerage
Cutaneous Stimulation

Decision-Making Support
Delegation
Delirium Management
Delusion Management
Dementia Management
Dementia Management: Bathing
Deposition/Testimony
Developmental Care
Developmental Enhancement: Adolescent
Developmental Enhancement: Child
Dialysis Access Maintenance
Diarrhea Management
Diet Staging
Discharge Planning
Distraction
Documentation
Dressing
Dying Care
Dysreflexia Management
Dysrhythmia Management

Ear Care
Eating Disorders Management
Electroconvulsive Therapy (ECT) Management
Electrolyte Management
Electrolyte Management: Hypercalcemia

Electrolyte Management: Hyperkalemia
Electrolyte Management: Hypermagnesemia
Electrolyte Management: Hypernatremia
Electrolyte Management: Hyperphosphatemia
Electrolyte Management: Hypocalcemia
Electrolyte Management: Hypokalemia
Electrolyte Management: Hypomagnesemia
Electrolyte Management: Hyponatremia
Electrolyte Management: Hypophosphatemia
Electrolyte Monitoring
Electronic Fetal Monitoring: Antepartum
Electronic Fetal Monitoring: Intrapartum
Elopement Precautions
Embolus Care: Peripheral
Embolus Care: Pulmonary
Embolus Precautions
Emergency Care
Emergency Cart Checking
Emotional Support
Endotracheal Extubation
Energy Management
Enteral Tube Feeding
Environmental Management
Environmental Management: Attachment Process
Environmental Management: Comfort
Environmental Management: Community
Environmental Management: Home Preparation
Environmental Management: Safety
Environmental Management: Violence Prevention
Environmental Management: Worker Safety
Environmental Risk Protection
Examination Assistance
Exercise Promotion
Exercise Promotion: Strength Training
Exercise Promotion: Stretching
Exercise Therapy: Ambulation
Exercise Therapy: Balance
Exercise Therapy: Joint Mobility
Exercise Therapy: Muscle Control
Eye Care

Fall Prevention
Family Integrity Promotion
Family Integrity Promotion: Childbearing Family
Family Involvement Promotion
Family Mobilization
Family Planning: Contraception
Family Planning: Infertility
Family Planning: Unplanned Pregnancy
Family Presence Facilitation
Family Process Maintenance
Family Support
Family Therapy
Feeding
Fertility Preservation
Fever Treatment
Financial Resource Assistance

Fire-Setting Precautions
First Aid
Fiscal Resource Management
Flatulence Reduction
Fluid/Electrolyte Management
Fluid Management
Fluid Monitoring
Fluid Resuscitation
Foot Care
Forgiveness Facilitation

Gastrointestinal Intubation
Genetic Counseling
Grief Work Facilitation
Grief Work Facilitation: Perinatal Death
Guilt Work Facilitation

Hair Care
Hallucination Management
Health Care Information Exchange
Health Education
Health Policy Monitoring
Health Screening
Health System Guidance
Heat/Cold Application
Heat Exposure Treatment
Hemodialysis Therapy
Hemodynamic Regulation
Hemofiltration Therapy
Hemorrhage Control
High-Risk Pregnancy Care
Home Maintenance Assistance
Hope Instillation
Hormone Replacement Therapy
Humor
Hyperglycemia Management
Hypervolemia Management
Hypnosis
Hypoglycemia Management
Hypothermia Treatment
Hypovolemia Management

Immunization/Vaccination Administration
Impulse Control Training
Incident Reporting
Incision Site Care
Infant Care
Infection Control
Infection Control: Intraoperative
Infection Protection
Insurance Authorization
Intracranial Pressure (ICP) Monitoring
Intrapartal Care
Intrapartal Care: High-Risk Delivery
Intravenous (IV) Insertion
Intravenous (IV) Therapy
Invasive Hemodynamic Monitoring

Kangaroo Care

Labor Induction
Labor Suppression
Laboratory Data Interpretation
Lactation Counseling
Lactation Suppression
Laser Precautions
Latex Precautions
Learning Facilitation
Learning Readiness Enhancement
Leech Therapy
Limit Setting
Lower Extremity Monitoring

Malignant Hyperthermia Precautions
Mechanical Ventilation
Mechanical Ventilatory Weaning
Medication Administration
Medication Administration: Ear
Medication Administration: Enteral
Medication Administration: Eye
Medication Administration: Inhalation
Medication Administration: Interpleural
Medication Administration: Intradermal
Medication Administration: Intramuscular (IM)
Medication Administration: Intraosseous
Medication Administration: Intraspinal
Medication Administration: Intravenous (IV)
Medication Administration: Nasal
Medication Administration: Oral
Medication Administration: Rectal
Medication Administration: Skin
Medication Administration: Subcutaneous
Medication Administration: Vaginal
Medication Administration: Ventricular Reservoir
Medication Management
Medication Prescribing
Meditation Facilitation
Memory Training
Milieu Therapy
Mood Management
Multidisciplinary Care Conference
Music Therapy
Mutual Goal Setting

Nail Care
Nausea Management
Neurologic Monitoring
Newborn Care
Newborn Monitoring
Nonnutritive Sucking
Normalization Promotion
Nutrition Management
Nutrition Therapy
Nutritional Counseling
Nutritional Monitoring

Oral Health Maintenance
Oral Health Promotion
Oral Health Restoration
Order Transcription
Organ Procurement
Ostomy Care
Oxygen Therapy

Pain Management
Parent Education: Adolescent
Parent Education: Childrearing Family
Parent Education: Infant
Parenting Promotion
Pass Facilitation
Patient Contracting
Patient Controlled Analgesia (PCA) Assistance
Patient Rights Protection
Peer Review
Pelvic Muscle Exercise
Perineal Care
Peripheral Sensation Management
Peripherally Inserted Central (PIC) Catheter Care
Peritoneal Dialysis Therapy
Pessary Management
Phlebotomy: Arterial Blood Sample
Phlebotomy: Blood Unit Acquisition
Phlebotomy: Cannulated Vessel
Phlebotomy: Venous Blood Sample
Phototherapy: Mood/Sleep Regulation
Phototherapy: Neonate
Physical Restraint
Physician Support
Pneumatic Tourniquet Precautions
Positioning
Positioning: Intraoperative
Positioning: Neurologic
Positioning: Wheelchair
Postanesthesia Care
Postmortem Care
Postpartal Care
Preceptor: Employee
Preceptor: Student
Preconception Counseling
Pregnancy Termination Care
Premenstrual Syndrome (PMS) Management
Prenatal Care
Preoperative Coordination
Preparatory Sensory Information
Presence
Pressure Management
Pressure Ulcer Care
Pressure Ulcer Prevention
Product Evaluation
Program Development
Progressive Muscle Relaxation
Prompted Voiding

Prosthesis Care
Pruritus Management

Quality Monitoring

Radiation Therapy Management
Rape-Trauma Treatment
Reality Orientation
Recreation Therapy
Rectal Prolapse Management
Referral
Religious Addiction Prevention
Religious Ritual Enhancement
Relocation Stress Reduction
Reminiscence Therapy
Reproductive Technology Management
Research Data Collection
Resiliency Promotion
Respiratory Monitoring
Respite Care
Resuscitation
Resuscitation: Fetus
Resuscitation: Neonate
Risk Identification
Risk Identification: Childbearing Family
Risk Identification: Genetic
Role Enhancement

Seclusion
Security Enhancement
Sedation Management
Seizure Management
Seizure Precautions
Self-Awareness Enhancement
Self-Care Assistance
Self-Care Assistance: Bathing/Hygiene
Self-Care Assistance: Dressing/Grooming
Self-Care Assistance: Feeding
Self-Care Assistance: IADL
Self-Care Assistance: Toileting
Self-Care Assistance: Transfer
Self-Esteem Enhancement
Self-Hypnosis Facilitation
Self-Modification Assistance
Self-Responsibility Facilitation
Sexual Counseling
Shift Report
Shock Management
Shock Management: Cardiac
Shock Management: Vasogenic
Shock Management: Volume
Shock Prevention
Sibling Support
Simple Guided Imagery
Simple Massage
Simple Relaxation Therapy

Skin Care: Donor Site
Skin Care: Graft Site
Skin Care: Topical Treatments
Skin Surveillance
Sleep Enhancement
Smoking Cessation Assistance
Socialization Enhancement
Specimen Management
Spiritual Growth Facilitation
Spiritual Support
Splinting
Sports-Injury Prevention: Youth
Staff Development
Staff Supervision
Subarachnoid Hemorrhage Precautions
Substance Use Prevention
Substance Use Treatment
Substance Use Treatment: Alcohol Withdrawal
Substance Use Treatment: Drug Withdrawal
Substance Use Treatment: Overdose
Suicide Prevention
Supply Management
Support Group
Support System Enhancement
Surgical Assistance
Surgical Precautions
Surgical Preparation
Surveillance
Surveillance: Community
Surveillance: Late Pregnancy
Surveillance: Remote Electronic
Surveillance: Safety
Sustenance Support
Suturing
Swallowing Therapy

Teaching: Disease Process
Teaching: Foot Care
Teaching: Group
Teaching: Individual
Teaching: Infant Nutrition
Teaching: Infant Safety
Teaching: Infant Stimulation
Teaching: Preoperative
Teaching: Prescribed Activity/Exercise
Teaching: Prescribed Diet
Teaching: Prescribed Medication
Teaching: Procedure/Treatment
Teaching: Psychomotor Skill
Teaching: Safe Sex
Teaching: Sexuality
Teaching: Toddler Nutrition
Teaching: Toddler Safety

Teaching: Toilet Training
Technology Management
Telephone Consultation
Telephone Follow-Up
Temperature Regulation
Temperature Regulation: Intraoperative
Temporary Pacemaker Management
Therapeutic Play
Therapeutic Touch
Therapy Group
Total Parenteral Nutrition (TPN) Administration
Touch
Traction/Immobilization Care
Transcutaneous Electrical Nerve Stimulation (TENS)
Transport
Trauma Therapy: Child
Triage: Disaster
Triage: Emergency Center
Triage: Telephone
Truth Telling
Tube Care
Tube Care: Chest
Tube Care: Gastrointestinal
Tube Care: Umbilical Line
Tube Care: Urinary
Tube Care: Ventriculostomy/Lumbar Drain

Ultrasonography: Limited Obstetric
Unilateral Neglect Management
Urinary Bladder Training
Urinary Catheterization
Urinary Catheterization: Intermittent
Urinary Elimination Management
Urinary Habit Training
Urinary Incontinence Care
Urinary Incontinence Care: Enuresis
Urinary Retention Care

Values Clarification
Vehicle Safety Promotion
Venous Access Device (VAD) Maintenance
Ventilation Assistance
Visitation Facilitation
Vital Signs Monitoring
Vomiting Management

Weight Gain Assistance
Weight Management
Weight Reduction Assistance
Wound Care
Wound Care: Closed Drainage
Wound Irrigation

APPENDIX D

ABBREVIATIONS

α	alpha
β	beta
°	degree
° C	degrees Celsius, degrees centigrade
° F	degrees Fahrenheit
%	percent, percentage
<	less than
>	greater than
AAA	abdominal aortic aneurysm
abd	abdomen, abdominal
ABGs	arterial blood gases
ACE	angiotension-converting enzyme
ADH	antidiuretic hormone
ALT	alanine aminotransferase
ANA	antinuclear antibody
APTT	activated partial thromboplastin time
ARDS	adult respiratory distress syndrome, acute respiratory distress syndrome
ARF	acute renal failure
ASA	acetylsalicylic acid, aspirin
ASCVD	arteriosclerotic (or atherosclerotic) cardiovascular disease
ASHD	arteriosclerotic (or atherosclerotic) heart disease
AST	aspartate aminotransferase
ATN	acute tubular necrosis
AV	atrioventricular
BP	blood pressure
BS	blood sugar, blood glucose
BUN	blood urea nitrogen
C	Celsius, centigrade
C&S	culture and sensitivity
CABG	coronary artery bypass graft
CAD	coronary artery disease
cAMP	cyclic adenosine monophosphate
CAVH	continuous arteriovenous hemofiltration

CAVHD	continuous arteriovenous hemodialysis, or hemodiafiltration
cc	cubic centimeter
CHF	congestive heart failure
CI	cardiac index
CK, CPK	creatine kinase, creatine phophokinase
cm	centimeter
CNS	central nervous system
CO	cardiac output
CO_2	carbon dioxide
COPD	chronic obstructive pulmonary disease
CPAP	continuous positive airway pressure
CRRT	continuous renal replacement therapies
CSF	cerebrospinal fluid
cTnI	cardiac specific troponin I
cTnT	cardiac specific troponin T
CV	cardiovascular
CVA	cerebrovascular accident, stroke
CVP	central venous pressure
CVVHD	continuous venovenous hemodialysis, or hemodiafiltration
DI	diabetes insipidus
DIC	disseminated intravascular coagulation
DKA	diabetic ketoacidosis
DLV	differential lung ventilation
DTRs	deep tendon reflexes
ECG	electrocardiogram
EDH	epidural hematoma
EF	ejection fraction
ETT	endotracheal tube
F	Fahrenheit
FIO_2	fraction of inspired oxygen
FRC	functional residual capacity
Fx	fracture
GCS	Glasgow Coma Scale
GFR	glomerular filtration rate

GI	gastrointestinal		mmol	millimole
GVHD	graft-versus-host disease		MODS	multiple organ dysfunction syndrome
h, hr	hour		MSOF	multisystem organ failure
Hct	hematocrit		NANDA	North American Nursing Diagnosis Association
HELLP	hemolysis, elevated liver enzymes, low platelets		NIC	nursing interventions classifications
HF	heart failure		NIF	negative inspiratory force
HHS	hyperosmolar hyperglycemic state		NMB	neuromuscular blockade
HI	head injuries		NOC	nursing outcomes classification
HITT	heparin-induced thrombopenia and thrombosis		NPO	nothing by mouth
HIV	human immunodeficiency virus (AIDS)		NS	normal saline
Hmg	hemoglobin		NTG	nitroglycerin
HOB	head of bed		O_2	oxygen
HR	heart rate		OD	overdose
HTN	hypertension		OPCAB	off-pump coronary artery bypass
I&O	intake and output		OTC	over-the-counter
IAB	intra-aortic balloon		PA	pulmonary artery
IABP	intra-aortic balloon pump		PAT	paroxysmal atrial tachycardia
ICP	intracranial pressure		pCO_2, $PaCO_2$	partial pressure of arterial carbon dioxide tension
IE	infective endocarditis		PCWP	pulmonary capillary wedge pressure
ITP	idiopathic thrombocytopenic purpura		PE	pulmonary embolism
IV	intravenous		PEEP	positive end-expiratory pressure
IVF	intravenous fluids		pH	hydrogen ion concentration
IVP	intravenous push		PIH	pregnancy-induced hypertension
kg	kilogram		pO_2, PaO_2	partial pressure of arterial oxygen tension
LDH	lactic dehydrogenase		Postop	postoperative
LFTs	liver function tests		PPD	purified protein derivative (TB testing)
LMWH	low molecular weight heparin		PRN, prn	as needed
LOC	level of consciousness		PS	pressure support
LR	lactated Ringer's		PSV	pressure support ventilation
LVSW	left ventricular stroke work		PT	prothrombin time
LVSWI	left ventricular stroke work index		PTCA	percutaneous transluminal coronary angioplasty
m^2	square meter		$PtiO_2$	oxygen saturation of peripheral cerebellar tissues
MAO	monoamine oxidase			
MAOI	monoamine oxidase inhibitor		PTT	partial thromboplastin time
MAP	mean arterial pressure, mean arterial blood pressure		PVC	premature ventricular contraction
			PVR	peripheral vascular resistance
mEq	milliequivalent		q	every
MH	malignant hyperthermia		RF	renal failure
MI	myocardial infarction		RL	Ringer's lactate
MIDCAB	mininimally invasive direct coronary artery bypass		ROM	range of motion
			RVSW	right ventricular stroke work
ml	milliliter		RVSWI	right ventricular stroke work index
mm Hg	millimeters of mercury			

SB	Sengstaken–Blakemore tube
SCUF	slow continuous ultrafiltration
SGOT	see AST
SGPT	see ALT
SIADH	syndrome of inappropriate antidiuretic hormone
SIMV	synchronized intermittent mandatory ventilation
SIRS	systemic inflammatory response syndrome
$SjvO_2$	oxygen saturation of the jugular venous bulb
SL	sublingual
SMV	synchronized mandatory ventilation
SVR	systemic vascular resistance

SVT	supraventricular tachycardia
TEE	transesophageal echocardiography
TOF	train of four
TPN	total parenteral nutrition
TPR	total peripheral resistance
u/L	units per liter
U/O	urinary output
UA	urinalysis
UTI	urinary tract infection
VAD	ventricular assist device
VMA	vanillylmandelic acid
VS	vital signs
V_T	tidal volume

INDEX

Note: **Bold** type indicates main entries which are nursing diagnoses.

NOTES

License Agreement for Delmar Learning, a division of Thomson Learning, Inc.

Educational Software/Data

You the customer, and Delmar Learning, a division of Thomson Learning, Inc. incur certain benefits, rights, and obligations to each other when you open this package and use the software/data it contains. BE SURE YOU READ THE LICENSE AGREEMENT CAREFULLY, SINCE BY USING THE SOFTWARE/DATA YOU INDICATE YOU HAVE READ, UNDERSTOOD, AND ACCEPTED THE TERMS OF THIS AGREEMENT.

Your rights:

1. You enjoy a non-exclusive license to use the software/data on a single microcomputer in consideration for payment of the required license fee, (which may be included in the purchase price of an accompanying print component), or receipt of this software/data, and your acceptance of the terms and conditions of this agreement.

2. You acknowledge that you do not own the aforesaid software/data. You also acknowledge that the software/data is furnished "as is," and contains copyrighted and/or proprietary and confidential information of Delmar Learning, a division of Thomson Learning, Inc. or its licensors.

There are limitations on your rights:

1. You may not copy or print the software/data for any reason whatsoever, except to install it on a hard drive on a single microcomputer and to make one archival copy, unless copying or printing is expressly permitted in writing or statements recorded on the diskette(s).

2. You may not revise, translate, convert, disassemble or otherwise reverse engineer the software/data except that you may add to or rearrange any data recorded on the media as part of the normal use of thesoftware/data.

3. You may not sell, license, lease, rent, loan or otherwise distribute or network the software/data except that you may give the software/data to a student or an instructor for use at school or, temporarily at home.

Should you fail to abide by the Copyright Law of the United States as it applies to this software/data your license to use it will become invalid. You agree to erase or otherwise destroy the software/data immediately after receiving note of termination of this agreement for violation of its provisions from Delmar Learning.

Delmar Learning, a division of Thomson Learning, Inc. gives you a LIMITED WARRANTY covering the enclosed software/data. The LIMITED WARRANTY follows this License.

This license is the entire agreement between you and Delmar Learning, a division of Thomson Learning, Inc. interpreted and enforced under New York law.

LIMITED WARRANTY

Delmar Learning, a division of Thomson Learning, Inc. warrants to the original licensee/purchaser of this copy of microcomputer software/data and the media on which it is recorded that the media will be free from defects in material and workmanship for ninety (90) days from the date of original purchase. All implied warranties are limited in duration to this ninety (90) day period. THEREAFTER, ANY IMPLIED WARRANTIES, INCLUDING IMPLIED WARRANTIES OF MERCHANTABILITY AND FITNESS FOR A PARTICULAR PURPOSE, ARE EXCLUDED. THIS WARRANTY IS IN LIEU OF ALL OTHER WARRANTIES, WHETHER ORAL OR WRITTEN, EXPRESS OR IMPLIED.

If you believe the media is defective please return it during the ninety (90) day period to the address shown below. Defective media will be replaced without charge provided that it has not been subjected to misuse or damage.

This warranty does not extend to the software or information recorded on the media. The software and information are provided "AS IS." Any statements made about the utility of the software or information are not to be considered as express or implied warranties.

Limitation of liability: Our liability to you for any losses shall be limited to direct damages, and shall not exceed the amount you paid for the software. In no event will we be liable to you for any indirect, special, incidental, or consequential damages (including loss of profits) even if we have been advised of the possibility of such damages.

Some states do not allow the exclusion or limitation of incidental or consequential damages, or limitations on the duration of implied warranties, so the above limitation or exclusion may not apply to you. This warranty gives you specific legal rights, and you may also have other rights which vary from state to state. Address all correspondence to: Delmar Learning, a division of Thomson Learning, Inc., 5 Maxwell Drive, P.O. Box 8007, Clifton Park, NY 12065-8007. Attention: Technology Department.

SYSTEM REQUIREMENTS

The CD-ROM version will be developed to run on client systems with the following minimum configuration:

- Operating System: Microsoft Windows 98 SE, Windows 2000, Windows XP
- Processor: Pentium PC 120 MHz or higher
- RAM: 64 MB of RAM or better
- Free Drive Space: 25 MB free disk space
- CD-ROM Drive—necessary for installation only
- Internet Connection Speed: 56K or better in order to view web links provided in program but is not required.
- Screen Resolution: 800 × 600 pixels or better
- Color Depth: 16-bit color (thousands of colors) or 24-bit color (millions of colors)
- Sound card: N/A

SET UP INSTRUCTIONS

To install the program, simply run the "X:\setup.exe", where X is the drive letter of you CD-ROM drive. Follow the on screen prompts to complete the installation. You may also:

1. Double click My Computer
2. Double click the Control Panel icon
3. Double click Add/Remove Programs
4. Click the Install button and follow the on screen prompts from there.